The Mental Health Matrix

A Manual to Improve Services

There have been major changes to mental health services internationally in recent years, revolving around the concept of care in the community. Although speed of change and precise service mechanisms differ between countries, there is nevertheless increasingly widespread consensus on key components essential to adequate care provision. This in turn provides an opportunity to develop a widely acceptable framework to direct future developments. This book proposes a simple model that can be used as a guide to increased clinical effectiveness through focused evidence-based reform. Using a time/space framework, it is intended to act as a practical manual to assess strengths and weaknesses in services, and to be useful to care providers, trainees and planners.

PROFESSOR GRAHAM THORNICROFT is Professor of Community Psychiatry and Director of the Section of Community Psychiatry (PRiSM) at the Institute of Psychiatry in London and undertakes a range of research in the field of mental health service evaluation. He has published widely in this area, including editing *Measuring Mental Health Needs* (1992), *Emergency Mental Health Services in the Community* (1995), *Mental Health Outcome Measures* (1996), *Mental Health Service Evaluation* (1996), *Commissioning Mental Health Services* (1996), *London's Mental Health* (1997), *Mental Health in our Future Cities* (1998), and *Managing Mental Health Services* (1999).

PROFESSOR MICHELE TANSELLA is Professor of Psychiatry at the University of Verona and also Director of the WHO Collaborating Centre for Research and Training in Mental Health and Service Evaluation, Verona. He is currently vice-president of the International Federation of Psychiatric Epidemiology and an active member of many committees including the Executive Committee of the European Network for Mental Health Service Evaluation (ENMESH). Amongst a distinguished list of publications he is author of *Annotated Bibliography of Psychiatric Epidemiology* (1992) and editor of both *Mental Health Outcome Measures* (1996) and *Making Rational Mental Health Services* (1997).

The Mental Health Matrix

A Manual to Improve Services

GRAHAM THORNICROFT
& MICHELE TANSELLA

Foreword by
PROFESSOR SIR DAVID GOLDBERG

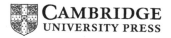

CAMBRIDGE
UNIVERSITY PRESS

PUBLISHED BY THE PRESS SYNDICATE OF THE UNIVERSITY OF CAMBRIDGE
The Pitt Building, Trumpington Street, Cambridge CB2 1RP, United Kingdom

CAMBRIDGE UNIVERSITY PRESS
The Edinburgh Building, Cambridge CB2 2RU, UK   http://www.cup.cam.ac.uk
40 West 20th Street, New York, NY 10011–4211, USA   http://www.cup.org
10 Stamford Road, Oakleigh, Melbourne 3166, Australia

First published 1999

Printed in United Kingdom at the University Press, Cambridge

Typeset in Lexicon 9.35/13pt (from the Enschedé Font Foundry) in QuarkXPress [SE]

A catalogue record for this book is available from the British Library

Library of Congress Cataloguing in Publication data

Thornicroft, Graham.
The mental health matrix : a pragmatic guide to service
improvement / Graham Thornicroft & Michele Tansella.
  p.   cm.
Includes bibliographical references and index.
ISBN 0 521 62155 0 (hb)
1. Mental health planning.   I. Tansella, Michele.   II. Title.
RA790.5.T49   1999
362.2–dc21   98–38431   CIP

ISBN 0 521 62155 0 hardback

We dedicate this book to

AMALIA THORNICROFT
CALUM THORNICROFT
HEIDI LEMPP
CAROLE TANSELLA
CHRISTA ZIMMERMANN-TANSELLA

Contents

Contributors

Alain D. Lesage, MD, M. Phil., FRCP(C)
Centre de recherche Fernand-Seguin
and Hôpital Louis-H. Lafontaine
7331 Hochelaga
Montréal (Québec)
CANADA
H1N3V2

Povl Munk-Jørgensen, MD, DrMS
Head of Department, Associate Professor
Department of Psychiatric Demography
Institute for Basic Psychiatric Research
Psychiatric Hospital in Aarhus
Aarhus University Hospital
Skovagervej 2
DK-8240 Risskov
DENMARK

Alan Rosen
Director, Royal North Shore Hospital &
    Community Mental Health Services
St Leonards
New South Wales 2065
AUSTRALIA
Associate Professor & Clinical Senior
    Lecturer
Universities of Sydney and Wollongong
AUSTRALIA

Michele Tansella
Professor of Psychiatry
Instituto di Psichiatria
Universita di Verona
Ospedale Policlinico
37134 Verona
ITALY

Graham Thornicroft
Professor of Community Psychiatry
Institute of Psychiatry
Kings College London
De Crespigny Park
London SE5 8AF
UK

Toma Tomov
Professor of Psychiatry
Head, Department of Psychiatry
Medical University
Sofia
BULGARIA
Director
Bulgarian Institute for Human Relations
New Bulgarian University
Sofia
BULGARIA

Richard Warner, MB, BS, DPM
Medical Director
Mental Health Center of Boulder County
1333 Iris Avenue
Boulder
Colorado 80304–2296
USA
Clinical Professor of Psychiatry and
    Adjunct Professor of Anthropology
University of Colorado
USA

Foreword

PROFESSOR SIR DAVID GOLDBERG
Institute of Psychiatry, King's College London

This volume represents a watershed in writing about the mental illness services, in that the authors are proposing a model that brings together a public health concern with the health of populations, with an insistence on remembering that services must also be judged by their effectiveness in dealing with disorders at a patient level. It was all there before they wrote it, but no-one has previously put it together so elegantly. Space and time are fairly obvious dimensions to choose for a model; what they have achieved is to produce a simple model that neatly serves as a framework for comparisons between different services, and illuminates the way in which planning at different levels of the model relates to events at other levels. It is especially ingenious to use the 'time' dimension to indicate time with respect to the treatment of illnesses, rather than merely indicating the historical passage of time. This gives the whole model greater power, which the authors have exploited brilliantly. Nothing will ever be quite the same again; it is a book certain to be widely read and quoted.

One point needs further clarification. Models can be predictive, they can be explanatory, they can be heuristic, or they can be descriptive. In Chapter 17 misgivings are expressed from the Nordic countries that the model is not specific, which implies that no predictions follow from it. First and foremost, this is a descriptive model, which helps to ensure that like is compared with like, by carefully disentangling the nine divisions in the proposed matrix. However, as the authors point out, the model can also be used as a tool to improve services in a particular place, so that features of a mental health system become better understood, or lead to priorities for improving services. However, the model is here being used as a tool: it makes no predictions or suggestions itself. It may even be that the present vogue for community care will pass, and that we will return to a more institutional approach in the future: even if that were to happen, the present model would serve as a framework for considering changes in the system.

Older readers of the book may be faintly troubled by the implication (in Chapter 3, the historical context) of unbroken progress towards more desirable services, with the achievements of the 'middle period' being seen as mere preludes to the great symphony now occurring. The rehabilitation services that were set up in that period should not be seen as a transitional step – merely a way of emptying the asylums. The principles that were set up then are good now, even if time has moved on, and they now need to be adapted to a changed world. The widespread closures that have occurred in rehabilitation workshops, in day centres and facilities for those with long-term disability in England, were carried out to save money and to balance budgets – not because they were no longer needed.

Towards the end of the book the authors leave their metaphor of the 3×3 matrix, and use another from the card table. The three ACEs are highly desirable aspects of each level of their model (see Table 11.4). However, three ACEs disturbed me somewhat, and I fell to brooding about what the fourth ACE might be. It was clearly something that the authors preferred not to think about.

With diffidence – as befits someone whose function in the deck is to be a mere joker (surplus to requirements, or simply replacing a missing card?) – let me suggest that the fourth ACE is Austerity, Criticism and Enmity. It is worth saying a few words about each.

Austerity is the main force opposing change and improvements to the mental health services. Unlike the old asylums, the budgets of community-orientated services are fatally easy to prune; and it is difficult to be innovative when your service is facing progressive reductions to its budget with each succeeding year. Criticism stands for the criticism that is made of junior staff when things go wrong: in England blame is now habitually devolved downwards, so that planners at both national and local levels are rarely or never held to be responsible for individual disasters, even though their decisions have often resulted in situations that cannot be handled well at patient level, given the level of resources available. This devolution of blame makes life easy at the top; but it is at the expense of a demoralised, burnt out work force, which in deprived inner city areas cannot attract staff in sufficient numbers. Judicial enquiries into homicides by patients consider only the 'patient level' of the present model – never the decisions made at national or local levels that have made work at the patient level so difficult. Enmity exists, in suitably muted forms, between workers working for different masters, or between different disciplines. Another kind of enmity is represented by sometimes ill-informed criticisms of the service in the media. In England, there are often tensions between health and social services; between managers and the work force, and between different professional groups. The British government asks for partnerships, but it is doubtful whether real common ground can be found between those working for different organisations with separate budgets. The best examples of well-functioning mental health services are to be found in those American cities where there is a common purchaser of both health and social care – able to commission services from either, as well as from NGOs and user groups.

However, these are minor points. This book fizzles with excitement, as familiar concepts and findings are shown in a new light, by being measured against the framework now described so clearly. Readers will find Figure 13.3, 'Well targeted services', a good example of this facility that the authors have to throw new light on old problems.

The model is timely, as broadly similar events are occurring in many countries. The new model provides a language for comparisons between regions of the world – and these are demonstrated by the ease with which it has been applied in the five chapters that bring the book to a close.

Preface

LEON EISENBERG, MD
Department of Social Medicine, Harvard Medical School

Graham Thornicroft and Michele Tansella have written an altogether remarkable monograph. *The Mental Health Matrix* is lucid, written in such simple and spare language as to make its concepts transparent, free of cant and of special pleading. For all these reasons, it should have a profound impact on the provision of mental health services; that is, *if* it is read by the practitioners, the policy makers and the politicians who need to understand its basic principles. Thornicroft and Tansella present no new data; what they provide are new ways to determine what data are needed across domains and to assess available data to permit evidence-based, integrated conclusions.

Amidst the clamour of cost-containment, they have managed to do the unique. They highlight the importance of a *population-based* approach to mental illness, because of its health benefits, at the same time that they make the care of the *individual patient* the focus for clinical planning. In the United States, at least (and I suspect, this is not solely an American disease), 'population medicine' is a slogan often used to rationalise cost control by limiting services that might have benefited individual patients. Such rhetoric is absent from this volume. Better care can be less expensive care when ineffective high cost procedures and episodic interventions are replaced by integrated services, but the goal must be the provision of care that benefits patients rather than investors or managers (or mental health workers!).

Indeed, so profound is the proposed way of looking at services and so different is it from what each of us is accustomed to, whether we be clinicians, public health workers or designers of social policy, that I urge its use as a study guide for interdisciplinary working groups. The subtitle of the book is *A Manual to Improve Services*; that is precisely what it provides. Its concluding sections set forth illuminating case studies that apply the matrix model to areas as different as Australia, Canada, Eastern Europe, the Nordic countries and the United States.

The authors suggest the model can help in 'understanding the possible causes and effects of episodes of severe violence committed by psychiatric patients'. They contrast a narrow focus on the clinician, on the one hand, with a more inclusive analysis of case load, staff training and national investment in services, on the other. Let me pursue this typology through a specific illustration of misplaced blame and its social consequences.

The tragedy in question took place in July 1986 on a ferryboat between Staten Island and New York City. A homeless 43-year-old Cuban refugee, responding to command hallucinations, slew two passengers and wounded nine others. The tragedy was transmuted into public outrage when the newspapers discovered that Gonzalez had been seen four days earlier in the emergency room of a teaching hospital. Although the psychiatric house officer who saw him recognised that he was wildly psychotic, he was unable to find a bed for the patient at his own university hospital or any of the seven other in-patient units he telephoned. The patient was uninsured and without funds. The news report of an inability 'to find a bed' was an inability to find a *free* bed. The state agency piously concluded that the house officers performance 'did not meet professional standards' and that there had been 'inadequate supervision'. The diagnosis of clinical failure obfuscated the real problem: pathology in national and state policy.

The public consequences were enormous; within two weeks, the number of patients brought to psychiatric emergency rooms in New York City increased by 50%; the number admitted led to such overcrowding that patients had to be transferred by bus and van to remote backup state mental hospitals. Despite that manoeuvre, psychiatric emergency admissions spilled over into unused medical and surgical beds in municipal hospitals. The crisis did not abate until almost a year later when public services settled back into their ante-bellum status.

Were the ferry murders a sentinel event in an epidemic of homicidal psychoses? Clearly not. The 'epidemic' was panic among the gate keepers. The police brought verbally abusive homeless persons to emergency rooms, no longer willing to gamble on their harmlessness. House officers on emergency duty would no longer sign out potentially violent patients without evaluation by a senior physician, resulting in long queues in the emergency room. Staff psychiatrists opted to be on the 'safe side' by hospitalising patients they would have sent back to the streets before the ferry murders.

The fundamental problem did not lie with the resident's clinical judgement, but with the failures at the national, state and local levels. Because the United States is the only country in the world without universal health insurance, lack of coverage precluded private hospitalisation and placed the patient in a queue for public care. State/federal fiscal relationships had made it advantageous to states to downsize public hospital capacity in order to shift payments for the mentally ill from state to federal budgets. At the local level, the pathology included the homelessness of thousands of mentally ill patients because public housing is inadequate and because aftercare and rehabilitation services are insufficient. Preventing avoidable hazards to ordinary citizens demands an address to these issues.

If the principles of *The Mental Health Matrix* are widely understood, the groundwork will have been laid for comprehensive public mental health services. However, understanding will not in itself suffice. To actualise what is possible 'in principle' requires a social strategy and the political will to make change happen.

Acknowledgements

We are pleased to acknowledge the valuable contributions towards this book by Julie Grove, David Goldberg and Mike Slade at the Institute of Psychiatry in London, Eric Byers at the Maudsley Hospital, and Graziella Nicolis at the Department of Medicine and Public Health, Section of Psychiatry in Verona. In addition we have enjoyed a productive and enjoyable relationship with our commissioning editors at Cambridge University Press, Richard Barling and Jocelyn Foster.

PART I **The context**

Geographical Dimension

Temporal Dimension

	(A) Input Phase	(B) Process Phase	(C) Outcome Phase
(1) Country/Regional Level	1A	1B	1C
(2) Local Level (catchment area)	2A	2B	2C
(3) Patient Level	3A	3B	3C

Figure 1.1 Overview of the matrix model

1
Aims, concepts and structure of the book

1.1 **The purpose of the book**

The reform of mental health services is now a prominent issue in most economically developed countries and also in several countries of Central and Eastern Europe. Although the speed and the precise local detail of these changes vary between countries, there is a clear need for an overall conceptual framework, which can assist both those leading and those who are affected by these changes. In a sense this book acts as a guide, providing a map of the territory and a compass to orientate the direction of reform.

The process of re-modelling mental health services is a reform in two senses: it is a profound change in the values informing how treatment and care should be provided to people suffering from mental illness, and it is also a radical structural change in the physical shape and pattern of services. This book seeks to provide an overall conceptual model, and acts as a pragmatic manual to help those who are involved in changing mental health services and those who wish to learn from evidence and experience accumulated elsewhere.

In this volume, we shall selectively present evidence for the clinical effectiveness of community-based mental health services, including the results of research studies, such as randomised controlled trials. We shall also include a range of other types of evidence, such as knowledge based on the experience which has accrued from good clinical practice, especially in those areas not yet subjected to formal evaluation.

A clear limitation of this book is that it does not include information from large parts of the world, including Africa, Asia and South America. We believe that the situation in less economically developed countries needs to be separately addressed by those with the relevant direct personal experience. At the same time we hope that the framework and the methodology we propose in this book will be of some assistance to others undertaking that task (Ben-Tovim, 1987; Desjarlais *et al.*, 1995).

1.2 **A conceptual framework: the 'matrix model'**

We believe that a conceptual model is necessary to help formulate service aims and the steps necessary for their implementation. To be useful such a model should be simple. We have therefore created a model with only two dimensions (each of which has three levels), which we call the 'matrix model'.

Our aim is that this model will help people to diagnose the relative strengths and weaknesses of services in their local area, and to formulate a clear course of action for their improvement. Such a service development plan will involve judgements about the risks and benefits of competing alternative courses of action. We also expect that the matrix model will assist in producing a detailed step-by-step approach which is clear and flexible enough to be relevant to different local circumstances.

The two *dimensions* of this conceptual framework, which we call the matrix model, are the geographical and the temporal (see Figure 1.1). The first of these refers to three *geographical* levels: (1) country/regional, (2) local and (3) patient. The second dimension refers to three *temporal* phases: (A) inputs, (B) processes and (C) outcomes. Using these two dimensions we construct a 3 × 3 matrix to bring into focus critical issues for mental health services.

We have chosen to include the geographical dimension in the matrix model because we believe that mental health services should be primarily organised at the local level. This level can act as a 'lens' to focus policies and resources most effectively for the benefit of individual patients. In our view decisions at this local level should be informed both by the larger-scale public health context and by the smaller scale of direct clinical encounters.

We have selected a temporal axis as the other organising dimension. This is because although we consider that outcomes are the most important aspect of service evaluation, nevertheless these outcomes can only be interpreted in the context of their prior temporal phases, namely inputs and processes.

The matrix model allows us for the first time to use these two dimensions simultaneously, and the consequent 3 × 3 framework is intended to clarify the analysis of problems and solutions in developing mental health services.

Such a conceptual framework both sets the boundaries within which useful explanatory models can be articulated, and gives a context for the definitions of key terms, which are particular to a given historical period (Kuhn, 1962). A conceptual framework for health service research, for example, is important to help avoid two types of risk: general descriptions referring to large areas, which are difficult to use in any particular site; and data from a specific service, from which it is difficult to extrapolate. This framework can be useful because it facilitates the bridging of information between different levels of analysis. Indeed, in practice the lack of a conceptual map of this kind, both to analyse problems in the functioning of mental health services and to locate specific interventions, often produces inappropriate responses to dysfunctional services, as described in examples reported in the next section.

This model is not intended in any way to be prescriptive, but has to be taken as an explanatory tool, first for understanding and then for action to improve services. Those readers who want to use the book for practical purposes need to adapt this matrix model in ways that maximise its relevance to each local situation. These situations vary so much that a rigid explanatory system will not be useful in this respect. Mental health care is different from those medical specialities which continue to be more hospital based, such as surgery, in which treatment protocols and guidelines may be applied in a more exacting manner.

We therefore encourage readers to adjust this model to suit their own situation, and we consider that the success of this model will be measured by how far it is useful in practice.

1.3 Examples of the use of the matrix model

The application of the matrix model will be the central theme of this book. We present here three early examples of the use of the matrix model. The first illustration refers to how the model can assist in understanding the possible causes and effects of episodes of severe violence committed by psychiatric patients. In practice the causes of such incidents are often described primarily at the patient level (the patient and the direct care staff), but the consequences seldom remain at that level, and may affect both the local and country levels. Characteristically these extreme adverse events are multi-causal and so the use of a clear multi-level framework, such as the matrix model, allows many concurrent factors at different levels in the mental health service system to be taken into account. In other words, when the analysis is complex, then the response must be commensurate to that degree of complexity.

For instance, in an inquiry into an individual adverse outcome, namely an incident of severe violence committed by a patient (Cell 3C in Figure 1.1), we may need to analyse the precursors to the event in terms of the lack of a local method to establish and maintain maximum clinical case loads (Cell 2B) for community-based staff, an inadequate degree of targeting of most severely disabled patients (Cell 2B), and poor local staff training (Cell 2A), in the wider context of low national rates of investment in mental health services (Cell 1A). As a consequence the required responses should be placed at precisely those locations (Cells) where the weaknesses have been recognised.

This method of analysis can therefore allow the formulation of a more complete preventative strategy which combines actions at more than one level. This can reduce two risks: over-specification and over-generalisation. On one hand, conceptualising the problem only at the patient level can more easily lead to the attachment of blame to individual clinicians. In effect this reduces complex multi-level causal influences to only the patient level. On the other hand, there is a risk of over-generalisation, that is to attach to the whole psychiatric system (at the country level) the blame for failing to prevent such tragic events, and of therefore failing in all aspects of the service.

This use of the matrix model is to identify key contributory factors in such sentinel events, and to direct an inter-related series of responses to address policy, organisational and clinical weaknesses at their appropriate levels.

A *second example* of using the matrix model refers to how information from services in one site, both from direct visits and from published descriptions, can be translated to be relevant to another. What people do in practice is to adapt experience from other centres and information from the research literature to make a diagnosis of the relative strengths and weaknesses of services in their local area, and to formulate a course of action for their improvement. Without a conceptual framework, this process, essentially one of translation, often presents difficulties in deciding which aspects of 'foreign' data are relevant to local circumstances, and also knowing how to implement the service requirements identified from the system diagnosis.

The outcome of such a local translation process may lead to several possible courses of action. Commonly the information conveyed consists of visible local service inputs, including physical and staff resources (part of Cell 2A in Figure 1.1), and some limited process details on the style of working and clinical contact rates (Cell 2B), along with limited data on outcome variables at the patient (Cell 3C) or local levels (Cell 2C). What we need in fact is a standardised account of the small number of most relevant features in every cell of the matrix, so as to understand more fully any particular local service which demonstrates good practice, and to appreciate how best to transfer such practice to other settings.

An example of the translation of one service component from North

America to Britain is the introduction of case management (CM) and assertive community treatment (ACT). At the national level, there has been a prioritisation of the severely mentally ill (Department of Health, 1994) which has encouraged CM and ACT; at the local level specific procedures (called the Care Programme Approach) have been established to require the allocation of case managers to patients and the organisation of regular clinical review meetings; while at the patient level widely differing interpretations of CM have been made in practice.

The *third example* is how the matrix model can help in understanding why some clinical interventions of proven efficacy have not been implemented on a widespread basis (the gap between efficacy and effectiveness), while other forms of treatment, which have not been subjected to proper evaluation, have become common (claimed effectiveness in the absence of both proven efficacy and proven effectiveness).

Family psycho-social interventions for patients with schizophrenia and their carers, for example, are now established as being of proven efficacy (Mari & Streiner, 1996; Dixon & Lehman, 1995). These psychosocial family interventions have seven components: (a) construction of an alliance with relatives who care for the person with schizophrenia; (b) reduction of adverse family atmosphere (that is, lowering the emotional climate in the family by reducing stress and burden on relatives); (c) enhancement of the capacity of relatives to anticipate and solve problems; (d) reduction of expressions of anger and guilt by the family; (e) maintenance of reasonable expectations for patient performance; (f) encouragement of relatives to set and keep to appropriate limits whilst maintaining some degree of separation when needed; and (g) attainment of desirable change in relatives' behaviour and belief systems. Such psycho-social interventions are applied extremely rarely in routine clinical practice. To implement these complex components requires co-ordination of inputs and processes at the patient level (Cells 3A and 3B) and at the local level (Cells 2A and 2B). From this perspective a new treatment has a decreasing likelihood of widespread dissemination if it requires changes in inputs and processes at more than the patient level. More examples of the application of the matrix model will be provided throughout the book.

1.4 The structure of the book

This book will draw upon both theoretical and practical contributions. When possible we have structured each chapter by presenting first our own interpretation of the most useful theoretical framework available, followed by practical examples from service planning or from clinical practice. In this way we attempt to bring a greater degree of synthesis and coherence to each step of our argument.

We cannot deny that our paradigm is European, and to be more precise stems from Western Europe, and we are aware that this has profoundly influenced our way of conceptualising mental health care. For this reason we have asked five colleagues to add a wider, critical international perspective on re-forming mental health services, in relation to Australia, Canada, Central and Eastern European countries, Nordic European countries, and the United States.

We also use special feature boxes with relevant quotations, for ease of retrieval for the reader, and because we see these quotations as the essence of the concepts that we employ, and because to paraphrase the originals would only diminish their clarity and impact.

The fields of mental health research and practice are littered by jargon, in a way that may often be confusing for those from different traditions, even in translating from American to English! To avoid as far as possible such confusion we have included a glossary to explain our own understandings of the meanings of key terms.

In spite of the fact that we have attempted to make balanced and fair use of the available research evidence, at the same time we are not neutral. We therefore need to make explicit for the reader our own bias. While we have both undergone a medical training, we place ourselves in the traditions of epidemiological psychiatry, and public health medicine. From these traditions we value the importance of an evidence-based approach. In addition we believe, from our own experience, in the importance of a direct interplay between research and clinical practice, which should be mutually beneficial. Indeed we consider that the medical model alone (without taking into account contextual social, psychological and economic factors) is insufficient to understand the full complexity of mental disorders, their antecedents and their serious consequences in terms of disability and suffering.

Community, mental health services and the public health

2.1 The meaning of 'community'

Health professionals are familiar with the importance of taking a clinical history so that a detailed appreciation of the past can lead to a richer interpretation of the present. The same 'historical' approach used to translate symptoms into diagnoses is applicable to the translation of words into useful concepts. In this manual, before discussing community mental health services we need to address at the outset the question: what is the meaning of 'that overused word community' (Acheson, 1985).

Table 2.1 shows five definitions of 'community', selected from the *Concise Oxford Dictionary*. The first two meanings ('all the people living in a specific locality', 'a specific locality, including its inhabitants'), include both the people in a particular area and that locality itself. These lead us to our view that mental health services are often best organised for defined local areas, for all local residents, and that research upon such services will necessarily include consideration of the size and characteristics of the population at risk (the denominator). We shall return to what has been called 'the science of the denominator' when we discuss the 'local level' in Chapter 5 (Henderson, 1988).

The third definition ('body of people having a religion, a profession, etc., in common') is consistent with our argument when we consider disaggregated sub-groups of the total population who may be at higher risk for particular mental disorders, or whose needs for services are distinct. Such groups may include immigrants, people who are homeless or those exposed to particular environmental or biological risk factors such as bereavement or pregnancy.

Finally, the fourth and fifth definitions of 'community' refer to the *fellowship of interests* and to the *general public* respectively. This wider community of citizens can be seen to delegate responsibility for the care of mentally ill people to the mental health services: in effect an unwritten contract exists

Table 2.1. *The definition of 'community'*

Community
1 all the people living in a specific locality
2 a specific locality, including its inhabitants
3 body of people having a religion, a profession, etc., in common (*the immigrant community*)
4 fellowship of interests, etc.; similarity (*community of intellect*)
5 the public

Source: Concise Oxford Dictionary, Oxford University Press, 1993

in which the public agree to fund and support (or fail to oppose) those services which contract to provide treatment. But beyond this, there is an additional level of covert public expectation – that services will provide a public service not only by treating, but also by removing or containing those who pose a risk to the public safety or to the public peace of mind. The boundaries limiting the categories of deviant behaviour for which mental health services have a legitimate obligation vary, but what persists are the subtle balances between control and treatment, and between the rights of the individual and those of this wider public.

Intriguingly the word 'community' becomes increasingly complex upon closer inspection. The sense conveyed by the term 'community care', for example, presumes that a functioning social entity exists in a local area, as conveyed by the wealth of associations contained in the *Oxford Thesaurus*. This positive aura for the term may relate to a 'remembered community', which is a symbolic, idealised concept, but which in fact may never have existed (Banton *et al.*, 1985). This notional 'remembered community' has four characteristics: a small and manageable size; the interpenetration of communication and experience of its members; a shared sense of membership or belonging; and participation in a common cause. In any particular local area, some or all of these characteristics may be absent. We need to be cautious in allowing any sense of fetish to become attached to the word 'community' and we propose that it is time to move from an ideological to a more pragmatic approach in the field of 'community' psychiatry.

2.2 Re-appraising the value of 'common'

The etymological root of 'community' in fact originates in the Latin *communitas* meaning 'common'. As Table 2.2 shows, the *Concise Oxford Dictionary* offers five definitions of 'common', all of which may be relevant to

Table 2.2. *Definitions of 'common'*

Common
adjective
1 occurring often (*a common mistake*)
2 ordinary; of ordinary qualities; without special rank or position (*no common mind; common soldier; the common people*)
3 shared by, coming from, or done by, more than one (*common knowledge; by common consent; our common benefit*)
4 belonging to, open to, or affecting, the whole community or the public (*common land*)
5 derogatory, low-class; vulgar; inferior (*a common little man*)

Adapted from: *Concise Oxford Dictionary*, Oxford University Press, 1993

the central themes of this book. The *first definition* is 'occurring often', and there are the following implications for the commonness of the mental disorders. Their widespread occurrence means that they will have a very substantial impact on every community and in every type of society. Further, the nature of each local community and each social environment is known to be closely related to risk of mental illness and the likelihood that an illness will become chronic. Equally, since mental disorders are so widely distributed, it is reasonable to plan responses to these disorders based upon the assumption that many core services should be commensurately decentralised.

The *second meaning* of common is 'ordinary', which may refer to the need to provide routine care, support and treatment in everyday 'real world' clinical settings, and to address the ordinary, practical problems that patients cannot solve alone. Indeed the focus of this book as a whole is upon the application of knowledge gained from research conducted in experimental settings to routine clinical practice. In this way we intend this guide to be common, even if it is not ordinary!

A similar concept can apply to the *third meaning* of 'common': 'shared by, coming from, or done by, more than one', which can also refer to an aspect of community-based services, namely the multi-disciplinary teamwork. These issues are expanded upon in Chapters 11 and 12.

A *fourth meaning* of 'common' is 'belonging to, open to, or affecting, the whole community or the public'. This meaning is also important because it may be linked to one aspect of community-based mental health services, namely their easy access by the whole local community or by all members of the public. Indeed, more generally, we believe that each member of the public has a legitimate entitlement to health care, regardless of ability to pay, and that it should not be considered as a market commodity.

The roots of 'common' offer an intriguing *fifth interpretation*, that is 'derogatory, low-class; vulgar; inferior, a common little man'. This will be familiar to staff working in community mental health services who may feel valued less than their hospital-based colleagues. A further purpose of this book is to argue that the services given to patients in community settings are no less valuable than those delivered in hospitals. Perhaps more important in relation to this definition is the fact that many patients who suffer from severe mental disorders stay within or proceed to join the lowest socio-economic status category.

> ' The only way by which any one divests himself of his natural liberty and puts on the bonds of civil society is by agreeing with other men to join and unite into a community.'
> J. LOCKE 1632–1704
> *Second Treatise of Civil Government* (1690) Chapter 8, Section 95

2.3 Defining 'community care' and 'community mental health'

Having discussed the meanings of 'community' and its etymological roots, how then should *'community care'* be defined? The term 'community care' was first officially used in Britain in 1957 (Report on the Royal Commission on Mental Illness and Mental Deficiency), and its historical development has been traced by Bulmer (1987), who has offered four interpretations. It may mean: (i) care outside large institutions, (ii) professional services provided outside hospitals, (iii) care by the community, (iv) normalisation or ordinary living. Later usages include (v) care in one's own home, and (vi) the full range of social care services, although as Knapp (1996) stressed, the breadth of the latter is now narrowing with the growing discussion of the concept of long-term care.

Taking into account these roots of 'community', how can *community mental health services* best be defined? Table 2.3 presents a selection of key definitions which have appeared over the last 35 years.

Taking these previous contributions into account we propose here our own definition:

> A *community-based mental health service* is one which provides a full range of effective mental health care to a defined population, and which is dedicated to treating and helping people with mental disorders, in proportion to their suffering or distress, in collaboration with other local agencies.

Table 2.3. *Changing definitions of community mental health services*

G. F. Rehin & F. M. Martin (1963)
'any scheme directed to providing extra-mural care and treatment...to facilitate the early detection of mental health illness or relapse and its treatment on an informal basis, and to provide some social work service in the community for support or follow-up.' (quoted in Bennett & Freeman, 1991).

M. Sabshin (1966)
'the utilisation of the techniques, methods, and theories of social psychiatry, as well as those of the other behavioural sciences, to investigate and meet the mental health needs of a functionally or geographically defined population over a significant period of time, and the feeding back of information to modify the central body of social mental health and other behavioural science and knowledge.'

R. Freudenberg (1967)
'community psychiatry assumes that people with mental health disorders can be most effectively helped when links with family, friends, workmates and society generally are maintained, and aims to provide preventive, treatment, and rehabilitative services for a district which means that therapeutic measures go beyond the individual patient.'

G. Serban (1977)
'community psychiatry has three aspects: first, a social movement; second a service delivery strategy, emphasising the accessibility of services and acceptance of responsibility of mental health needs of a total population; and third, provision of best possible clinical care, with emphasis on the major mental health disorders and on treatment outside total institutions.'

D. Bennett (1978)
'community psychiatry is concerned with the mental health needs not only of the individual patient but of the district population, not only of those who are defined as sick, but those who may be contributing to that sickness and whose health or well-being may, in turn, be put at risk.'

M. Tansella (1986)
'a system of care devoted to a defined population and based on a comprehensive and integrated mental health service, which includes out-patient facilities, day and residential training centres, residential accommodation in hostels, sheltered workshops and in-patient units in general hospitals, and which ensures, with multi-disciplinary team-work, early diagnosis, prompt treatment, continuity of care, social support and a close liaison with other medical and social community services and, in particular, with general practitioners.'

G. Strathdee & G. Thornicroft (1997)
'the network of services which offer continuing treatment, accommodation, occupation and social support and which together help people with mental health problems to regain their normal social roles.'

Integral to this definition is our view that a modern community-based mental health service may be designed as an *alternative* and not complementary to the traditional more custodial pattern dominated by large mental hospitals and out-patient clinics offering follow-up care usually limited to medication management (Tansella & Zimmermann-Tansella, 1988). In other words the newer system of care discussed in this book is designed to replace and not supplement the former institutional arrangements. The difference between these two views is further clarified in Chapter 13.

2.4 The public health approach to mental health

'Psychiatry is forced to study groups and populations because it deals with individuals, not in spite of that fact.'
ØDEGAARD, 1962

2.4.1 Defining the public health approach

Before we explain the importance of the public health approach, we first need to define it and to understand its historical roots. According to Eisenberg (1984) the public health paradigm is rooted in the work of Virchow, who introduced the concept of 'social medicine' into Germany in 1848, and who proposed to reform medicine on the basis of four principles:

(i) the health of the people is a matter of direct social concern;
(ii) social and economic conditions have an important effect on health and disease, and these relations must be the subject of scientific investigation;
(iii) the measures taken to promote health and to contain disease must be social as well as medical;
(iv) medical statistics will be our standard of measurement.

'Die Artzte sind die natuerlichen Anwaelte der Armen und die soziale Frage faellt zum grossten Teil in ihre Jurisdiktion'

[Doctors are the natural advocates for the poor and the social questions fall for the most part in their jurisdiction]
RUDOLF VIRCHOW, *Medizinische Reform* 1948
Source: M. Shepherd (1983)

The current discipline of public health medicine has been classically defined by C. E. A. Winslow, as quoted in Hanlin and Picket (1984):

Public health is the science and the art of: (i) preventing disease,
(ii) prolonging life and (iii) organised community efforts for the sanitation of the environment, the control of communicable infections, the educa-

tion of the individual in personal hygiene, the organisation of medical and nursing services for early diagnosis and preventive treatment of disease, and the development of the social machinery to ensure everyone a standard of living adequate for the maintenance of health, so organising these benefits as to enable every citizen his birthright of health and longevity.

Holland and Fitzsimons (1990) provided a more succinct definition of public health as a practical speciality concerned with the application of research findings in an attempt to cure or prevent disease and to allocate resources appropriately. More recently, Beaglehole and Bonita (1997) have proposed an appropriate definition of public health as 'one of the collective efforts organised by society to prevent premature death, illness, injury and disability and to promote the population's health.' The interest of this definition is that it covers medical care and rehabilitation, health promotion, and the underlying social, economic and cultural determinants of health and disease.

The public health approach is primarily concerned with the health of populations. Although populations are self-evidently made up of individuals, the individual approach and the population approach are, in many ways, quite distinct. Measures of morbidity, explanations of possible causation and the consequent interventions may be entirely different or require alternative strategies. As Henderson (1996) has pointed out 'It is an appealing notion that populations, while they are undeniably made up of individuals and as far as we know no other component, take on properties of their own, much as molecules have attributes not found in their constituent atoms.'

> 'Psychiatrists, unlike sociologists, seem generally unaware of the existence and importance of mental health attributes of whole populations, their concern being only with sick individuals.'
> G. ROSE, 1993

In this book we propose that mental health practitioners adopt, in addition to the individual-health approach, the public-health approach, and we compare the two approaches in Table 2.4. In terms of the matrix model, we are suggesting that clinicians refer in their work to the individual, local and to the country/regional levels when deciding the appropriate level for their diagnoses and interventions.

We consider that the provision of a reasonable level of mental health care to the whole population is a legitimate expectation and that the overall responsibility to co-ordinate provision lies at the country/regional level.

Table 2.4. *Comparative characteristics of the public health and the individual health approaches to mental health*

Public health approach	Individual health approach
1 Whole population view	1 Partial population view
2 Patients in socio-economic context	2 Tends to exclude contextual factors
3 Can generate information on primary prevention	3 Less likely to generate information on primary prevention
4 Individual as well as population-based prevention (both secondary and tertiary)	4 Individual level only (secondary and tertiary prevention)
5 Systemic view of service components	5 Facilities / programme view of services
6 Favours open access to services	6 Access to services may be limited by age, diagnosis or insurance cover
7 Team work preferred	7 Individual therapist preferred
8 Long-term / longitudinal / life-course perspective	8 Short-term and intermittent / episodic follow-up perspective
9 Cost-effectiveness seen in population terms	9 Cost-effectiveness seen in individual terms

2.4.2 The meaning of the public health approach as applied to mental health

The first meaning of the public health approach as applied to mental health is that *services should be available to everyone in need, independent of their ability to pay*. A second meaning is that the *mental health of individuals is integrally linked with the wider social and economic health of their communities*. A strategy for promoting mental health throughout the whole population must therefore be of public concern and cannot be purely a private enterprise.

> ' the needs of the mentally ill cannot safely be entrusted to the 'invisible hand' of market forces ... mental health services should be based upon egalitarian principles, not simply as a moral imperative, but because a socially just system of provision is by far the most effective for a nation's health.'
> B. COOPER. (1995)

2.4.3 The public health impact of mental disorders

The public health impact of mental disorders can be judged according to the following criteria: (i) frequency; (ii) severity; (iii) consequences; (iv) availability of interventions; (v) acceptability of interventions; and (vi) public concern.

First, in terms of *frequency*, mental illnesses are common, disabling and expensive. This means that there are substantial public health implications for high incidence–low duration conditions, most notably affective and anxiety disorders. There is a different pattern of public health challenges from low incidence and high duration disorders such as schizophrenia and the affective psychoses. The public health impact will also be conditional upon the population at risk, which may well change in relation to demographic and socio-economic trends. For example, between 1981–1990, in many British cities there has been a net reduction of over 5% in the total population, but a net increase in the total population aged 18–30, which is the main age group at risk for the onset of psychotic disorders. This trend may be further amplified by differing birth rates among the ethnic minority groups which are at higher risk for psychotic disorders, such as among Black Caribbean and West African people in Britain.

A further consequence of demographic changes is that increasing numbers of people now live to an age when they become at risk of developing dementia. As discussed below, a further example of this point is given in the Global Burden of Disease study, which developed projection scenarios of mortality and disability, disaggregated by cause, age, sex and region of the world, and which confirmed the importance of demographic changes (Murray & Lopez, 1996a).

Second, as far as *severity* is concerned the burden of psychiatric morbidity can also be expressed in disruption to social functioning. Mental illness produces very considerable direct costs to health and social care services. In 1993, for example, 92 million working days lost in the UK were due to mental illness (18% of all working days lost) with a total estimated cost of £6.2bn pa. Of this productive loss, 49% was due to anxiety and stress, 27% depression, 16% psychotic disorders, 5% other psychiatric disorders, and 3% alcohol dependence (Kavanagh, 1994).

For schizophrenia alone, the estimated indirect annual UK cost of lost production is £1.7bn, and it is the single largest disease category in terms of NHS expenditure, accounting for 9% of in-patient health service expenditure (House of Commons, 1994). Expressed in terms of overall health service costs, the mental illnesses are again expensive. Total NHS expenditure in 1993–4 was £30.7bn of which total secondary health care expenditure was £20.7bn and of this, total specialist mental illness expenditure was £1.8bn (Mental Health Foundation, 1993).

In terms of *combined mortality and disability*, the World Bank estimates for different disorders the Global Burden of Disease (GBD) measured in disability-adjusted life years (DALY). DALYs can be considered as a standardised form of quality-adjusted life years (QALYs), and for particular conditions they can be defined as the sum of years of life lost because of premature mortality, plus the years of life lived with disability, adjusted for the severity of disability. Murray & Lopez (1997a) report that neuropsychiatric conditions account for 10.5% of the worldwide burden of DALYs, and exceeds the contributions of cardiovascular conditions (9.7%) and malignant neoplasms (5.1%).

In terms of mortality, mental health problems contribute 8.1% of all *avoidable life years lost*, compared, for example, with 9% from respiratory diseases, 5.8% contributed by all forms of cancer, and 4.4% from heart disease (Desjarlais *et al.*, 1995).

Depressive disorders are the most prevalent of the neuro-psychiatric disorders, constituting the largest proportion of community burden. Since the most common neuro-psychiatric disorders begin during adulthood, the demographic transition will result in a sharp increase in overall burden of such disorders, based upon projections using simple relational models. In terms of future trends unipolar major depression is expected to increase from 3.7% to 5.7% of total DALYs between 1990 and 2020, moving from fourth to second in the overall ranking of leading causes of DALYs in the world. This increase is entirely due to demographic changes, as the age-specific rates are projected to remain constant (Murray & Lopez, 1996a, b, 1997b). In parallel with this, it is estimated that the total number of cases of schizophrenia in 'less developed countries' will increase from 16.7 million in 1985 to 24.4 million in 2000 (Desjarlais *et al.*, 1995).

Third, mental disorders may have important *consequences*, both for the patient and their families. For the patient, these include suffering caused by symptoms, lower quality of life, the loss of independence and work capacity, and poorer social integration. For the family and the community at large there is an increased burden from caring, and lowered economic productivity.

In terms of the number of avoidable deaths, suicide is a major cause of death throughout the world, especially in the more economically developed countries, and can cause more deaths than road traffic accidents. In France in 1991, for example, 11 725 deaths were due to suicide, compared with 10 198 deaths due to road traffic accidents. There are considerable variations in suicide rates between different countries, and there is evidence that particular groups, especially young unemployed men and elderly people who are socially isolated are especially at risk of suicide.

Fourth, as far as the *availability* of interventions is concerned, the public health approach implies that mental health services should be made available, in proportion to need, to cure (by removing symptoms) or to decrease suffering (by minimising symptoms and disability). In addition, the treatments necessary to achieve these goals should not normally be provided entirely separate from other health services, but on the contrary should form an integral part of mainstream clinical practice (Cooper, 1995). Related to this is the balance between public services and private practice. We agree with the view of Sedgwick (1982) that it is a public responsibility to assess mental health needs in the interests of the population as a whole. On this basis, the scope of private practice may usefully complement public services provided that: (i) universal coverage, and (ii) the provision and availability of services of minimum acceptable standards are already assured. Sedgwick also expressed forceful views on the nature of psychiatry.

> ' it funnels money, skills and careers away from the severe and chronic ... problems of the lower socio-economic orders (who cannot foot the bill or speak the language of the more affluent private sector) and into the less chronic, less severe but financially rewarding and culturally voguish difficulties of the well-heeled.'
> P. SEDGWICK
> Psychopolitics (1982)

Fifth, in relation to *acceptability and public concern* about interventions, the following factors are relevant: public perceptions of mental illnesses as health problems, their perception as problems which have solutions, whether the solutions are seen to be of proven effectiveness, the frequency, nature, severity and persistence of side-effects, and the risks of abuse of particular types of treatment, for example, in drug misuse.

Moreover, there is another way in which public concern demonstrates the public health impact of mental disorders. Observed abnormal behaviour associated with mental disorders, compared with that related to physical illnesses, is more likely to provoke public concern and to be perceived as posing a public risk, because it is more often unpredictable, and because it is more difficult to understand. The degree of personal suffering associated with mental disorders is also less often understood than for physical illnesses, and instead of receiving sympathy the mentally ill may induce concern. Indeed there is only a very weak relationship between the concern registered by the public for particular mental disorder conditions and that assessed by professionals. For example, severe depression is largely unrecognised by the public and provokes little reaction, but is seen by professionals as one of the most common causes of suffering and severe disability, and one which may lead to suicide in about 10% of cases.

2.4.4 **Prevention as an essential component of the public health approach**

The public health approach offers a further distinct advantage in that it includes explicit consideration of the *prevention* of disorders, not only their treatment. Although there is relatively little evidence on how to effect the primary prevention of mental disorders, the wider associations between social context and mental illnesses are well established. The quality of a person's social environment, for example, 'is closely linked to the risk for suffering a mental illness, to the triggering of an illness episode, and to the likelihood that such an illness will become chronic.' (Desjarlais *et al.*, 1995).

Poverty does appear to be the central mediating factor in many of these complex relationships. The association between low income and poor health, which is well established, may be either direct or indirect (Lynch, 1996). In fact the cumulative impact of poverty may produce sustained effects upon physical, cognitive, psychological and social functioning (Lynch *et al.*, 1997). The effects of hardship were shown in terms of activities of daily living as well as for clinical depression. They found, however, little evidence for causation, meaning that episodes of illness caused subsequent economic hardship.

Indeed poverty, economic inequities and social marginalisation have been shown to be risk factors for a range of mental disorders. Research into these associations is particularly challenging since the 'causation' of mental illnesses cannot be seen as a simple linear consequence of aetiological factors (for example, unemployment causing depression). Rather, to the best of our understanding, a multitude of interacting influences bear upon the likelihood of a mental illness starting, becoming severe or remaining chronic (Thornicroft, 1991).

Traditionally prevention distinguishes three levels: primary, secondary and tertiary (Goldberg & Tantam, 1991; Newton, 1992; Sowden *et al.*, 1997). *Primary prevention* refers to measures which stop the genesis or expression of the disorder. *Secondary prevention* refers to early detection of cases, usually by screening, where early treatment can significantly improve the course and outcome of the disorder. *Tertiary prevention* includes measures designed to reduce disabilities which are due to the disorder (Breakey, 1996). This framework is more useful in branches of medicine in which causes are well identified, the time between the action of the causal factor and the onset of symptoms is relatively short, there is a single primary aetiological factor, and screening procedures are simple, effective and acceptable. Only the last of these criteria commonly applies to most functional mental disorders.

The model proposed by the Institute of Medicine (1994), 'the Intervention Spectrum for Mental Health Problems', may have more heuristic value. It considers the three phases of prevention, treatment and maintenance as a continuum, and divides prevention into three sectors: *universal, selected* and *indicated*.

Universal interventions are directed at the entire population, and for the reasons already discussed, are relatively less important at this stage in our knowledge about how to prevent mental illnesses.

Selected interventions are targeted to individuals at risk, and since risk factors are more often identified than causes, in future we can expect increasing attention will be paid to such selected measures.

Indicated interventions are directed to individuals at high risk or to those with early features of illness. This can be termed the *high-risk strategy* which attempts to reduce in people identified with one or more risk factors for mental disorder, either the risk factor itself or its impact. This is the perspective most often taken in medical and psychiatric thinking, which as Henderson (1996) correctly pointed out 'is also politically appealing because it segregates those who are afflicted or susceptible, while the rest of society is left alone to enjoy its presumed normality.' A recent review on the effects of programmes of mental health promotion to high risk groups, both children and adults, has been published by Sowden *et al.* (1997).

In contrast, Rose (1992) has described the value of the *population-based strategy*. The power of this strategy is that 'a large number of people exposed to a small risk commonly generates many more cases than a small number exposed to a high risk' (Rose, 1993). In relation to mental disorders, this stimulating analysis would lead to an attempt to decrease the level of exposure to psycho-social or biological risk factors not for high-risk individuals but for the whole community. In Rose's words (1993) the 'visible part of the iceberg (prevalence) is a function of its total mass (the population average), and one cannot be reduced without the other'.

The consequence of this population-based strategy is to focus preventive measures on the control of the mass determinants of population prevalence and incidence rates. This view, which without doubt is innovative, is not uniformly applicable to all mental disorders, and implies continuous distributions of both morbidity and risk factor(s). This model, therefore, according to current knowledge, would apply to disorders which appear to be continuously distributed throughout the population, such as depressive disorders, but not to other disorders, such as schizophrenia, whose expression appears to be categorical. Interestingly, both continuous factors (such as age) and categorical factors (such as sex) may contribute or indeed interact in contributing towards the development of mental disorders.

2.5 **The purpose of the service**

Having defined the community-based service, and having discussed the relevance of the public health approach for such a service, it is useful now to establish the aims of the service as a whole. In other words: what is the purpose? It is relevant here to use the matrix model to describe the purpose at the country, local and patient levels.

The mental health service functions best conducted at the *country / regional level* are, in sequence:

   (i) to receive information from the local level (acting as a detector of problems as well as a routine monitor for trends);

  (ii) to aggregate these data to allow the analysis of particular problems, and to examine key associations (for example, between alcohol abuse and violence);

 (iii) to define a hierarchy of priorities;

 (iv) to ensure the formulation of a national strategic plan for service development;

  (v) to create and act upon an implementation programme to put the national strategy into practice (which may include the dissemination of exemplary practice);

 (vi) to compare the national plan with detailed information on the actual functioning of local services;

(vii) to set national standards.

The same feedback system applies to the contribution of the country / regional level to the formulation of a system of mental health laws, regulations and guidance.

The purposes of the mental health services which are best carried out at the *local level* can be described as:

  (i) to provide a reasonable range and quality and population coverage of mental health care;

 (ii) to collaborate openly with other local agencies to provide together a network of services, for example, primary-care liaison and consultation, and working closely with providers of housing and sheltered accommodation;

(iii) to conduct programmes of selected and indicated preventative interventions;

(iv) to maintain active surveillance of the service for early detection of trends and to identify clusters of factors which may generate hypotheses for subsequent aetiological or intervention research, which is the central concern of clinical epidemiology (Cooper, 1993).

At the *patient level* the primary purpose of the service is:

(i) to decrease suffering of the patient and the family and

(ii) to promote both recovery and restitution of social competence (Goldberg & Huxley, 1992).

Conflicts may occur between different concurrent and legitimate purposes of the mental health service. For example, there may be a direct conflict between an *individual's* need for confidentiality of information, and the *local* need for other agencies to be aware of which patients have a history of violence, and a national requirement for detailed service contact information for planning and policy purposes.

A second arena of possible manifest conflict is between the treatment choice (or treatment refusal) of an *individual* patient, and the expressed demands of family members or neighbours in the *local* area, when the patient's behaviour becomes, to them, unacceptably disturbed. In this case the mental health service may seek to fulfil two purposes simultaneously: to provide treatment and care for the patient, and to provide respite and protection for those affected by the patient.

A third area of conflict can occur between *nationally* influenced levels of unemployment and the associated limited work opportunities for many *individual* patients disabled by mental illness, with consequences for the need to provide sheltered occupation at the *local* level.

While conflicts are inevitable, solutions are not! Our intention is to show that the matrix model can assist in clarifying the conflicting views at the different levels, and can help in finding solutions. The extent to which we succeed will be judged by the reader.

3
The historical context

The aim of this chapter is to complete the Part I of this book by providing the historical context for the development of community mental health services. A more detailed description of the model follows in Parts II and III of the book. Following this, in Part IV we shall turn to the practical application of the model in the process of re-forming mental health services.

We present here only a highly selective account of the historical background for the following reasons. First, we are not historians and an extended historical appraisal is beyond our competence. Second, several excellent relevant historical analyses have now been published, to which we refer readers who seek more a detailed understanding (Jones, 1972; Scull, 1979; Levine, 1981; Gilman, 1996; Grob, 1991). Finally, we want to avoid the risk of being excessively absorbed by a contemplative appreciation of the past, at the expense of addressing the future.

3.1 **The matrix model and the development of mental health care**

The matrix model can be used as one framework to help understand the historical development of mental health services over the last 150 years. Several different approaches have been used in analysing these trends. The main forms of historical analysis are: socio-economic, political and clinical/technical. These approaches can all be placed (within the over-arching structure provided by the matrix model) in relation to *three historical periods*.

Period 1 describes the rise of the asylum between about 1880 and 1950; Period 2 is the decline of the asylum, from around 1950 to 1980; and Period 3 refers to the re-forming of mental health services, since approximately 1980. These three periods are summarised in Table 3.1. The dates applicable to each period have a wide 'confidence interval', and vary considerably, both between countries and between regions. One important consequence of viewing these changes in a longer-term perspective is to clarify that the current application of community-based services is a very recent historical phenomenon, and reflects a realisation of ideas that had been largely confined to the realm of debate for several decades.

The use of the matrix model, as we have indicated, implies the use of the two main dimensions. The first is the geographical, comprising the country/regional, local and individual levels, and the second is the temporal, including the input, process and outcome phases. It is useful to underline that different emphases have been given over these three historical periods to both dimensions. In terms of the geographical dimension, we see a process of decentralisation, with a move from the country/regional level to the local level of service provision, and more recently, in the third period, towards specifying individual treatment and care within the local service (see Table 3.2).

In terms of the second dimension of the matrix model (inputs, processes and outcomes), we suggest that the differential emphasis between the three historical periods is even more emphatic. In the *first period* (1880–1950) attention was given almost entirely to inputs, and it was assumed that the consequent processes and outputs would accrue proportionate to the inputs. The evidence is otherwise (Basaglia, 1968; Clare 1976; Martin, 1984; Tansella, 1986). Scandals have occurred at regular intervals, and regardless of the level of input from asylums. A series of inquiries, for example, into malpractice at several British hospitals for the mentally ill provided the occasion for a further critical evaluation of the function of psychiatric institutions. Martin (1984) has documented 14 investigations and inquiries in Britain from 1969 (Ely) to 1980 (Rampton). He sets out the recurring themes associated with established cases of ill-treatment: isolation of the institutions, lack of staff support, poor reporting procedures, a failure of leadership, ineffective administration, inadequate financial resources, the divided loyalties of trade unions, poor staff training and occasional negligent individuals. In the first period, desired outcomes were measured not in terms of individual patients within the institutions, but rather they were assumed to be public order and perceived public safety and security outside the asylum gates.

In the *second period* (1950–1980), as Table 3.2 indicates, increasing attention was given to the processes of treatment without sufficient emphasis upon the importance of measuring the outcomes of care. For example, in general adult psychiatry in this period there was a powerful emphasis upon the process of 'rehabilitation' (Shepherd, 1984, Bennett & Freeman, 1991). At that time, a commonly used concept was the 'step-ladder' model of

Table 3.1. *The key characteristics of three periods in the historical development of mental health systems of care*

Period 1 (1880–1950)	Period 2 (1950–1980)	Period 3 (1980–2000)
Asylums built	Asylums neglected	Asylums replaced by smaller facilities
Increasing number of beds	Decreasing number of beds	Decrease in the number of beds slows down
Reduced role for the family	Increasing but not fully recognised role of the family	Importance of families increasingly recognised, in terms of care given, therapeutic potential, the burden carried, and as a political lobbying group
Public investment in institutions	Public disinvestment in mental health services	Increasing private investment in treatment and care, and focus in public sector on cost-effectiveness and cost containment.
Staff: doctors and nurses only	Clinical psychologist, occupational therapists and social worker disciplines evolve	More community-based staff, and emphasis on multi-disciplinary team working
	Effective treatments emerge, beginning of treatment evaluation and of standardised diagnostic systems, growing influence of individual and group psychotherapy	Emergence of 'evidence-based' psychiatry in relation to pharmacological, social and psychological treatments.
Primacy of containment over treatment	Focus on pharmacological control and social rehabilitation, less disabled patients discharged from asylums	Emergence of concern about balance between control of patients and their independence

Table 3.2. *Geographical levels of the matrix model and the differental historical development of mental health systems of care*

Geographical levels	Period 1 (1880–1950)	Period 2 (1950–1980)	Period 3 (1980–2000)
Country / regional	Emphasis on concentration of undifferentiated patients (the indigent, mentally or physically handicapped, demented, and psychotic) in single remote mental hospitals, where patients were categorised by behaviour and sex	Larger asylums retain differentiated responsibility for the long-stay patients: including the more behaviourally disturbed, or treatment non-responsive, and mentally handicapped Differentiation of specialist wards / hospitals for forensic patients	Decreasing number of adult long-stay beds in health service facilities. Remaining regional level facilities focus on forensic services
Local		Beginning of psychiatric wards in general hospitals for acute patients, differentiated from day hospital, day centre, sheltered workshops, and other local rehabilitation facilities	Increasing number of community mental health teams and centres. Proliferation of local non-hospital residential facilities, including group homes, nursing homes, sheltered apartments, and supported housing schemes. Decreasing emphasis upon separate rehabilitation facilities
Individual			Design of individualised inter-agency treatment programmes involving, multi-disciplinary teams, voluntary organisations, GPs, social services, church and charities, etc. Less separation between treatment and rehabilitation, stress on secondary prevention of relapse, and also on improving quality of life. More evidence-based psychotherapies

rehabilitation, which meant that patients could be expected to benefit from service inputs by making a graduated return to full, normal functioning after an episode of mental illness. This humanitarian approach offered optimism to staff about patients who in Period 1 has been classified as 'untreatable', but it also confined many long-term psychotic patients to poorly paid work. Most notably, however, there was remarkably little research on the outcomes of these rehabilitative processes.

Related to this, in the second period, was the prevailing interest in developing a common language for classification and diagnosis which at the international level was well demonstrated by the outstanding efforts of the WHO Division of Mental Health (Sartorius & Janca, 1996). While this emphasis is understandable, and it was a necessary step to establish a shared international terminology, again there was a notable lack of attention to individual outcomes and to developing common outcome instruments which were reliable and valid (Thornicroft & Tansella, 1996). This imbalance between the attention to diagnoses for categories of patients, and the inattention to other treatment processes and to treatment outcomes for individual patients has been noticed and heavily criticised both by anti-psychiatrists and by other commentators in this second period (Laing, 1966; Basaglia, 1968; Cooper, 1974; Kovel, 1976; Sedgwick, 1982; Ingelby, 1981).

In the *third period* (1980 to the present) the full complement of phases along the temporal dimension are brought into focus (see Table 3.3). For the first time, the relationships between inputs, processes and outcomes can be considered as a whole, at the individual level. At the same time, we have already stressed the importance of considering also the other two geographical levels (country/regional and local) in terms of these inter-relationships, and such research is now beginning. This is confirmed by the current development of (i) standardised international measures of inputs and processes as well as outcomes, and (ii) newer statistical methodologies for multi-level and graphical modelling (Biggeri *et al.*, 1996).

3.2 **Period 1. The rise of the asylum (1880–1950)**

Period 1, the rise of the asylum, occurred between approximately 1880 and 1950 in many of the more economically developed countries. It is characterised by the construction and enlargement of large asylums, remote from their feeder towns, offering mainly custodial containment and the provision of the basic necessities for survival, to people with a wide range of clinical and social abnormalities. The predominant model used to explain the disorders of the inmates was that unknown biological causes

Table 3.3. *Temporal phases of the matrix model and the differential historical development of mental health systems of care*

Temporal phases	Period 1 (1880–1950)	Period 2 (1950–1980)	Period 3 (1980–2000)
Inputs	Attention primarily upon buildings. Poor staff selection and training, mental health and social welfare legislation to regulate the use of institutions	Building of occupational and rehabilitation centres, modernisation of legal and policy framework, development of liaison between psychiatry and other medical disciplines, establishment of newer allied disciplines, and sub-specialities within psychiatry. New anti-psychotic and anti-depressant medications	Community mental health centres built, individual, family and population-level needs assessments, home treatment teams, new anti-depressant and anti-psychotic medications, integrated pharmacological and psycho-social treatments, cognitive-behavioural treatment, self-help and patient advocacy, modernisation of mental health legislation in some countries. Enhanced attention from mass media. Emphasis on the control of public expenditure
Processes		Influence of psychodynamic theory on mental health services at zenith. Decreasing length of in-patient stay and appearance of 'revolving door' pattern of service use. Reduced bed numbers in asylums, but hospital costs not reduced. Diversion of acute patients to acute hospitals. Attention to group processes in 'therapeutic milieu', therapeutic communities, and group psychotherapy. Monitoring patterns of service contact using case registers	Focus on continuity of care over time, by the same team, and/or co-ordination between different agencies, using, for example, case management. Targeting services toward more disabled patients. Greater attention to risk assessment. Development of audit of clinical practice. Growth of evaluative research as a tool to improve clinical practice. Introduction of market principles (separation of purchaser and provider roles, designed to improve quality through competition)
Outcomes			At the country and local levels limited use of indicators (mortality, suicide and homelessness rates). At the individual level standardised outcomes measures in research studies, and in some clinical services, rated by staff, service users and their families

were responsible. The subsequent discovery of pellagra and the psychiatric manifestations of syphilis confirmed this view. The asylums therefore acted as repositories for those considered untreatable.

In economic terms, this required considerable investment and many large institutions were built in the last two decades of the nineteenth century. Indeed the choice of remote sites fitted both the need to remove this perceived threat to the public safety, and was also consistent with then current views of mental hygiene, which held that recovery was facilitated by restful country settings. One consequence of this choice of geographical location was the subsequent professional segregation of psychiatrists and nurses from the main body of clinical practice, and from the centres of professional status in the metropolitan, university teaching hospitals.

> **asylum** *noun*
>
> 1 sanctuary; protection, esp. for those pursued by the law (*seek asylum*).
>
> 2 *historical.* any of various kinds of institution offering shelter and support to distressed or destitute individuals, esp. the mentally ill.
> Source: *Concise Oxford Dictionary* (1993)

The characteristics and stages of this progressive growth in hospital beds have been subject to detailed analyses (Jones, 1972; Hunter & McAlpine, 1974; Grob, 1991). Three themes were apparent throughout these developments: namely clinical, humanitarian and economic considerations. In 1842 the English Poor Law Commissioners, for example, reported that 'It must, however, be remembered that with lunatics, the first object ought to be their cure by means of proper medical treatment' (Poor Law Commission, 1842). Indeed it was clinical effectiveness which was used to justify the extra cost of asylums compared with the work houses.

There was also an important moral aspect to the debate regarding the asylum. At one extreme was the view represented by the utilitarian Chadwick, who was Secretary to the Poor Law Commissioners until 1847, that the greater good was served by incurring the least burden on the pockets of the sane (Finer, 1952). Indeed, this view was reinforced later in the nineteenth century by a progressive disillusionment with the ability of the asylums to improve the condition of the majority of patients (the 'untreatable'), along with a tendency towards block treatment in hospitals. Patient populations were vastly in excess of their original planned size. In 1850, for example, each hospital had an average of 297 patients – by 1900 this had risen to 961. Dr Granville, writing in 1877 about the doubling in size of the Hanwell Asylum in West London to nearly 2000 patients, lamented the loss of 'that special character which arises from dealing with a limited number of cases directly' (Granville, 1877).

Thirdly, the economic argument was also given early prominence. In 1838 Edward Gulson, Assistant Poor Law Commissioner, gave evidence to the House of Commons Select Committee on the Poor Law Amendment Act. He recommended a transfer of power over lunatics from the county asylums to the Poor Law Commissioners, 'where they would be kept at one half or a third or a fourth of the expense at which they are now kept'. These three guiding imperatives, the clinical, the moral and the financial, therefore combined in a subtle and continuing interplay, the effects of which were manifest in the late nineteenth century as the establishment and overgrowth of the asylums.

> '**Gli infermieri non devono tenere relazioni con le famiglie dei malati, darne notizia, portare fuori senz'ordine lettere, oggetti, ambasciate, saluti: ne' possono recare agli ammalati alcuna notizia dal di fuori, ne' oggetti, ne' stampe, ne' scritti.**'
>
> (**Norma di regolamento in un ospedale psichiatrico**)
>
> '**Nurses must not have relationships with families of patients, pass on information, take out of the hospital without orders letters, objects, messages, greetings: nor are they not allowed to bring to patients any news from outside, or objects, or printed material or notes.**'
>
> (**From a list of regulations in a psychiatric hospital**)
>
> Quoted in '*Morire di Classe*' F. Basaglia & F. Basaglia Ongaro (eds), 1969.

It is important to note that although we suggest that the three historical periods have occurred consecutively, the times at which they began and finished in different countries have varied greatly. In Italy for example, psychiatric bed numbers were stable until 1963 (Tansella *et al.*, 1987), and then diminished precipitously after the legislation introduced in 1978, so it is reasonable to conclude that in Italy Period 2 began about a decade later than in England.

In addition to differences in timing, there are also considerable cross-national variations in the contours of each historical period. In Italy the segregation of mental health professionals, together with their patients during Period 1, was balanced by specific areas in which psychiatrists gained power at this time. Asylum doctors, and in particular the director of the 'manicomio' (asylum), were the only staff authorised to confirm the admission or discharge of patients, were fully responsible for the hospital budget, and had responsibility for all disciplinary matters for staff and patients. These clinician-administrators were effectively charged with maintaining the proper control of those excluded from their local communities.

Notably, until the Italian mental heath law of 1978, the responsibility for both public and private asylums lay not with the Health Ministry but with the Ministry of Internal Affairs and its local prefectures (Canosa, 1979).

Similarly, until 1968 everyone who had been admitted to a psychiatric hospital had their names entered by a tribunal into a national judicial register, which was a lifelong assignment (which persisted also after hospital discharge), and this was considered a shameful family stigma which meant the permanent loss of many civil rights, including voting, and the ownership of property and land. The tribunal which confirmed psychiatric admissions had to nominate a legal guardian to act in the legal interests of such patients.

While we propose here a somewhat fixed sequence of historical periods, we wish to emphasise that there will necessarily be some blurring in practice in two directions. On one hand there will be prefigurative elements in earlier stages which act as sentinels or precursors for later more substantive or more generalised trends. Examples of prefigurative community-orientated service developments are given by Talbott (1996). He details a series of early innovative services *a l'Americaine*, beginning with the first alternative farm of St. Anne in 1855, followed by, for example, mass boarding out schemes in the late 19th century, travelling clinics in the early years of this century, and 'vocational rehabilitation' projects, which began just before our notional end of Period 1 in 1955.

On the other hand, later developmental stages will often retain remnants of earlier times, for example a few remaining large and remote vestigial institutions in which poor material and treatment conditions are redolent of a previous period. In Japan, for example, the number of beds in 1960 was 95 067, and this increased to 172 950 in 1965. By 1993 there were 1672 psychiatric hospitals which contained 362 963 beds, a degree of in-patient provision far higher than in most economically developed nations, and is similar to the levels seen in England 40 years ago. There has been a slight decrease in bed numbers since 1993 (Shinfuku *et al.*, 1998).

In terms of the matrix model, these inter-penetrating time scales indicate that changes at one geographical level may take many years to filter up or down to other levels. For example, a change of national policy, such as the prioritisation of the severely mentally ill in England and Wales remains incomplete more than six years after its introduction (Department of Health, 1990).

3.3 Period 2. The decline of the asylum (1950 – 1980)

The rationale for deinstitutionalisation and the justification for the transfer of long-stay patients from the larger psychiatric hospitals are based on sociological, pharmacological, administrative and legal changes (Jones, 1972; Scull, 1984; Brown, 1985; Busfield, 1986; O'Driscoll, 1993). From the mid 1950s an increasingly forceful sociological opinion emerged, both within and without the psychiatric profession. This view criticised the ill effects of prolonged stay within the large psychiatric institutions. Barton (1959) described institutional neurosis' as a disease in its own right … characterised by apathy, lack of initiative, loss of interest'. He confidently asserted that 'rehabilitation solves these problems'. Extending this, Goffman (1961) formulated the concept of the 'total institution', central to which was 'the handling of many human needs by the bureaucratic organisation of whole blocks of people'. Wing & Brown (1970) reinforced this view with their description of the 'institutionalism' of chronic patients. From their study of long-stay patients in three British hospitals, they accepted the hypothesis that 'the social conditions under which a patient lives (particularly poverty of the social environment) are actually responsible for part of the symptomatology (particularly the negative symptoms)'.

Treatment patterns were also changing rapidly. Within three years of the formulation of chlorpromazine in 1952, its use as an anti-psychotic agent was widespread (Jones, 1972). The decline of asylums is often reported in associations with the 'anti-psychotic drugs revolution'. While we fully recognise the usefulness of these drugs, their importance should not obscure other revolutionary innovations in patient care. Industrial Therapy Organisations, for example, were set up (Early, 1978; Wing, 1960), therapeutic communities were developed (Clark, 1974), day hospitals appeared (Bierer, 1951), and hostels and half-way houses were established.

As far as anti-psychotic drugs are concerned, it was evident from the outset that while their impact on psychiatric practice was considerable, the view that the coincident fall in the resident population of mental hospitals was directly due to their introduction was subject to considerable controversy. At the first International Congress of Neuro-Pharmacology Sir Aubrey Lewis reported that 'British figures regarding mental hospital populations impose caution in giving the pharmacological action of these new drugs most of the credit for the undoubted fall that has occurred in the absolute number of people resident in certain mental hospitals' (Lewis, 1959). Shortly afterwards, Shepherd and colleagues (1961) published a statistical account of the changes in an English county mental hospital before and after the introduction of the psychotropic drugs in 1955, which proved that the impact of pharmacotherapy was very small, and suggested that the non-specific benefits of new drugs may already have been attained by other measures, such as more medical personnel, changing criteria for discharge, increased acceptance of the mentally ill by families and by the community, and the expansion of rehabilitative practices and social facilities.

'Certainly if we had to choose between abandoning the use of all the new psychotropic drugs and abandoning the Industrial Resettlement Units and other social facilities available to us, there would be no hesitation about the choice: the drugs would go.'
SIR AUBREY LEWIS, 1959

The legal provisions relating to the mentally ill in Britain were unified in the Mental Health Act of 1959. This established Mental Health Review Tribunals, dissolved the Board of Control, and delineated the responsibilities of central and local government. The Act also extended the provisions of guardianship from the mentally deficient to all the mentally disordered, and allowed voluntary admission providing patients did not positively object to treatment, thereby facilitating a huge reduction in the proportion of compulsory patients (Jones, 1972).

The scandals referred to in Period 2 had further consequences. Such influences combined to allow the substitution of secondary aims, such as the establishment of routine ward practices, for the primary aim of delivering care to patients. The effect of such inquiries was to reinforce the developing polarisation of views: if the large institutions were self-evidently pernicious, it followed that community-based facilities must be commensurately desirable. This assumption was not based upon research evidence, but it was nevertheless directly incorporated into government policy, both in Britain and in the USA (Barham, 1992).

Financial considerations have also been especially important in fostering this transfer of care. In the United States, for example, the introduction of Medicaid in the 1960s promoted a rapid expansion of nursing homes with an associated transfer of financial responsibility, or 'cost shifting', from state to federal programmes (Scull, 1984; Mechanic, 1986; Levine, 1981; Lamb, 1994). In Britain, by comparison, mental health services had been committed to widespread hospital closure since 1955, and Government policy has most clearly reflected this organisational and clinical reality since 1975 (DHSS, 1975).

For much of this time deinstitutionalisation has been left undefined. In 1975 the then Director of the National Institute of Mental Health in the USA described three essential components of such an approach: the prevention of inappropriate mental hospital admissions through the provision of community facilities, the release to the community of all institutional patients who have received adequate preparation, and the establishment and maintenance of community support systems for non-institutionalised patients (Brown, 1975). Bachrach (1976) defined deinstitutionalisation more succinctly as the contraction of traditional institutional settings, with the concurrent expansion of community-based services.

In Italy, the maximum number of psychiatric beds occurred in 1963 (91868 residents, 1.61 per 1000 population), and by 1981 the number had more than halved (38358, 0.68 per 1000 population). During this same period the number of admissions grew steadily until 1975, three years before the reform of 1978, which made first admissions to traditional large mental hospitals illegal (in fact since 1982 all admissions to these institutions, both public and private, had been against the law). In this respect Italy is atypical compared with other Western European countries, which have continued to rely to some extent upon these longer-stay hospitals as a last resort.

The peak of psychiatric bed numbers for England as a whole occurred in 1954 and coincided with the introduction by Mr Kenneth Robinson of a Private Members motion to the House of Commons, 'That this House ... expresses its concern at the serious overcrowding of mental hospitals. . .' (Jones,1972). A reduction in numbers was seen as the only humane option. In the following year Houston (1955) wrote in the Lancet 'By incarceration we were aggravating the natural process of the disease. At last a new era is dawning and the doors of despair are being unlocked.' The predicted decline in numbers of psychiatric in-patients has continued progressively over the 40 years since that time (Tooth & Brooke, 1961). The average number of psychiatric beds occupied each day in 1985 in England and Wales, for example, was 64800 (Audit Commission, 1986), which represented, based upon the Annual reports of the Lunacy Commissioners, a return to the occupancy level last seen in 1895 (Scull, 1984). On the latest available information, there are now a total of 47296 psychiatric beds in England (Audit Commission, 1994).

> ' The average standard of psychiatric practice in Britain is abysmally low. Psychiatrists themselves are sometimes reluctant to make this admission, though the evidence is overwhelming. In an average mental hospital a long-stay patient is likely to see a doctor for only ten minutes or so every three months. ... Scandals about the ill treatment of patients in mental hospitals, including those of relatively good reputation, occur with monotonous regularity.'
> A. CLARE (1976)
> *Psychiatry in Dissent*

3.4 Period 3. Re-forming mental health services (1980 – 2000)

Those who criticise the deficiencies of current community mental health care sometimes forget the shortcomings of the institutional era. In a letter to the *Lancet*, towards the end of Period 2, a British psychiatrist indicted his frustration with the low quality of the services provided by long-stay institutions, 'I do not know whether the country can afford adequate staffing of psychiatric hospitals and rebuilding the majority of them. Without that I fear that inspection, inquiries and Ombudsmen will no more improve the psychiatric service than court marshals improve the morale of the army.' (Last, 1972). During Period 2, British Government policy, initially set out in the White Paper 'Better Services for the Mentally Ill' (DHSS, 1975), had established a target of 47 900 in-patient psychiatric beds, after the completion of the programme of closure of psychiatric hospitals – a bed reduction target which has now been met. At the same time, it is clear that the rate of hospital closure has outstripped the rate of establishing replacement residential and day-care services.

A comprehensive survey of psychiatric hospitals in England found that long-stay beds have been substituted by places in nursing and residential care homes, often managed by the independent sector (Davidge *et al.*, 1993). Similarly, after the first 30 years of the hospital closure programme, the 67 000 remaining psychiatric in-patients in 1984 represented 45% of the total target reduction over the decade (Social Services Committee, 1985). At that time the 6800 available residential places were 41% of the proposed target increase, and the 17 000 day hospital places were only 17% of the target figure. In day centres, the 9000 places showed an increase of only 16% toward the stated target of 28 200 (Thornicroft & Bebbington, 1989; Wing, 1992).

While 57 000 bed places have been lost, as well as the opportunities for day activities which were also available to many of these patients in hospital, relatively few residential or occupational places have been reprovided at the national level. Indeed the OPCS National Survey of Psychiatric Morbidity in 1994 found only about 10 000 psychiatric patients in NHS hospitals who had been in-patients for more than 6 months (Meltzer *et al.*, 1995).

In consequence there is now considerable debate about the numbers of psychiatric beds that are needed (Wing, 1971; Hirsch, 1988; Wing, 1992; Thornicroft & Strathdee, 1994; Faulkner *et al.*, 1994; Wing & Lelliot, 1994). The 1975 White Paper suggested targets of 50 District General Hospital beds per 100 000 of the population, and an additional 35 for the elderly severely mentally infirm and 17 for the 'new' long-stay patients. The 1985 House of Commons Social Services Committee report on Community Care noted that 'a smaller number of in-patients beds is now thought necessary for general psychiatric services since the average length of stay has continued to decline'. Even so, there is at present neither government policy nor a widespread professional consensus on how far bed closures should proceed.

Table 3.4. *Parallels between late 19th and late 20th century developments*

Phase	19th century	20th century
Optimism phase	mental hygiene movement	community mental health approach
Building phase	institutions – large, mental hospitals, operating as self-sufficient and isolated communities	decentralised community mental health centres & smaller residential and day-care facilities
Disillusionment phase	overcrowding of accumulating patients	scandals, inquiries and public reaction
Control phase	attempt to differentiate between 'curable' and 'incurable' patients	attempt to differentiate between 'safe' and 'risk' patients

Facilities for long-stay patients, now more often accurately described as long-term, are only one component of a full range of local provisions. Several estimates have been made of bed needs based upon reviews of the available literature on the levels of need and the variations in need across the main treatment and care categories (Wing, 1992; Strathdee & Thornicroft, 1992).

We do not wish to suggest to the reader that the historical development of mental health services is a consistent linear trend from the asylum to a community-based system of care. Multiple contradictions occur at each stage and any country will show examples of phases of evolution and involution. This has been well expressed by Goldman & Morrisey as 'cycles of care'. Indeed intriguing parallels in form, if not of content, appear when we compare the central themes of nineteenth and twentieth century mental health services, as summarised in Table 3.4.

As for the future, we shall resist the seduction of prediction, as Sartorius (1988) has put it '. . . the predictions of the future are usually statements of current desires; and the methods which are proposed to achieve goals in the future have the limitation of the past, when they were produced'.

PART II **The matrix model: the geographical dimension**

In Chapter 1 we introduced the central framework of this book, the matrix model. Since the two dimensions of this model need to be taken into account simultaneously, for the sake of clarity we shall begin by using Part II to outline the three geographical dimensions in general terms. However, in Part III we shall go on to describe each of the three temporal dimensions separately and also in relation to the first axis, and in this way we shall illustrate the importance of the interactions between the two dimensions by referring to the cells of the matrix model, which we call 1A to 3C, as shown in Figure 1.1, on page 2.

4

The country / regional level

4.1 **Defining the country / regional level**

By country we mean the level with a shared government at which mental health laws are established, any relevant minimum clinical standards are set, overall policy is formulated and which is often the level at which the training of professionals is organised. In some countries different regions or states, while sharing some regulations, may formulate their own policy directives and clinical practice guidelines, particularly in countries with a more federal or decentralised political structure. The issues relevant at this country / regional level can be considered in the following three domains: social and political, economic, and professional.

4.2 **Social and political domains**

In the social and political domain, there is the balance that exists in each country, on one hand between concerns for the duty of care to individual patients and the degree of importance attached to their civil liberties, and on the other hand the legitimate expectations of the wider public that mentally ill individuals should receive prompt and proper treatment and care and also that the wider community should be protected from disturbance and harm from patients.

To simplify the complex interactions which take place within the social and political domain, we think that it is useful to consider three aspects within this domain: perceptions by the public, perceptions by politicians, and their policy and legal consequences. Although we portray this as a linear association in Table 4.1, these are recursive pathways, and the chaining effects can be considered to start from any point. Even though there are multiple feedback loops between these three steps, we place them in this particular order because, in our view, step (A) is increasingly the prime driver of this sequence of perceptions and events.

Table 4.1. *Pathway from social and political perceptions to policy*

[A] Perceptions ⇒ of the Public	[B] Perceptions ⇒ of Politicians	[C] Policy & Legal Consequences
Influenced by [C] and by:	Influenced by [A] and by:	Influenced by [B] and by:
Personal experience	Personal and family	Macro-economic
Family experience	experience of politicians	situation
Word of mouth	Personal views of politicians	Other competing
Media accounts of events	Direct pressure of mass	business of
Media commentary	media	government
Lobbying / interest groups	Representations of	Consensus on necessary
Professional organisations	professionals	action
Visibility of issues, scale	Mediation of civil servants	Likelihood of results
(prevalence) of the	Evidence from research	before the next election
problems	Evidence from inquiries	
Social attitudes on civil		
liberties & public safety		

Within the scheme shown in Table 4.1, mental health policies (step C) will reflect the wider mood of the times along a continuum between acceptance and tolerance at one extreme, and exclusion and prejudice at the other. The larger social view of the adequacy of mental health services is influenced in turn by the policy and legislative framework. Other factors which bear upon composite social attitudes about what should be done in terms of mental health services are first of all, direct personal experience of mental illness. Because, as we have discussed earlier in this book, mental disorders are among the commonest types of suffering, then we can expect that up to a half of the adult population will have themselves experienced mental illness directly, or have had contact at close quarters with mental illness in a close relative.

Paradoxically, given the very common nature of such conditions, the prevailing stereotypes identified by survey on public attitudes to mental illness are overwhelmingly negative (Angermeyer & Matschinger, 1996). A full consideration of the many roles of the channels of mass media and public concerns about risk are beyond the scope of this book, and are covered elsewhere (Furedi, 1997). We do want to distinguish, however, between the twin roles performed by the mass media of factual reporting of mental illness related events, and their commentary or interpretation functions. As is the case for other news reporting, adverse events are more newsworthy than treatment or services successes. The bias is therefore always towards an unfavourable image of mental health services.

Politicians are interpreters of public opinion. They selectively translate perceptions of the public into policy and legal actions. This is a complex process, in which other influences can play an important role, such as the personal views and experiences of close political advisors, or the preferences of ministers for the views of patients or professionals. At each stage the mediating role of senior civil servants is often of central importance, especially in countries where there is a short length of stay and rapid discharge of their political masters! Where the government at the country/regional level is satisfied that changes should be introduced, either as policy guidance or as legal statutes, a series of barriers can still prevent their introduction (see C in Table 4.1).

Where public and political perceptions are convergent, and wider political circumstances at the country/regional level are favourable, their net effect will be embodied from time to time in new mental health regulations and laws. For instance, the Italian Law No. 180 in 1978 was approved at a point when the public mood was rather libertarian, and because of the role of active and enthusiastic psychiatrists, and at a political moment when the centre-left coalition, guided by the Christian Democratic Party, was receiving external support from the Italian Communist Party, presently called the Democratic Left Party (see Basaglia, 1968; Mosher & Burti, 1989; Tansella, 1991).

By comparison, in England the Mental Health (Patients in the Community) Act in 1995 was a statutory expression of a widely held public view that mental health staff had insufficient power to compel patients living in the community to accept treatment and supervision. This balance will be to a large extent context-specific. For example, the extent and speed of political reactions to such changes in the public mood (and their expression in the media) may be modulated by the presence of clinically trained personnel working on policy matters, who can act as conduits for the introduction of clinical values (see the three ACEs in Chapter 11)

Further, the frequency with which new law and policy directives appear will vary considerably between countries. In countries in which such new regulations appear less frequently, clinicians may feel less constrained by such remote control, may have a greater opportunity properly to consolidate new policies, but may also show far greater heterogeneity in their clinical practice and quality of care.

To a large extent mental health services more sensitively and subtly reflect the climate of social opinion than most other areas of medical practice, which includes human rights, the position of minority ethnic groups, the problems of marginalised groups, the poor, prisoners, and migrants. All these issues affect the balance between therapy and control. The point of balance reached at any particular historical time in each country will closely reflect wider prevailing public attitudes on how far civil liberties should outweigh risk containment (Furedi, 1997).

4.3 **The economic domain**

Economic issues acting at the country level also influence service organisation and development and clinical practice. In terms of public expenditure on mental health services, the overall level of economic development (along with the relative importance attached to mental health in relation to other medical specialities) has a profound effect upon the extent and quality of the clinical services available, and upon the capital expenditure available for the construction of health facilities and for their maintenance. The methods used to allocate health expenditure from central finance ministries to local regions, and then to individual local areas vary enormously, for example in the extent to which these allocation methods take account of local variations in general health or in psychiatric morbidity.

Equally, economic cycles of growth and recession, which may affect subgroups of the population in different ways, influence the direct funding of state mental health services (both capital and revenue), the provision of welfare benefits, and expenditure on mental health research, such cycles also have indirect effects mediated by levels of employment. Unemployment, for example, has established effects on suicide and on the onset, course and outcome of psychiatric disorders (Warr, 1987; Warner, 1994). The direct consequences of unemployment include higher rates of depression and suicide among affected individuals. The indirect effects are illustrated by how changing employment prospects in different stages of the economic cycle impact upon the course and outcomes for psychotic disorders, and may account for some of the variations between developed and developing countries.

Economic factors may also be expressed through the detailed ways in which welfare benefits are received by psychiatric patients. One indirect effect is that in many developed countries more secure entitlement to welfare benefits depends upon the registration of a patient as permanently disabled or as retired from the job market, which may reduce opportunities for implementing rehabilitation programmes to assist in graded recovery. A further consequence of permanent reliance on welfare benefits is that such patients will usually only have access to low-cost housing. Wider economic factors will in turn affect the availability and quality of such affordable housing.

4.4 **The professional domain**

The third set of issues acting at the country/regional level are concerns for the professions, including standards of care and agreed staffing levels, training, accreditation and continuing education. *Training* in many countries, for example, is based upon curricula developed when psychiatric services were hospital based. There is often a clear phase lag in which clinical practice moves ahead of the content of training courses, whose curricula are formulated at the country/regional level, and whose content tends to change more slowly than practice. Where universities and colleges are directly responsible for training and professional education, they need to be directly involved in current clinical practice. Similarly, the timeliness of decisions at the country level will affect the availability of sufficient numbers of staff with relevant clinical skills at the local level. Any consequent staffing vacancies will impact especially on mental health services which already have low staffing levels.

A second responsibility usually accepted by the professions at the country / regional level is the *examination and accreditation* of their members, through which minimum standards of professional competence are meant to be ensured. Traditionally this was largely a once-only process leading to a basic or higher professional qualification. Increasingly in more economically developed countries the medical and other health care professions are introducing discretionary or mandatory systems of continuing professional development (sometimes called continuing medical or professional education), which are intended to renew the knowledge base of practitioners on an ongoing basis.

A third duty for the professions is to participate in *long-term manpower planning*. The purpose of this is to estimate the required capacity for each profession in the future and to arrange for sufficient (and not excessive) numbers of trainees to qualify to match the estimated need. In Italy, for example, such forward planning is now being transferred from the country to the regional level. This process also illustrates an important wider point: the extent to which the key functions within the mental health system are mutually interdependent, and that these interdependencies cross the geographical levels. If a catchment area mental health service has been well planned at the local level, it may still provide a relatively poor quality of care if manpower planning at the country/regional level has been poorly carried out so that relatively few properly trained staff are available to fill vacancies. In this case a well functioning service reflects the successful completion of multiple functions at all three geographical levels.

A fourth function which is most often set at the country/regional level is the setting and monitoring of *minimum standards of care*. These may apply to the number of nurses expected to be present on an in-patient ward, the number of doctors for each standard catchment area, the production of agreed national formularies, the adoption of standard diagnostic systems, or the regulations governing the documentation of clinical contacts with patients. In each case the agreed standard or system which has been set only has meaning and value if (i) an effective parallel system exists to inspect clinical practice and to monitor the application of the norms, and (ii) a reliable method of feedback exists that will successfully modify the performance of a service which fails to meet any given standard.

The quality and the extent of the data collection system which is able to produce national statistics on mental health care provided by specialist services varies greatly between countries. However, even in countries with more advanced data systems there are two common weaknesses, namely that information is more often: (i) about hospital than community service contacts, and (ii) event-based than patient-based, for example recording total number of admissions per year rather than the number of individual patients who have been admitted, and whether the same patient has had multiple admissions in the same or in different hospitals. In Chapter 10 we shall examine in more detail how such data can be used for planning purposes.

4.5 Conclusions

For the present, what we wish to do in this chapter is to emphasise, particularly for readers who are involved with clinical work at the individual level or managerial work at the local level, the relevance to them of issues which are confined largely to the country/regional level. In a sense there is a type of organisational 'food-chain' in which the effects of country/regional level decisions cascade down, and so constrain what is possible at the lower geographical levels. In this way, for example, the clinical decisions of professionals in difficult cases are often coloured by the wider climate of social, political and economic opinion.

For the future, two issues are likely to grow in importance. In terms of professional training there will be an increasing mobility between countries of the health professions, along with a tendency to harmonise systems of professional accreditation, a trend already underway within the European Community, but also evident on a more global basis. Second, mental health care is following other areas of medicine in increasing the stress on evidence-based clinical practice. This trend can only be diffused from individual centres of excellence to routine practice if it is co-ordinated at the country/regional level. This implies central funding support for psychiatric research, for the conduct and dissemination of systematic reviews, and for clinical guidelines and treatment protocols, which can be produced locally. These will most likely be implemented within a professional culture under the aegis of organisations at the country/regional level, such as national associations of nurses, psychiatrists or psychologists.

While we agree with the importance of this trend we anticipate that there will be a need for the foreseeable future to complement the evidence base (see Chapter 10) with the ethical base (see Chapter 11) for mental heath services. One example of this complementarity will be to operationalise ethical principles into quantitiative outcome measures.

5
The local level

5.1 Defining the local level

By local level we mean the catchment area for which an integrated system of care for general adult mental health services can be provided. The population size will vary between countries and regions, but is generally between 50 000 to 250 000 total residents. In some countries the scale of the local level is smaller where a single generic team is the main service provider (as in South-Verona in Italy), whereas in other settings (for example in Victoria in Australia) the main unit of organisation driving the whole service is the 24-hour Crisis Assessment Team, leading to a larger-scale 'local level' of about a quarter of a million population.

Where local services are organised on the basis of catchment areas at the local level, these are often called sectors. The concept of the sector has permeated community mental health service development. Following the emergence of the first sectors in France in 1947, by 1961 over 300 had been established. In the USA the Community Mental Health Centres Act (1963) introduced the principle of a catchment area for each CMHC, and by 1975, 40% of the population had sectorised services. In Europe, throughout the 1970s sector development grew but sizes varied between countries (Lindholm, 1983). Germany has sector sizes in the range of 250 000, the Netherlands around 300 000, while the areas for the Scandinavian countries are smaller with Denmark averaging 60–120 000, Finland 100 000, Norway 40 000, and Sweden 25–50 000. Of all countries, however, Italy has most comprehensively adapted the concept by virtue of Law 180, passed in 1978, which established sectors in the range of 50–200 000 population. A further range of factors can also affect the choice of sector size and they are shown in Table 5.1.

5.2 Rationale for accentuation of the local level

Why do we place our main emphasis in this book upon the organisation of services at the local level? Why do we refer to the local level as the

Table 5.1. *Factors influencing sector size*

Factors in the population
1. Socio-demographic composition of population
2. Social deprivation indices
3. Ethnic composition
4. Age–sex structure
5. Knowledge of psychiatric morbidity
6. Existing service utilisation patterns
Factors in the organisation of services
1. Social services boundaries
2. Primary care organisation
3. Extent of sheltered housing
4. Number of old and new long-stay patients
5. Presence of a large institution
6. Presence of a district general hospital
7. Manpower and other resources parameters
Factors in the local area
1. Significant geographical structures
2. Inherent community structures
3. Presence of building sites or development

Source: modified from Strathdee & Thornicroft (1992)

'lens' to focus policies and resources at the country/regional level (see Chapter 4) effectively for the benefit of individual patients (see Chapter 6)?

The *first* reason for this focus is that it is usually the best level at which to consider the components of the general adult mental health system, their organisation and their integration with each other. A series of key questions arise at this level. Are services better organised with generic or separate specialised (acute versus rehabilitation, or all diagnoses versus diagnosis-specific) teams? How far, if at all, should in-patient and community services be organisationally integrated? Should the crisis and emergency functions, which will include night-time and weekend services, be separated from the routine clinical teams? Finally, are the main components of adult mental health services mutually substitutable, for example, does the creation of home treatment mental health teams reduce the requirement for in-patient beds? For all these questions little research information exists, and a dependence upon data from randomised controlled trials alone is unlikely to produce answers, unless applied in multiple, representative sites using long-term designs.

Second, the local level is usually the most relevant scale at which to formulate a service strategy which will take into account the following types of interface with the general adult psychiatric service: links with specialist mental health services such as old age, forensic, learning disabilities and substance misuse; those with general health services, including primary and secondary care services, such as family doctors and general hospital services; and the range of non-clinical services such as social service and housing departments, patient representative groups, local politicians, local newspapers and radio stations, and family, carer and voluntary groups. The reader will find a more detailed discussion of this in Chapter 13, where we shall describe the interfaces between the separate service components at the local level.

Third, knowing the socio-demographic characteristics of each local area can guide assessment of needs for services, and assist the siting of facilities, by using specific population indicators, both direct census variables and composite scores of social deprivation. In this respect a health indicator may be defined as a measure that summarises information relevant to a particular phenomenon, or which acts as a reasonable proxy for such a measure (Cook & Campbell, 1976). An alternative method of establishing local need, which we suggest should be considered if these more robust epidemiological data area not available, is to establish a local consensus of views from a wide range of interest groups. We shall expand upon these issues in Chapter 10, when we consider epidemiologically based measures or estimates of local needs as useful information for planning.

A *fourth* consideration is that an emphasis on the local level can reverse the trend which forced the deportation of patients away from their homes and their local communities and which was a characteristic of the period in which institutions were built for large catchment areas. The advantage of stressing local services is that the directionality is reversed: instead of forcing patients to move to remote sites, services are forced to move to the patients' local area.

Further intended benefits of planning and delivering services at the local level are shown in Table 5.2. In addition, there are some key characteristics of service delivery, such as accessibility, co-ordination and continuity of care, which we consider to be more achievable within the local context. We shall elaborate upon these and other principles fundamental to modern mental health services in Chapter 11.

5.3 Limitations of an emphasis upon the local level

There are also disadvantages to planning mental health services at the local level. *First,* it may not be cost-effective to develop expertise and

Table 5.2. *Claimed planning and operational advantages of organising services at the local level*

Planning advantages
1 High identification rates of patients
2 Feasible scale for clinical and social assessments
3 Appropriate and planned development of services
4 Assists development of a wide range of local service components
5 Improved knowledge and use of community resources
6 Greater budgetary clarity

Service delivery advantages
1 Minimise patients lost to follow-up
2 Individually tailored inter-agency patient care programmes
3 Facilitates home treatment
4 Improved identity of staff with locality
5 Clarity of functions of local teams
6 Facilitates inter-agency liaison training and working
7 Allows comparative research and evaluation

Quality of service advantages
1 Less use of crisis and in-patient facilities
2 Improved patient education and intervention
3 Greater support of relatives and carers
4 Defined responsibility for each patient
5 Improved communication for staff, patients & carers
6 Improved primary–secondary service communication

Source: Strathdee & Thornicroft (1992)

facilities for low prevalence disorders which receive better quality care at a higher regional or supra-regional level. For example, services for eating disorders or forensic patients may be better provided in specialist centres at the regional level to the populations of combined local catchment areas. On the other hand, where such sub-specialist services exist there may be a secondary effect that local catchment areas lose expertise to treat such conditions.

Related to this mainly *diagnostic* issue is the question of whether specialisation should take place *within* the local level, for example on the basis of the *degree of disability* or the *chronicity* of the condition. This usually refers to the dilemma of providing either generic and unitary adult mental health services, or separating the care of acute and chronic patients.

The separatists' view favours the creation of 'rehabilitation', or 'continuing care', teams on one hand, and 'acute', or 'crisis intervention' teams on the other hand. The argument for such a separation is that it allows dedicated resources to be secured for the longer-term and more disabled patients, who are at risk of relative neglect in generic services which tend to prioritise and concentrate time and treatment on more urgent cases. There is little evidence to draw upon in addressing this question, and our own view is that such separation tends to incur greater administrative costs for the two types of team, and adds a greater degree of complexity to the interfaces between the components of an already complex system. We therefore favour generic teams which explicitly balance acute and long-term care, and which can particularly provide continuity of treatment for long-term patients, who also episodically become acutely ill.

A *second* concern attached to the provision of local services is that the quality and capacity of services in different, even adjoining, local areas may vary enormously. This does introduce inequity, which may be mitigated to some extent *post hoc* by a small-scale migration of patients towards better resourced services. Such inequalities are better addressed *a priori* by co-ordinating the planning of local services at the regional level, and by methods of updating the distribution of health resources from time to time by explicitly taking into account not only overall population needs, but also other specific local factors, such as the referral and turnover rates of patients, and the composition of the case load of each local service in terms of severity mix.

A *third* issue is that local catchment area services may offer less freedom to patients, and reduced choice for referrers in the services to which they have access. As far as patients are concerned, this is an over-emphasised problem, since a well-organised local service can usually respect the wish of patients to change clinician by a reallocation within the same clinical team. In addition, it is occasionally necessary deliberately to refer a patient to a team serving another catchment area, for example if the patient is a member of staff in the local health services, or if a complex family includes more than one patient, and treatment will be clarified by providing distinct treatment to each patient in separate settings. In this case catchment area boundaries are better seen as somewhat fluid and pliable than as rigid and insurmountable.

A *fourth* local level concern is the degree to which the boundaries of the key agencies which deliver services to the mentally ill are coincident. The three most important boundaries are those for the mental health services, for primary care health services and for social services. The main point here is that most organisational questions become far easier if these boundaries are co-terminous. The less this is true the more complex are the multiple relationships necessary between partially overlapping agencies. In terms of planning, it is useful in addition to have geographically defined service catchment areas which exactly coincide with local government and census boundaries, so that the relevant population data can be easily obtained.

Related to the aim of reducing the geographical distance between patients and services is the question of how the same aim can be achieved in terms of social and economic status. It has long been recognised that those who suffer from mental illnesses often also suffer from profound reductions in their material standard of living, and that this is associated in less regulated societies with a progressive 'zoning' of their places of residence. In other words, people who are most disabled by mental illnesses can only afford to live in the poorest types of accommodation, so that ghettoisation occurs. In a sense, this is a different type of exclusion: formerly patients were confined to impoverished and separate institutions (*'marginalisation within the asylum'*), whereas more recently such patients are likely to be confined to impoverished areas which they share with others who do not have the economic means to afford anything better (*'marginalisation within the community'*).

Dear & Wolch (1987) see close parallels in these two types of marginalisation. They argue that professional care for the sick and needy has always proceeded from fundamental principles of isolation and geographical separation of such individuals. In their view, such isolation has four principal hallmarks: enclosure, partitioning, identification of functioning sites, and ranking. One extreme expression of the operation of such market forces, combined with public opposition to new mental health facilities and their manifestation through local government planning procedures, is the question of where to locate new services. A frequent response to this question is one of conflict avoidance by seeking uncontested sites, with the consequent concentration of patients and other marginalised groups into 'zones of dependence', which Dear & Wolch call 'service-dependent population ghettos'. This tendency is one of exclusion from the mainstream of social opportunities, and so runs directly counter to one of the central themes of this book: that patients with (especially severe) mental illness should not be marginalised and excluded from, but be welcomed and included within the challenges and richness of normal social life.

5.4 Key stakeholders at the local level

Working at the local level makes building links with key local figures both useful and inevitable. They will most often include not only family doctors, general hospital and other health service clinicians, but also social service and housing department staff, patients and their representatives, local politicians, local newspapers and radio stations, family members and carer groups. But a wider corona of stakeholders may also wish to have their presence and interests represented and respected. This wider set of constituencies may include: neighbourhood or residents' associations, local school staff, governors and parents, shopkeepers, local politicians, church ministers, and police officers. The importance of these stakeholders emerges particularly at times when plans are being developed to open new mental health facilities.

Faced with potential local opposition to a planned new mental heath service, staff are faced with a dilemma: should neighbours be kept in the dark about local developments or fully informed? An understandable concern by staff that local reactions may be hostile, uninformed and could sabotage community care projects, can lead them to tell neighbours as little as possible. However, it is possible to argue that neighbours will learn about new local developments sooner or later, and that their anger will be greater if they discover the truth at a late stage. Our experience has led us to the view that treating neighbours openly, as potential partners, and seeking their early informed consent for proposals at the planning stage is pragmatic, principled, and a proper base for mental health services that are fully integrated within their local communities.

5.5 **Conclusions**

Our emphasis on the primacy of the local level within the geographical dimension leads us to make explicit that the work of mental health services is more similar to primary care than most other specialist health services. This is so because what they have in common is not only a responsibility for a given (and usually geographically defined) patient population, but also a longitudinal perspective in assessing and treating patients (which hospital specialists with a typically cross-sectional or episodic approach will not be able to develop). Moreover, they will both adopt a clinical perspective which regards treatment and rehabilitation as a continuum rather than as conceptually and practically distinct. As some other areas of medicine, such as rheumatology, metabolic diseases or geriatrics, develop systems of service for patients with chronic or relapsing and remitting conditions, we expect that these skills will become more widespread in future.

On a more cautionary note, in some particular areas the local level, as we conceptualise it here, may not exist in terms of the organisation of services. Most European countries have an administrative infrastructure which organises health, social and other public services for defined geographical areas. However, health systems with a greater degree of deregulation, such as that in most parts of the United States, may more weakly reflect the public health approach, without which a meaningful and efficient integration of services, which we consider to be the central purpose of the local level, becomes extremely difficult to achieve. For the reasons given in this chapter, we are drawn to the conclusion that *locality* is the central organising theme for the efficient planning, organisation and delivery of mental health treatment and care.

6
The patient level

6.1 Defining the patient level

By patient level we refer to the therapeutic domain which may include treatment, care and support for individual patients, or for groups of patients, who share common characteristics or problems, as well as interventions for the members of their wider social networks, including their families and carers. This level is traditionally considered to be the only proper territory of the clinician. As we have already argued, the practice, as well as the outcome, of clinical psychiatry strongly depends upon the characteristics of the other two geographical levels, and it is therefore important for clinicians to be aware of how processes at these higher levels may positively or negatively influence their clinical work. This may especially be the case for clinicians who tend to concentrate their attention solely upon the patient level.

6.2 The significance of the patient level

In this chapter we shall introduce the key elements (shown in Table 6.1) which are intended, when used together, to create the framework for clinical interventions at the patient level. As far as the first element is concerned, choosing the most effective clinical interventions, information on the evidence for treatments for individual patients is outside the scope of this book, and we refer the reader to the extensive relevant literature (see for example: Sartorius et al., 1993; Murray et al., 1997). We would emphasise three points: (i) the research evidence in the field of mental health is concentrated almost entirely within the individual patient level, and has mostly accumulated from groups of unrepresentative patients, but is applied to whole populations of those affected; (ii) even within this level the evidence base generally applies to single clinical interventions rather than to treatment combinations, or to the other aspects of patient care that we discuss below, and (iii) whatever the evidence base, clinical practice always lags

Table 6.1. *Key elements for delivering effective clinical interventions at the patient level*

1 Choosing the most effective clinical interventions
2 Seeing the patient as a partner in treatment
3 Using the patient's family as a resource
4 Recognising the whole range of needs for each patient
5 Adopting a longitudinal approach
6 Promptness both in offering and withdrawing interventions

behind, and often very far behind (Geddes & Harrison, 1997). Salient issues at this level will include the personality, psychopathology, and disabilities of individual patients; the nature of family and group dynamics; patients' expectations and satisfaction with services; and their treatment compliance.

6.3 **The limitations of attending to the patient level**

In traditional clinical practice doctors see the particular patients who come to their attention and they mainly base their views about the characteristics of morbidity upon these experiences. This is a view which only considers the patients receiving care (enumerator) and takes no account of the total population at risk (denominator). In psychiatry, the preferred professional perspective has long been the view seen from the mental hospital base: it is one which includes single episodes of treatment, only for those affected individuals known to the physician.

This traditional hospital-based view commits four errors. *First* it disregards the denominator and so cannot estimate the proportion of true morbidity which is treated. *Second*, it cannot judge how far treated cases are representative of all prevalent cases and therefore of selection biases in the treatment process. *Third*, it excludes consideration of the patient's wider social context. *Fourth*, it tends to emphasise only the current episode of care. By comparison, the usual perspective of the family doctor and of other primary care practitioners is not only cross-sectional but also longitudinal and contextual. It is this view which is promoted by widening the perspectives of mental health professionals to include other levels of both the geographical and temporal dimensions of the matrix model. We shall elaborate upon the temporal dimension later in this chapter (in section 6.7), and for the present our point is simply that the inclusion of reference to other geographical levels allows clinicians to take account of the denominator, and so to reduce clinical bias.

Two important consequences flow from this epidemiologically

informed approach: the *first* is that the number of known cases can be compared with estimated overall morbidity to gauge how far the capacity of the mental health service is appropriate to the scale of need. The *second* consequence is that this approach allows judgement of how far known cases represent either all prevalent cases, or all cases in a defined group identified for treatment targeting.

While fully weighing the importance of interventions at the individual patient level, in our view this perspective is necessary but not in itself sufficient. Our argument is that the full potential of this level can only emerge when it is understood in relation to the other geographical levels.

6.4 **Seeing the patient as a partner in treatment**

We believe that it is unnecessary to convince the reader of the importance of involving the patient in his or her own treatment, so instead we shall present here ways in which this can be done. The first step in establishing a therapeutic relationship between clinician and patient that is one of a joint approach against the effects of the disorder is to provide understandable and useful information to the patient on the disorder, its probable course and prognosis, and on treatment options. This is for ethical reasons in that patients have a right to comprehensible information, and for evidential reasons in that it increases compliance with treatment recommendations (Haynes *et al.*, 1996).

When patients are informed in this way, it becomes possible to see them as *negotiators* in their own treatment. This allows, for example with psychotic patients who have experienced adverse effects of anti-psychotic medication and who are reluctant to take more, a number of therapeutic options: to agree a dose of medication as a mid-point between those initially proposed by both sides; to specify a dose range within which the patient has day-to-day discretion over the precise dose taken; or to plan jointly that no medication will be taken on a regular basis unless specific symptoms occur, such as previously identified early warning signs of relapse, which can be formalised as an advance directive.

This negotiating position applies equally to others types of treatment, such as participation in activities at a day centre programme or in applying for employment. It is often necessary to reduce our expectations in order to meet patients' desires or preferences. The issue is the balance between the need to be directive in prescribing treatment recommendations (especially for patients who need clear guidance) with a readiness to modify prescriptions in answer to patients' own preferences. This kind of flexibility may need to vary over time even for the same patient.

Such a negotiating stance is pragmatic since, in our own clinical experience, it is likely to increase the likelihood of patients adhering to a medication regime. But there are also wider ethical reasons for such a partnership approach. Recent research in the USA indicates that patients' perceptions of coercion during in-patient treatment are less when they report that they (i) have had an opportunity at some time during the admission to give a full account from their own point of view of the admission, and (ii) have felt that their account has been taken seriously by staff. These two factors are referred to by the MacArthur Network researchers as 'procedural justice', and indicate that when patients report that they have been treated respectfully in these two particular ways, they consequently find their treatment more acceptable, even if the admission has been compulsory, or if they have received enforced medication at some stage during their in-patient treatment.

We therefore suggest that each treatment programme be tailored to an individual patient as a dynamic process which takes into account the social context of the patient (for example, important life events), clinical recommendations, and patient preferences.

Certain forms of psychotherapy, especially behavioural and cognitive-behavioural treatments, have made explicit and have systematised such active patient participation. At the other extreme are interventions such as electro-convulsive therapy and psycho-surgery, which at the time the procedure takes place are entirely without the active participation of the patient.

The process of informing patients and subsequently negotiating a treatment plan is time consuming, and may be seen as wasteful by clinicians. Our view is that in fact this is a type of investment in the future, which will usually save time at a later stage, most typically when a patient's condition relapses, at which point agreeing any treatment plan is likely to be far more difficult. It is our clinical impression that this more inclusive approach to patient involvement in treatment decisions does lead to improved compliance, which for most conditions has been estimated at about 50% of prescribed medication (Haynes *et al.*, 1996), and that this renders relapse less likely. Patient participation may therefore be seen as both principled and pragmatic.

6.5 **Using the patient's family as a resource**

The family members of an individual suffering from mental illness may be a valuable resource to work alongside mental health services. Specific techniques for working with such families and methods of measuring their involvement and the impact of caring have received substantial

Table 6.2. *Common concerns of relatives of mentally ill people*

- What will happen when the parent / carer dies?
- Worry about suicide and aggressive behaviour
- Concern about underactivity by patients
- Needing information on the condition and any genetic implications
- Grief about the loss of expected child and adult
- Information on whether early life events have caused the present disorder
- Expert advice about welfare benefit entitlements
- Updated information about treatment options and developments

attention in the recent literature (Kuipers & Bebbington, 1991; Schene *et al.*, 1994). In this section our aim is not to repeat this work, but to establish the credentials of the family to be included within the clinical *dramatis personae*, and to enumerate the prerequisite conditions for such involvement to take place, especially in relation to the most common concerns which families experience, some of which are summarised in Table 6.2.

There are three particular misunderstandings which are relatively common in practice and prevent clinicians and families from collaborating effectively to help patients: (i) the belief of clinical staff that families are the cause of mental illness, (ii) the reluctance of clinical staff to recognise the mental health problems of carers themselves, and (iii) the interpretation by staff of clinical confidentiality to limit the information which they give to families.

The *first* type of error leads some to believe that patients' families are directly responsible for the onset of the disorder, or for episodes of relapse. While there is evidence that relapses of schizophrenia may follow exposure to a family atmosphere which rates highly for 'expressed emotion' (a concept which combines hostility, emotional over-involvement and criticism), there is no evidence that anything families do causes the disorder *de novo*, and therefore no grounds on which to consider that the family should be held blameworthy. Indeed where the family may be a contributory factor to the risk of relapse the common error is for staff to blame the relatives rather than to reframe this positively as an opportunity to help the family behave in a way that reduces the risk of relapse.

The *second* error is to neglect the changing mental health status of family members, which may fluctuate in relation to variations in the mental state of the patient. In most cases this association co-varies in the same direction, in other words deterioration occurs at the same time for both the patient and for relatives. Less frequently it is observed that the family shows signs of distress or suffering when the patient shows symptomatic improvement and increases his or her autonomy more rapidly than the family can accept. In both situations to ignore or to delay recognition of what is happening in the family environment can lead to two types of mis-interpretation. On one hand, clinical staff may misunderstand signals from the patient, such as reports of depressed mood, which indicate dis-tress within the family. For example, complaints by parents to a relatively inactive schizophrenic son, may be taken by staff out of context and be attributed to the symptoms to the patient alone, rather than located within the set of relationships within the family as a whole. Treatment in this case is likely to be ineffective. On the other hand, staff may misunderstand signals from family members, for example, concern by the parents of a mentally ill daughter that they cannot keep her at home for much longer may be interpreted by staff as a withdrawal of care by unsympathetic parents, rather than as a request for respite care, or for a higher degree of practical support to the family.

The *third* error of mental health services is to treat the issue of confiden-tiality in a way that is damaging to both the patients and relatives. It is common for staff to refuse to inform relatives about the diagnosis and the course and outcome of the condition, about current treatment and about treatment options, on the grounds that such information is confidential, and cannot be disclosed to third parties without the consent of the patient. While this is both a legal requirement and a hallmark of good clinical prac-tice, staff often fail to recognise that relatives cannot act on an informed basis to support the patient if they are specifically excluded from access to the relevant facts. One way to reconcile these apparently contradictory needs is for clinicians to raise this issue explicitly with each patient and to try to reach agreement on three matters: which categories of clinical infor-mation the patient agrees can be passed to named family members at any time, which types of information should be kept confidential and not dis-closed to any third party at any stage, and which categories may be disclosed to specific relatives in the future only under specified conditions, for example should the patient relapse and require compulsory admission to hospital (Szmukler & Bloch, 1997). A less formal but more common method to convey agreed information to family members is to arrange regular con-sultations at which both the family and the patient are present.

6.6 Recognising the whole range of patient needs

Modern clinical practice needs to consider biological, psychological and social factors at the same time, as well as their interaction. We may con-sider these factors as mainly internal (biological and psychological) or mainly external (social). In practical terms, at the patient level, the relative weight of these aspects may vary in different clinical conditions, even if it is the theoretical orientation of the clinician that often explains the differential attention they receive.

In such disorders as dementia, for instance, biological aspects are considered (given the current state of our knowledge), of greater salience than social or psychological variables, and this view affects diagnostic and therapeutic interventions. However, in conversion disorders psychological and social factors are now considered to predominate over biological variables, and this suggests a preferential use of psychological treatments over biological therapies. From a practical point of view, whatever the variables involved in the pathogenesis of a particular disorder, for individual patients we have to recognise the whole range of their needs and to offer a series of different therapeutic possibilities. This implies co-operation between different members of the clinical team and the availability of various therapeutic skills within the same mental health service. This does not always happen in clinical practice, either because members of different disciplines will only aim to identify patients needs which they consider to be within their own sphere of competence, or because they are not able to respond to identified needs for lack of appropriate skills or resources. An example of the range of needs to be considered is provided by the Camberwell Assessment of Need (CAN) (Phelan *et al.*, 1995) (see Table 6.3).

6.7 **Adopting a longitudinal approach**

As mentioned earlier in section 5.5, one of the specific characteristics of a mental health service is to draw upon both the cross-sectional and longitudinal perspectives in everyday clinical practice. In dealing with individual patients this means considering both perspectives in taking the history, in writing the case notes, in making diagnostic formulations, in making a prognosis, in formulating a care plan, and in establishing the correct pace at which the treatment should be given. While this longitudinal perspective is better achieved within a single clinical team, as a powerful tool for providing continuity of care, when an efficient communication system is in operation, the perspective can be maintained across different agencies or treatment teams, and this implies that clinical records or at lest clinical summaries will follow the patient and be made available to the current responsible clinicians.

The significance of such operational details is that they can (and in our view should) be arranged to maximise *continuity of care* to patients, and that

Table 6.3. *Areas of need included in the CAN (Camberwell Assessment of Need)*

Accommodation
Occupation
Specific psychotic symptoms
Psychological distress
Information about condition and treatment
Non-prescribed drugs
Food and meals
Household skills
Self care and presentation
Safety to self
Safety to others
Money
Childcare
Physical health
Alcohol
Basic education
Company
Telephone
Public transport
Welfare benefits

this is best provided by a continuing therapeutic contact with a single mental health service. When this is not possible, then the longitudinal perspective can only be sustained when new staff members can use *continuity of recorded information,* which then acts as proxy of *continuity of contact* and *longitudinal personal knowledge*. We shall elaborate upon this theme of continuity in section 11.2.2.

6.8 **Offering and withdrawing care in prompt measure**

In the training of mental health professionals considerable emphasis is placed on using treatments appropriately. In the use of one form of treatment, medication, for example, this means paying detailed attention to the dosage, and to the time and route of administration. In this way medication is titrated to maximise the therapeutic effects while minimising unwanted effects. The same attention should also be accorded to non-pharmacological interventions when dosage, timing and the means of delivery can affect the outcome.

In terms of *dosage,* as with drugs, so for other forms of interventions the *minimum effective dose* should be given. This 'dose' will vary both for different individuals, and also within individuals over time, according to the changes in clinical condition or context. Among more severely disabled patients, giving more than the necessary dose or duration of day care, for example, can induce a counter-therapeutic dependency on services and hinder the development of autonomy. Another example of inappropriately excessive care would be a prolonged period of in-patient treatment which can decrease the performance of everyday living skills of progressively institutionalised patients.

In relation to *timing*, good clinical practice demonstrates the capacity to provide services that can both rapidly increase and rapidly decrease in intensity according to the condition of the patient. Often, however, it is the case that services are simply unable to respond in a timely fashion at all, or are only able to increase their input quickly, but are slow to withdraw the amount of care during the patient's recovery. In this period, therefore, an over-provision of treatment may take place. This is wasteful of resources and may induce dependency in patients.

In terms of the means of *delivery of care*, mental health services should make every attempt to ensure that in their intervention for patients they choose in each situation the *least restrictive alternative*. For example, a commitment to decrease the use of compulsory admission to hospital may necessitate the provision of realistic alternative services offering high degrees of support to patients at times of acute crisis, in settings which patients will accept on a voluntary basis, such as their own homes if intensive domicilliary treatment teams are available, or to other facilities such as crisis centres or respite houses.

6.9 Conclusions

In this chapter we have outlined a framework for *style* of treatment interventions made at the patient level. In conclusion we wish to indicate a parallel framework that can be applied to the *content* of these interventions. One such framework is provided by evidence-based medicine (EBM), which reflects the maturation of methods and techniques for testing treatment efficacy, such as randomised clinical trials. This approach can usefully be supplemented by using data provided by structured clinical practice. This issue will be further discussed in Chapter 19.

PART III **The matrix model: the temporal dimension**

Part III will deal with health care measures and indicators which we consider in the phases of the temporal dimension: input, process and outcome. We shall use the term 'measures' to denote direct assessments, and 'indicators' as indirect assessments (or reasonable proxies) that summarise information relevant to a particular phenomenon. Like other instruments used for health services evaluation, such measures and indicators should have adequate validity, reliability, sensitivity and specificity (Jenkins, 1990). Since direct measures are difficult to collect, indirect proxy variables are more common and such performance indicators have been defined as 'operationally-defined indirect measures of selected aspects of a system which give some indication of how far it conforms to its intended purpose' (Glover & Kamis-Gould, 1996).

The distinction and balance between inputs, processes and outcomes within mental health services are far from clear-cut for three reasons. *First,* there is no consensus on the definitions of these terms, and their use in the literature is widely variable. The consequence of this is that it is often the case that the three temporal phases are used in a confused way so that processes (such as numbers of admissions) are used *as if* they were outcome variables. *Second,* these three categories of variables are inter-connected and need to be seen as different aspects of the wider, dynamic mental health care system. In this case, outcomes cannot be considered in isolation, and in fact patients will often want acceptable care processes *and* outcomes, so that attention to outcomes alone will miss a part of what is valued by the recipients of care. *Third,* the paradigm which best fits the tripartite sequence of input, process and outcome, is that of an acute episode of illness and its consequent medical care, such as an uncomplicated infection, or a straightforward surgical intervention such as an appendectomy. This is because the acute illness paradigm assumes (i) clear start and end points for the episode, (ii) that outcomes are directly related to treatment inputs and to the processes of their delivery (or as Donabedian put it in 1992, outcomes are the states or conditions attributable to antecedent health care), and (iii) that outcome is simply the difference (or health gain) between health status before and after treatment. Many mental disorders, however, especially those treated by specialist mental health services, are chronic, relapsing and remitting conditions, which do not fit a simple acute illness paradigm.

The structure of the following three chapters attempts to respond to these challenges. In each chapter, we shall first define the relevant phase of the temporal dimension (input in Chapter 7, process in Chapter 8 and outcome in Chapter 9). Then we shall examine the main characteristics of each temporal phase at the three levels of the geographical dimension (country/regional, local and patient). By using the matrix model in this way, we shall try to add a greater degree of clarity to understanding the working of mental health services.

It is interesting to consider how perspectives on the importance of these three phases differ at the three geographical levels. From a *patient's perspective*, within a national health insurance system (patient level), the rank order of importance is likely to be: (i) outcome (amelioration of symptoms or degree of recovery), (ii) process (quality of care received) and (iii) input (indirect taxation costs or fees for services). From a *managerial point of view* (local level), this rank order is often reversed, and priorities are seen to be (i) inputs (service cost containment or reduction), (ii) processes (offering services acceptable to patients and avoiding complaints), and (iii) outcomes. From a *public health perspective* (country/regional level) the priorities are more often (i) service efficiency (the ratio of outcome benefits to input costs), and (ii) process. Also the criteria used to judge each of these phases may differ between these three levels, being more subjectively based at the patient level and more evidence-based at the other two levels.

7
The input phase

7.1 **Defining the input phase**

We define as *inputs* 'the resources which are put into the mental health care system'.

Defined in this way, *inputs* are those elements which are injected into the total mental health service system, and which need to be distinguished from the activities which take place within that system in providing mental health care, which we describe in the next chapter as the *process* phase. These resources enter the system at the three geographical levels, and may be further categorised as visible or invisible.

The *visible inputs* consist mainly of staff and facilities. In psychiatry, as compared with other medical specialities, a relatively small contribution towards visible inputs at present is expenditure on medication, supplies, equipment and investigations. Visible expenditure on staff includes the numbers, the mix of different disciplines (such as psychiatrists, psychologists and nurses) and their relative distribution across the service as a whole.

Often forgotten are the *invisible inputs* which activate the visible system inputs, and which potentiate the effective functioning of the service network. Without these invisible factors the visible inputs may be rendered largely ineffective. Indeed, the influence of these invisible inputs usually only becomes manifest when they are absent, unrecognised or disregarded. One example is the importance of establishing good working relationships between specialist and general health services, and between health and social services, for the joint care of people with long-term and severe mental illness.

Such invisible system inputs include: the experience, qualifications and training of staff. Training will regularly update staff to avoid skill degradation, and to enhance the degree of match between their abilities and the style of working in each particular service. A second category of invisible inputs includes the legal and policy framework within which the service is authorised to operate, and which, as described above, may change on a frequent basis. A third type of invisible input is the organisational arrangements which shape how the process of care takes place. Particular examples

Table 7.1. *Categories of input to mental health services*

Visible inputs

Budget
- absolute amount of money allocated to mental health services
- proportionate allocation in relation to total health expenditure or
- other indicators

Staff
- numbers of staff at each level
- mix of professions

Buildings and facilities

Equipment / technology for investigation, diagnosis and treatment

Invisible inputs

Working relationships
- between health and social services
- between specialist and general health services

Policies and regulations
- laws
- organisational arrangements and quality standards
- treatment protocols and guidelines

Media representations of mental health issues

Public attitudes to mental health issues

---

of these inputs are operational policies at the local level, and quality standards which may operate at local or country levels.

From the whole range of visible and invisible service inputs, often the only elements to be quantified in health service research studies are the number and use of psychiatric beds. Equally the response to any system failure, which is commonly a complex product of inadequacies or dysfunctions in many service components, is often reduced to a question of how many (more) beds are needed. Invisible inputs, therefore, usually remain excluded from consideration, even in the most sophisticated attempts to evaluate mental health services.

Inputs in themselves are of indirect but not of direct importance. We believe that the primary purpose of activities within a mental health service should be to contribute towards the delivery of effective treatments to individual patients (cell 3C of the matrix model of Figure 1.1). Therefore inputs are important only in so far as they contribute towards improved outcomes for individual patients. Even so, financial inputs, for example, because they are relatively easy to quantify, are often used as indicators of system performance, and it is common for governments to describe increased expenditure on mental health services *as if* this is identical with better achieving the aims

Geographical Dimension

Temporal Dimension

	(A) Input Phase	(B) Process Phase	(C) Outcome Phase
(1) Country/Regional Level	1A · expenditure on mental health services and budget allocation · mental health laws · government directives & policies · planning for training of mental health staff · treatment protocols & guidelines	1B	1C
(2) Local Level (catchment area)	2A · local service budget and balance of hospital and community services · assessment of local population needs · staff numbers and mix · clinical and non-clinical services · working relationships between services	2B	2C
(3) Patient Level	3A · assessment of individual needs · demands made by patients · demands made by families · skills & knowledge of staff · content of clinical treatments · information for patients/carers	3B	3C

Figure 7.1   Overview of the matrix model, with key issues at the input phase

of the service. It is not. The vital point therefore is whether inputs contribute towards measurable and improved outcomes. If they do, then it is necessary to calibrate such improvements against the extra units of input, so that competing demands for funds can be rationally compared in terms of their cost-effectiveness, to allow evidence-based decisions for funding priorities.

In this chapter we shall illustrate the main categories of mental health services, a wider range of these inputs are shown in Table 7.1, and we shall discuss them in relation to the three geographical levels, as illustrated in Figure 7.1.

7.2 **Inputs at the country/regional level**

Since the structure of mental health services varies very considerably between countries, the influence of the country/regional level will vary accordingly. In countries where there is a form of national health service, there is usually a higher degree of centralisation of control and direction. Here we shall concentrate our discussion upon three categories: budget, staff and policies.

In terms of *budget allocations*, there are often huge variations between and within countries in their absolute and relative allocations for health services. At the national level, in 1995 the total expenditure in OECD (Organisation for Economic Co-operation and Development) countries, as a percentage of the gross domestic product varies from 14.5% (USA) to 6.5% (Denmark)(OECD, 1997). Within these figures it is interesting to note that in countries which have a significant national health service, such as Norway, Denmark and Britain, more than 80% of this expenditure is on public services, while, on the other hand, the USA spends only 44% of total health costs on the public sector.

Within countries there are also substantial *variations in budget inputs*. In England in 1992, for example, the average amount spent on mental health by health districts per head of total population varied between £13.25 and £164.41, more than a 12–fold variation. In relative terms, in the same year the percentage of the district health budget dedicated to mental health services varied between 6.6% and 21.7%, a more than three-fold difference. While we shall argue in Chapter 10 that the population level needs of different areas are very different because the prevalence of severe mental illness is far higher in socially deprived areas, what is important is that the variation in actual and relative expenditure in England bear almost no relation to any reasonable estimate of need. Current spending is in fact usually closely connected with historical patterns of expenditure, and in particular is greater near the sites of current or previous large asylums.

A related point is the distinction between the *absolute* and the *relative budget* allocations to any unit or level. While the total budgetary 'cake' is usually fixed annually for mental health services, it is possible, by focusing attention in financial discussions only upon changes in proportionate expenditure, to miss opportunities to increase the absolute amount spent. For example, in the period after a major mental health scandal, or just after a new government or minister for health has come into office, there may be a brief opportunity to increase the priority attached to mental health.

In allocating funds from the country to the local level, a very difficult balance needs to be struck. This balance is between, on the one hand, the design of an overall funding formula which distributes funds to the whole country/region in relation to population needs (when financial allocation is not made using other criteria or at random!), and on the other hand allowing sufficient flexibility so that adjustments can be made for exceptional factors which substantially change the required service capacity. Such specific factors may include: international immigrants, refugees or asylum seekers, the presence of a major rail terminus or port which delivers patients from other areas, or the concentration in one area of large numbers of shelters for the homeless or hostels for the mentally ill. A reasonable system to allocate service funding in relation to need will therefore allow such factors to be considered.

In relation to the *input of staff*, this is the main resource input to the mental health service, and we shall discuss staffing in more detail in Chapter 12. In the context of the country/national level, it is important to understand that staffing has a longer 'lead-time' than other inputs. This is, first, because the time necessary to train some mental health professionals may be up to 10 years. Second, the time needed to recognise shortfalls in the numbers of professionals and alter training capacities may also take several years. Third, the period from the completion of training to becoming fully productive may be longer than for some other areas of medicine since, to some degree, the effectiveness of each clinician depends upon their detailed knowledge of particular patients under their care, and this holds to a greater extent than, for example, in surgery.

What is shared in common at the country/regional level is that *policy inputs* are set which influence each lower level of practice. These higher level policies can take a number of forms: statutes which have the force of law, official guidance which may be obligatory or discretionary, and codes of practice by the professions which codify reasonable clinical practice. The non-statutory measures (such as official circulars and recommendations) tend to be revised more often but to have less impact.

Changes over time at this level will also take place slowly. In Italy, for example, there were new mental health laws in 1904, 1968 and 1978: three times in a century. In England new mental health acts were introduced on only four occasions during this century. In relation to changes in scientific knowledge, clinical practice, and to wider social and ethical trends, such legal changes occur very slowly. It could therefore be said that the law lags behind clinical practice, which in turn lags behind science. On the other hand, it is sometimes the case that central governmental guidance is issued or updated too often. Major changes in service structure or practice will often take several years to perfuse throughout the relevant country or region. If a new directive appears before the last one has been consolidated then there is a real possibility that overlapping and partially completed directives contribute to a chaotic policy bottleneck.

Policy may therefore be made too slowly or too rapidly. A judgement on the rate at which new polices can be positively absorbed in any particular setting thus depends upon a clear feedback path, from ordinary clinical sites to policy makers, about the readiness of clinicians and service managers for the next iteration of change.

7.3 Inputs at the local level

Knowing how to use the budget available at the local level most effectively for the benefit of patients requires some understanding of the actual ways in which current funds are spent. In most economically developed countries the majority of services to the mentally ill are provided by local health or social services. The line of demarcation between the two is one of the recurrent dilemmas (or points of friction) facing planners and politicians. In Britain, for example, less than 10% of total expenditure on mental health services is by social services departments. In Sweden, by comparison, a recent law has transferred responsibility and funds for longer-term patients in hospital, who no longer require active medical treatment, from the health to the social service authorities. This measure is designed to be an incentive for social services to move such patients from hospital to cheaper and more appropriate residential care as soon as possible.

The first important input issue that arises at the local level is the balance of expenditure between hospital and community services. In the last quarter of a century, in most economically developed countries, this shifting balance has been in one direction – from hospital to community. Second, it is important to set local targets for the desired percentage of the budget to be spent on community services at the end of each cycle of change. Third, the time period needed to achieve each cycle should preferably be set in advance, to maintain sufficient impetus to the change process while maintaining at least a reasonable quality of care. Fourth, it is usually necessary to account for transitional (double-running) costs while the community services are established and before significant savings accrue from bed reductions. In most economically developed countries deinstitutionalisation starts with over three-quarters of total mental health expenditure going to hospital services. In 1995, for example, the hospital mental health budget in the USA fell below 50% for the first time.

Two important points need to be recognised here. Those managing such a process need to ensure that funds follow the patients, otherwise clinical activity shifts rapidly from hospital to community sites but over two-thirds of the budget typically remains at the hospital. Second, during decentralisation there is the ever-present risk that monies will leak out of the mental health system and into other areas of medicine unless the budget holders are extremely astute and guard against such financial predation.

At the next lower (local) level it is often useful to distinguish between direct clinical services, clinical support services, and non-clinical support services (see Table 7.2). Traditionally all these three categories were provided at the hospital site, and in psychiatry these were often in total institutions, and in some places continue to be. It is important for mental health services to receive as much non-clinical support when decentralised as when they were centralised. What is interesting is that the interfaces with all these support services become much more complicated when they are no longer co-located in one site. Although we have developed a conceptual understanding of the provision of community mental health services, we have no language for community-orientated support services, without which the direct clinical services cannot continue to provide care of any quality.

To allow comparison of inputs at the local level we need a common currency of meaningful units. While hospital services traditionally use the total number of available *beds* as the prime indicator of the scale of the input, community services do not as yet have even such an over-simplified unit of measurement. It is unlikely that for community services only one indicator will be sufficient to describe such complex systems. Rather we shall need an array of quantitative and qualitative indices.

In relation to the range and scope of services, the European Service Mapping Schedule (Johnson *et al.*, 1997) is one of the first examples of such a standardised measure, and can be applied to all those service components which we describe in more detail in Chapter 13. In terms of staffing, it is necessary to compare particular types and grades of staff input and for the number of clinical sessions actually worked for direct clinician–patient contact rather than the number of whole time equivalent staff employed. These inputs can be expressed in terms of a standard denominator, for

Table 7.2. *Direct clinical and support services (Clinical and Non-clinical) as mental health service inputs*

Direct clinical services	Support services (clinical)	Support services (non-clinical)
In-patient services	**Pharmacy**	**Information technology and computing**
Out-patient services	*providing medication, advice and other related supplies to the direct clinical services*	*provision of routine service activity data and support for computers and software*
Day care services		
Community mental health and home treatment services	**Pathology and laboratory sciences**	**Medical records**
	providing analysis of physical investigations for mental health services	*usually centralised archives of patient clinical case notes*
Residential services in the community		
	Radiology, EEG and neurophysiology	**Transport and portering**
	Patient advocacy and legal advice	**Catering**
	Usually providing legal services to patients, relatives or staff concerning involuntary treatment and appeals, informed consent, or professional indemnity	**Cleaning**
		Works and building
(for details of these service components see Chapter 13)	**Residential placement services**	**Supplies**
	Arranging accommodation to facilitate discharge, especially for long-term patients	**Quality & Clinical Audit**
		Continuing Education
		Planning
		Staffing

Source: (Adapted from Reynolds & Thornicroft, 1999)

Table 7.3. *Comparisons of sessions of staff time per week in South Verona and South Manchester community mental health services (numbers and rates per 10 000 population)*

Professional group	South Verona (Average no. of sessions per week)		South Manchester (Average no. of sessions per week)	
	For the study population	For a population of 10 000 adult inhabitants	For the study population	For a population of 10 000 adult inhabitants
Psychiatrists	22	12	6.5	5
Psychiatrists in training	20	11	5.2	4
Psychologists	10	6	13.2	11
Social Workers	10	6	10	8
Community Nurses	50	28	23	19
Ward Nurses	45	26	87	72
Hostel nurses or 'operatore di assistenza'	12.7	7	0	0
Occupational Therapists	0	0	21	17
Total	169.7	96	165.9	136

(*Source:* Gater *et al.*, 1995)

example per 10 000 population total served. One example of this approach is shown in Table 7.3. What is interesting is that the absolute total number of sessions in the two sites are very similar, but in terms of the rates of sessions available for all grades of staff per 10 000 population, the South Manchester service has a greater input than in South Verona.

7.4 Inputs at the patient level

One of the central themes of this book is that the primary purpose of mental health services at the country/regional and at the local levels is to deliver services to individual patients which are of benefit to them in terms of outcome. We can therefore conceive of the patient level as a final common pathway for all inputs from higher levels, discussed previously in this chapter. We shall describe in this section three types of input specific to the individual patient level: the skills and knowledge of staff, the content of treatment, and the delivery of proper information to patients and their carers.

Regarding the *skills and knowledge of staff*, as we describe in more detail in Chapter 12, it is expertise rather than experience which is of central importance as an input (Roth & Fonagy, 1996). In most branches of medicine it is considered that if clinicians fail to update their technical skills for more than five years, then their expertise is almost completely out of date. We believe this also to be true for psychiatry, even though it is common for practitioners in this field to act as if the half life of psychiatric knowledge is longer, or even infinite! Our main point is that those who practice only on the basis of the knowlege they learned during their undergraduate and postgraduate training will soon become obsolescent. This is the case, first of all, in terms of diagnostic practice, which has become progressively more operationalised and specific during the last 20 years. In terms of therapeutics, such a risk for the decay of knowledge and skill is most apparent in the area of psycho-pharmacology. It is also true for the psychotherapies, especially regarding the currently rapidly expanding evidence that cognitive behavioural methods can be effective for some affective and psychotic disorders. The implication is that continuing medical education and continuing professional development are essential inputs to keep staff knowledge and skills updated.

The second type of individual level input is the *content of treatment*. In this book we shall not give a detailed account of specific types of treatment, but rather how they should be organised to be available to patients. The recent advent of evidence-based medicine (EBM) (L'Abbe *et al.*, 1987, Chalmers *et al.*, 1993, Cochrane Database of Systematic Reviews, 1996; Sackett *et al.*, 1996), which as applied to mental health services has been termed 'evidence-based psychiatry' (de Girolamo, 1997), means that for the first time mental health practitioners can decide upon the most effective treatments on offer for specific diagnostic patient groups, rather than base services upon personal opinions or upon staff preferences for which services they choose to provide. This new approach therefore implies that diagnostic skills of a high standard become more important than before, that the treatments given are based upon the most recent knowledge about effectiveness from EBM sources, and that when specific treatment skills are not available to particular groups of patients in any local area, that they are made available either by referring to other services which include such specific treatments, or, in the longer term and at the local level, by training staff in the necessary clinical techniques.

The third type of individual patient input is *information.* There is an increasing concern about the need to provide information to patients before obtaining their consent to perform investigations or to provide treatments. In this context we refer to information about diagnosis, course and outcome of the condition, about the types of treatment available, and about the wanted and unwanted effects of these treatments. The reasons for this interest are *legal* (for example, to warn patients about the adverse effects of drugs), *ethical* (it increasingly becoming routine clinical practice to allow the patient to make informed choices) or *evidential*, since patients who are well informed about treatments are more likely to be satisfied with the service and therefore to adhere to treatment recommendations.

Although this need is now widely acknowledged, the practice of conveying information to patients and their families is still usually rather informal. The evidence from general health care suggests that information is most effectively transferred if a stepwise procedure is followed by clinicians.

(i) Ask if the patient wants any information at all.

(ii) Make a list of the specific questions the patient wants answered.

(iii) Take the questions one at a time and for each one ask what the patient already knows.

(iv) Confirm or challenge correct or misinformed statements by the patient.

(v) Offer a short series of statements in answer to each question.

(vi) Ask if this is sufficient detail or if the patient wants further elaboration for each point.

(vii) Tell the patient that you would like to know if you have been able to answer each question by asking them to summarise what you have said.

(viii) Either confirm correct statements by the patient, or rephrase your own presentation of information if the patient has misunderstood or not retained the key points at all.

(ix) Repeat this sequence for each of the topics the patient has selected.

Within general medicine, specific issues will influence how and when information can be conveyed. For example, with brain-damaged patients there may be impaired capacity to understand information, also for patients with terminal illness, for patients whose mental condition varies because of toxic confusional states, or those who have specific sensory deficits such as blindness or deafness. Within psychiatry also a number of specific issues may complicate information transfer, for example, patients whose symptoms reduce their degree of insight, the selectively negative interpretation of information made by those who are severely depressed, or the reduced attentiveness of patients who are preoccupied by delusions, or hallucinations.

What is striking, however, is that within the field of psychiatry interest in the information needs of patients and their families is based mainly upon legal and ethical grounds. In spite of extensive research upon information needs and treatment adherence in health care, such evidence usually makes relatively little impact upon routine clinical practice (Masur, 1981; Mann, 1993). This situation will change in future if clinicians act more in accordance with research evidence than they have in the past.

8
The process phase

8.1 Defining the process phase

The *Concise Oxford Dictionary* defines process as 'a course of action or proceeding, especially a series of stages in manufacture or some other operation' or as 'the progress or course of something.'

We define as *process* 'those activities which take place to deliver mental health services'.

In relation to the theme of this book, the *process phase* therefore refers to a wide range of clinically related procedures which occur in the mental health service system. In fact, we consider the process of care as the shell within which the active ingredients of treatment (inputs) are delivered to patients.

The distinction between inputs and processes is important but is often not clear cut. On one hand, it should be recognised that these processes are the vehicle for the delivery of care, and are not the substance of the treatment itself (Shepherd & Sartorius, 1989). On the other hand, these processes (non-specific contextual factors) also contribute indirectly towards patient outcomes, through many psychological mechanisms. For example, increased patient satisfaction with services may improve consequent treatment adherence. We therefore see the content of specific treatments (inputs) as of primary importance, and the process of care as a second order issue. The balance between these two sets of factors will vary. In situations where there is a limited knowledge base about what are the effective treatments for a particular clinical condition, or where known effective treatments are simply not available in a given local area, then process issues tend to assume greater relative importance.

A distinction also needs to be made between the acute phase of an illness and the chronic phase, in three senses. *First,* research evidence on treatment effectiveness is more available for acute than for chronic conditions. *Second,* those with chronic symptoms may already, at least in part, have failed to respond to treatment for the acute phase of their condition. *Third,* these chronic cases are those which are differentially referred to specialist mental health services, as they have not responded fully to treatment from primary care clinicians.

*Geographical
Dimension*

Temporal Dimension

	(A) Input Phase	(B) Process Phase	(C) Outcome Phase
(1) Country/Regional Level	1A	1B · performance/activity indicators (eg admission rates, bed occupancy rates, compulsory treatment rates · clinical guidelines and treatment protocols · minimum standards of care	1C
(2) Local Level (catchment area)	2A	2B · monitoring, service contacts and patterns of service use · audit procedures · pathways to care & continuity · targeting of special groups	2C
(3) Patient Level	3A	3B · subjective quality of treatments · continuity of clinicians · frequency of appointments · pattern for care process for individual patients	3C

Figure 8.1 Overview of the matrix model, with examples of key issues in the process phase

The variables most often chosen as descriptors of these processes are not those providing direct data about how services operate, but those which are more readily available. Although the importance has long been recognised of an adequate and reliable system to classify the process of care, it is notable that this has not been achieved in any widely agreed way. Even at the highest level of aggregation, to allow inter-country comparisons of services, no common currency exists to define and measure process variables. We next go on to examine each of the three geographical levels of the matrix model in relation to the process phase, and Figure 8.1 illustrates the key themes relevant to this chapter.

8.2 **Process at the country/regional level**

The goals of monitoring care processes at the country/regional level include: to evaluate equity in the provision of care within the country or region, to allow international comparisons, to identify areas of relative over- and under-provision, to describe secular trends in service delivery, and to establish whether effective practice is being implemented. We shall illustrate these processes with three examples: the collection of service activity data, the formulation of treatment guidelines and protocols, and the creation of minimum standards of care.

The content and quality of *data on mental health services* which are routinely collected in different countries are enormously variable, and at present prohibit meaningful international comparisons. The data which are collected usually refer to hospital care, although it makes a decreasing contribution towards the whole range of services delivered for mental health. There is therefore an historical time lag which means that the available data are usually only partially relevant to current mental health service or policy issues.

Exceptionally, as in Denmark, a national psychiatric case register exists which builds a longitudinal record of patterns of hospital care for individual patients. More usually, national data sets record episodes of care, and are therefore suitable mainly for large-scale questions which can be answered by aggregated data, such as trends in hospitalisation rates, or compulsory admission rates. In England, for example, a series of mostly hospital-specific data items are routinely collected, some of which are illustrated in Table 8.1. By comparison, a national minimum data set is presently at the piloting stage, which aims to establish a common set of definitions of care episodes that take as the basic unit of care the period of treatment in the community between case reviews.

A second illustration of process issues relevant at the country/regional

Table 8.1. *Examples of mental health variables in the UK health service indicators*

Mental illness episodes which started within the previous year where residents were not treated within district
Percentage of residents who are compulsorily detained in hospital
Ratio of first admissions for residents aged 75+ to total population of that age group
Percentage of admitted patients who are compulsorily admitted to hospital
Percentage of admitted patients who are compulsorily treated in hospital
Admission rate to mental health facilities per 100 000 total population
Number of compulsory hospital admissions per 10 000 total population
Percentage of all admissions that are first ever admissions
First contact by community psychiatric nurses per 1000 total population by age

Source: Glover, 1996

level is the formulation of *clinical guidelines and protocols*. These two words are often used as synonyms, while it is more accurate to refer to guidelines as either diagnostic or therapeutic, while protocols should only refer to therapeutic procedures. The *Concise Oxford Dictionary* defines a guideline as 'a principle or criterion guiding or directing action', and it defines a protocol as 'the rules, formalities, etc. or procedure, group, etc.'.

There is an increasing tendency to align clinical practice with the recommendations contained within clinical guidelines and protocols. Their aim is to improve clinical practice by reducing the variability between an evidence-based (or expert-consensus based) recommendation of best practice and what actually occurs in clinical encounters. At the country/regional level it is appropriate to construct overall treatment guidelines, especially in collaboration with the relevant professional bodies, which can subsequently be modified to fit specific local circumstances and so be relevant at the local level. One example is the British Royal College of Psychiatrists' 'Defeat Depression' campaign.

The third example of process issues at the country/regional level is the setting of *minimum standards of care*. The monitoring of compliance with such standards may be undertaken by unitary organisations with statutory inspectorate functions, or by systems of accreditation which compare actual clinical practice with pre-established criteria for minimum acceptable levels of care. While the formulation of these standards is often at the country/regional level, their application is almost entirely at the local level. One example of such minimum standards is the British Parliamentary Bill proposed by MIND in 1995, which is summarised in Table 8.2.

Table 8.2. *Proposed community care (Rights to Mental Health Services) bill*

NATIONAL MINIMUM STANDARDS FOR COMMUNITY CARE SERVICES

1 The Secretary of State shall by regulations establish national minimum standards for each of the community care services referred to in section 1 above and shall keep such standards under regular review.

2 The standards mentioned in subsection 1 above shall include –

    (a) the minimum levels of provision to meet the needs of those assessed for services under this Act, their range, quality and diversity and accessibility to those who may be in need of them; and

    (b) the minimum standards for emergency services

3 The Secretary of State shall direct health authorities and National Health Service trusts to secure the provision of community care services to meet the standards established under subsection 1 above.

Source: MIND, 1995.

8.3 **Process at the local level**

We shall discuss here four examples of the processes of mental health care which are relevant at the local level: (i) case registers and other local information systems; (ii) audit procedures; (iii) the pathways of patients to and through care, and how far services offer continuity; and (iv) the targeting of specialist services to more disabled groups of patients.

Compared with the country / regional level, process data gathered at the local level using *case registers* can be more detailed, and more sophisticated. By co-ordinating data monitoring by different mental health institutions in the local area it is possible to obtain cumulative information and anchor them to identified individual patients. The availability of personal computers is making such case registers, or similar equivalent systems, more widespread. The types of data which can be collected using this system at the local level are listed in Table 8.3. Such process measures can be used for *monitoring* more in depth care processes over time, but such use is descriptive only. *Evaluating* care is a more complex exercise, and although process variables are usually used as if they were meaningful alone, for evaluation purposes they are incomplete without reference to their associated inputs and outcomes.

Our second example of process at the local level is process *audit*. Medical audit has been defined by the Department of Health (1989) as 'the systematic, critical analysis of the quality of medical care, including the procedures used for diagnosis and treatment, the use of resources, and the resulting outcome and quality of life for the patient'. In the context of peer review, 'a frank discussion between doctors, on a regular basis and without

Table 8.3. *Definitions of variables which may be used to describe the process of care at the local level*

- **Annual treated incidence** Total number of patients who had a first-ever contact with a psychiatric service during the specified year
- **Annual treated prevalence** Total number of patients who had a contact with psychiatric services during the specified year
- **One day treated prevalence** All patients in contact with psychiatric service on census day, together with patients with a current episode of care (i.e. those who had a psychiatric contact both before and after the census day, with less than 91 days between contacts)
- **Long-term patients on one day** All patients not continuously hospitalised during the previous year (i.e. not long-stay),who, on census day had been in continuous contact with one or more psychiatric services during the previous 365 days or longer, with less than 91 days between each contact
- **In-patient prevalence** Total number of patients who spent at least one day in hospital in the specified year
- **First ever admissions** Total number of first-ever hospital psychiatric admissions in the specified year
- **Readmissions** Total number of hospital psychiatric readmissions in the specified year
- **Total admissions** Total number of hospital psychiatric admissions with a date of admission in the specified year[1]
- **Mean number of beds occupied per day** Mean number of beds occupied in each day
- **Mean length of stay** Mean duration of stay for all admissions starting in the specified year
- **Admission rates for patients in contact with the services** In-patients prevalence divided by total treated prevalence, expressed as a percentage
- **In-patient care priority index for a specific diagnostic group** Total number of days spent in hospital per patient in the specified year for a particular diagnostic group as a ratio of the same figure for patients with all diagnoses
- **Day hospital prevalence** Total number of patients who had at least one contact (or visit) at day hospitals or at rehabilitation groups of community mental health centre in specified year
- **Mean day-hospital contacts** Mean number of day-hospital contacts per day-patients in the specified year
- **Day hospital care priority index** Total number of days spent in day hospital for specific diagnostic groups in the specified year as a ratio of the same quantity for patients with all diagnoses
- **Out-patient and casual contacts prevalence** Total number of patients who had at least one out-patient contact at hospital, community psychiatric clinics (including contacts made with psychiatrist in GP surgeries – for UK only), general hospital liaison and accident and emergency departments in the specified year[2]

Table 8.3. (*cont.*)

- **Mean out-patient and casual contacts** Mean number of out-patient and casual contacts per patient treated at this level of care in the specified year
- **Out-patients priority index for specific diagnostic groups** Total number of out-patients and casual contacts per patient in the year for a particular diagnostic group as a ratio of the same figure for patients with all diagnoses
- **Home visits and community contacts prevalence** Total number of patients who had at least one visit made to their home or to homes of their friends or relatives, or visits to patients temporarily with other agencies, or visits to premises of voluntary organisations or to social services premises, by psychiatrists, nurses, psychologist, and other psychiatric staff in the specified year[2]
- **Mean home visits and community contacts** Mean number of home visits and community contacts per patient treated at this level of care in the specified year
- **Home visits priority index for specific diagnostic groups** Total number of home visits and community contacts per patient in the specified year for a particular diagnostic group as a ratio of the same figure for patients with all diagnoses

---

Notes:
[1] If a patient was admitted more than once in the specified year, each admission is included in the figure for total admissions.
[2] Only direct face-to-face contacts are included. Any contacts made by telephone are excluded from the counts.
Source: Gater *et al.*, 1995

fear of criticism, of the quality of care provided as judged against agreed standards' (Wing *et al.*, 1992). Robinson (1991) has described the various methods of audit, some of which involve process measures, while others focus on outcome measures, and we refer here to the former. The most common method is criterion-based audit of case notes in which *a priori* standards are applied in a review of documentation and to the process of care.

 A third way in which local level care processes can be conceptualised is in terms of patients' *pathways* to and through mental health services. The term pathway describes the routes taken by patients in making a first contact with health services, and the subsequent sequence of contacts within an episode of care. These sequences are highly dependent upon the availability of services locally, and also upon historical patterns of referral and treatment between agencies. As we shall discuss in detail in Chapter 13, we view mental health services as an inter-related series of components, which can be seen to act together as a hydraulic whole, so that the pressure of morbidity is distributed throughout the system.

A similar metaphor can be applied to the wider set or agencies which

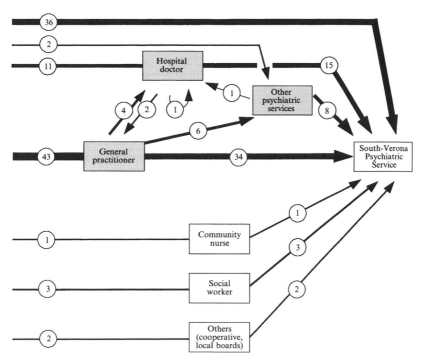

Figure 8.2 Pathways diagram for 116 residents of South-Verona referred to the Community Psychiatric Service. Percentages of this population taking each step on the pathway. The grey background indicates the medical sources of referral. From Balestrieri *et al.* (1994) with permission.

contribute towards the whole local system of care, and through which individual patients need to navigate to receive specific items of care. Interfaces between services therefore act as filters within the wider system, and an analysis of patients' pathways can reveal key local system weaknesses, such as points at which referrals fail to connect, or areas of wasteful overlap, where several agencies concurrently provide similar services. Another key feature of local services is the distinction between planned and unplanned contacts, and a recent study in South Verona found that patients whose first ever contact was unplanned had more care, both planned and unplanned, in the subsequent year (Tansella & Micciolo, 1998).

Such local processes are influenced by local inputs (for example, budget allocations) by country/regional level inputs (for example, governmental directives and policies), which influence these pathways, either facilitating or inhibiting movement. In particular, the pathway between primary and secondary care services is usually one with the densest patient traffic. The balanced distribution of cases of mental disorder between the local primary and secondary levels of care, and the efficient two-way operation of this pathway are crucial to the degree of fluidity or stasis of the system as a whole. One example of such an approach is the WHO study of pathways to care (Gater *et al.*, 1991; Balestrieri *et al.*, 1994), which is illustrated in Figure 8.2.

It is not only important to see which pathways patients take, but also to assure that they receive care as long as they need it, without periods of discontinuity and without an incoherent and conflicting pattern of contacts. The preferred pathway is characterised by continuity of care, and in Chapter 11 we shall define two types of continuity offered by different services or within the same service: cross-sectional (at one point in time) and longitudinal (across time).

Although continuity has until recently been discussed in a speculative rather than an operationalised way (Johnson *et al.*, 1997), there have been two recent attempts to quantify it for research purposes. Bindman *et al.* (1997) assessed the adequacy of written communication between primary and secondary care services for patients suffering from severe mental illness. Sytema *et al.* (1997) have proposed two measures of continuity namely the time between discharge from hospital and first subsequent outpatient contact, and the number of different types of mental health services used after hospital discharge.

The fourth issue which we shall discuss in relation to the process of care at the local level is *targeting*. There is now widespread agreement among professionals, managers and voluntary agencies on the groups of patients who should receive priority for specialist mental health services. Broadly, people who are most disabled by mental illness should be afforded the highest priority, and services should be provided in relation to need. There is evidence that in some areas resources are not currently matched to need, and that some very vulnerable individuals may be consequently neglected. It is therefore important in planning and providing specialist mental health services to have a clear view about how to put this policy into practice.

The most disabled group of psychiatric patients are often referred to as 'severely mentally ill' (SMI), but there is as yet no widely agreed definition of SMI. Four of the most useful definitions are given in Table 8.4. While different definitions of SMI are used by policy makers, researchers, clinicians, users and between disciplines and agencies, in many local areas the definition is reached pragmatically, often based on agreed priorities (Powell & Slade, 1996). Such a pragmatic approach may be based upon an analysis of factors which are associated with patients most likely to use acute hospital beds, as shown in Table 8.5.

Table 8.4. *Definitions of the severely mentally ill*

---

1. Goldman, (1981)

(i) *Diagnosis*: patients diagnosed according to DSM-III-R criteria with these 3 conditions:

Schizophrenia and schizo-affective drug	(ICD9 295)
bipolar disorders and major depression	(ICD9 296)
delusional (paranoid) disorders	(ICD9 297)

(ii) *Duration* at least one year since onset of disorder

(iii) *Disability* sufficient disability to seriously impair functioning of role performance in at least one of the following areas: occupation, family responsibilities, or accommodation

2. McLean & Liebowitz (1989)

At least one of the following must be present:

(i) two or more years contact with services

(ii) depot prescribed

(iii) ICD9 295.x or 297.x

(iv) 3 or more in-patient admissions in the last 2 years

(v) 3 or more day-patient episodes in the last 2 years

(vi) DSM-III highest level of adaptive functioning in the past year refer C or more

3 National Institute for Mental Health (1987)

(i) *Diagnosis* of non-organic psychosis or personality disorder

(ii) *Duration,* operationalised as a two-year history of mental illness or 2 years or more of treatment.

(iii) *Disability,* operationalised as including at least 3 of:
(a) vulnerability to stress; (b) disability that prevents self-sufficiency and causes dependency; (c) limited ability to obtain needed assistance; (d) social behaviour demanding intervention by mental health system or courts; (e) impaired activities of daily living and basic needs; (f) impaired social functioning; (g) limited and impaired performance in employment; or (h) limited and impaired performance in non-work (e.g. leisure and homemaking).

4. Audit Commission (1994), derived from Patmore & Weaver (1990)

(i) Psychotic diagnosis, organic illness or injury *and*
previous compulsory admission *or*
aggregate one year stay in hospital in past five years *or*
three or more admissions in past five years

(ii) Psychotic diagnosis, organic illness or injury *or*
any previous admissions in past five years

(iii) No record of Hospital admissions and
no recorded psychotic diagnosis, organic illness or injury

Table 8.5. *Characteristics of patients most likely to use acute hospital beds*

Socio-demographic factors	Young
	Male sex
	Lower socio-economic class
	Black
	Live alone or in unsupported accommodation
	Have no carer
Clinical factors	Diagnosis: schizophrenia, manic-depression, other psychoses
	Vulnerability to suicidal or forensic behaviours
	Concomitant physical morbidity
	Dual diagnosis – concurrent alcohol or drug abuse
Previous service use	Recently discharge from psychiatric hospitals/institutions
	Multiple previous admissions
	Minimal insight or control over their illness
	Poor collaboration with medication and other treatment strategies
	No trusting relationship with carers or professionals
	Previous compulsory hospital admission

8.4 **Process at the patient level**

At the individual level, it is striking that the question of what processes happen in meetings between mental health staff and patients in routine clinical encounters is almost unresearched. Although in most other medical specialities very detailed attention is paid to the content of the therapeutic process, in terms of the specific treatments used, and the dose, combination, timing and adherence to agreed protocols, by contrast the content of most mental health service contacts is a black box. The reasons for this may include a reluctance to address the difficulties of constructing adequate assessment measures of 'talking treatments' (except for research into behavioural and cognitive-behavioural treatments), and a marked emphasis in psycho-dynamically orientated psychiatry upon the importance of the confidential nature of the clinical session. Moreover, the relative isolation throughout most of the last century of psychiatry from other medical disciplines has rendered it less open to scrutiny and inspection. This trend has, to some extent, been reversed in the last ten years.

The importance of the process of care at the individual level can be seen from the perspective of the patient as well as the clinician. From the point of view of the patient, the process of care is significant *per se*, not only in relation to the outcome. This is because of the value attributed by patients to the 'shell' of treatment. This shell includes: the treatment setting, the quality of the clinician–patient relationship, the ease of access, the degree of satisfaction related to treatment, the quality and quantity of information received, and the feeling of being understood – these all contribute to a composite view by the patient of how well they are treated. For example, from the patient's perspective the concept of continuity of care often refers to a preference to see one trusted clinician, offering treatment and care, rather than different professional members of staff on each occasion.

Another aspect of process of care at the patient level is the frequency of clinical contacts, for example at an out-patient clinic. The appraisal of the proper interval between appointments may be different from the patient and the clinician perspectives, but surprisingly there is no appropriate research evidence to assist the decision about when to offer the next appointment. Such decisions therefore usually reflect the capacity of the local service, or traditions within each service. The exceptions to this tendency are practitioners of talking therapies: dynamic psychotherapists characteristically see patients at least three times a week, cognitive-behavioural therapists usually offer sessions every one or two weeks, and systemic family therapists will most often see each family once a month. Considering the vast cost implications of different treatment schedules, it is remarkable that so little research has been done to establish the most efficient rhythm of care. By comparison, there has been far more research attention paid to the relationship between length of stay for in-patient treatment (also a process measure) and clinical outcome, and this has been investigated especially according to diagnosis-related groups (DRGs). Our most striking personal impressions from visiting different clinical services is that the patient populations are often remarkably similar, but that the processes of care are widely different.

At the patient level, the chronological history of the previous process of care can inform future clinical care. For instance a case register or other computerised clinical information system can be used not only for administrative or research purposes, but also for the provision to the clinical teams of lists of severely mentally ill patients who have been in contact and are to be reassessed at regular intervals to ensure better continuity of care and improved practices. For this purpose a combination of several variables, such as diagnosis, number of hospital admissions, number of episodes of illness, total number of contacts over a given period, occupational status, multiple agency use, can be easily used to identify, from the pattern of the process of their care, individual patients who are in a particular high risk category, for example, for risk of readmission to hospital or of rapid relapse of schizophrenia (Tansella & Ruggeri, 1996).

9

The outcome phase

9.1 **Defining the outcome phase**

Outcome is defined in the *Concise Oxford Dictionary* as 'a result, a visible effect'. This sense that an outcome is the final step of a sequence of events is reinforced by the synonyms given for outcome in the *Oxford Thesaurus*, as shown in Table 9.1.

Outcomes are generally considered to be changes in functioning, in morbidity or in mortality (Thornicroft & Tansella, 1996). These outcomes are attributable to the treatment and care received, which themselves can be analysed as input and process variables. Outcomes are therefore a complex product of multiple influences, and they can be considered at the three geographical levels of the matrix model (Figure 9.1 shows such possible outcomes). The difficulties associated with defining and collecting outcomes data have meant that input and process variables have often been used as proxies for outcomes, a categorical error (Jenkins *et al.*, 1994).

Outcome can be considered from two points of view. The first is the *broad definition*, which refers to changes in any variable, for example a politician may describe an increase in investment in mental health services (input) as a favourable outcome. Similarly, a service re-reorganisation, following a monitoring exercise, may lead to an increase in the average frequency of out-patient contacts with patients (process), which the patients and clinicians may see as a positive outcome. Second, the *narrow definition*, refers only to the health status of an individual patient, or of aggregations of individual patient data, and implies measures taken at least at two time points, before and after a clinical intervention. In this chapter we shall deal with 'outcome' in terms of the second, narrow definition.

We shall describe the most common types of outcomes at the three geographical levels of the matrix model, as indicated in Figure 9.1, to show that the most appropriate forms of these data, and their availability, vary according to the differing information needs. If the question is whether mental

Geographical Dimension *Temporal Dimension*

	(A) Input Phase	(B) Process Phase	(C) Outcome Phase
(1) Country/Regional Level	1A	1B	1C · suicide rates · homelessness rates · imprisonment rates · special enquiries
(2) Local Level (catchment area)	2A	2B	2C · suicide rates · outcomes aggregated at local level · physical morbidity
(3) Patient Level	3A	3B	3C · symptom reduction · impact on care-givers · satisfaction with services · quality of life · disability · needs

Figure 9.1 Overview of the matrix model, with examples of key issues in the outcome phase

Table 9.1. *Synonyms for outcome*

Decision, determination, effect, end, event, fate, fruit, issue, judgement, pay-off, product, purpose, repercussion, resolution, result, solution, upshot.

health care is improving in a particular country or not (country/regional level), then the units of analysis which offer meaningful information will be different from that needed by a catchment area mental health service manager or administrator (local level), and from that required by a clinician (patient level) (see Table 9.2).

In the past process measures, or even input measures, were used *as if* they were outcome indicators. This was not only because of confused defini-tions, but also because the ability to define and measure outcomes in mental health care was not well developed. Substantial progress in this field has been made in recent years, and we shall therefore include in the final section of this chapter a methodological discussion on both the instruments to be used for outcome assessment and on types of research design appropriate for outcome evaluation.

9.2 **Outcome at the country/regional level**

In epidemiology the classic outcome measures at the population level are mortality and morbidity. While these have also been used in epi-demiological psychiatry as outcome measures, the use of such indicators taken from general medicine for psychiatry needs careful translation. This is because the conditions under investigation in cardiology or oncology have a direct causal association with death, while in psychiatry the estab-lished higher mortality rates (Allebeck, 1989) are indirectly associated with mental illness, most often through suicide or risks from patients' lifestyles. Second, morbidity indicators used as outcome measures in mental health need to be seen in a modest context: psychiatry so far has not been able to effect primary prevention for any form of severe mental illness.

 Mental health services are therefore almost entirely concerned with sec-ondary prevention (reducing symptom relapse) and tertiary prevention (reducing the suffering consequent upon symptoms). In this case, the rele-vant outcomes in the mental health field can be subsumed within the head-ings of impairment (primary symptoms), disability (consequent reduced ability to perform specific skills) and handicap (limited social role perfor-mance), as formalised by the WHO *International Classification of Impairments,*

Table 9.2. *Outcome measures suitable for the three geographical levels*

Outcome measure	Geographical dimension		
	Country level	Local level	Patient level
Lost occupation	√	√	√
Physical morbidity	√	√	√
Suicide and parasuicide in the general population	√	√	
Suicide and parasuicide in psychiatric patients	√	√	√
Homelessness	√	√	√
Special enquiries and reports	√	√	√
Standardised mortality ratios among current and former patients		√	
Symptom severity		√	√
Impact on care givers		√	√
Satisfaction with services		√	√
Quality of life / subjective well being		√	√
Disability / social role performance		√	√
Met needs for care		√	√
Global ratings of function		√	√

Table 9.3. *National mental health targets set for Britain in 1992*

To improve significantly the health and social functioning of mentally ill people

To reduce the overall suicide rate by at least 15% by the year 2000 (from 11.1 per 100 000 population in 1990 to no more than 9.4)

To reduce the suicide rate of severely mentally ill people by at least 33% by the year 2000 (from the estimate of 15% in 1990 to no more than 10%)

Disabilities and Handicaps (ICIDH, World Health Organization, 1980), or outcomes may deal with other consequences of health services provision, such as service satisfaction or impact on care givers.

Directly in relation to the population level, a frequently used outcome measure is *suicide rate*. Indeed rates of suicide have been judged in Britain to be so important that they have been included as two of the three national mental health targets in the Health of the Nation framework (Department of Health, 1993), as shown in Table 9.3.

Rates of homelessness among the mentally ill (or rates of mental illness among the homeless) can also be used as an outcome indicator of the

Table 9.4. *Most common themes from special mental health service enquires in London (in order of frequency)*

Adequacy and allocation of resources
Poor communication between agencies (especially between health and social services, between mental health and housing departments, and between specialist mental health services and GPs)
Poor assessment of risk of violence
Problems in discharge of patient from hospital (especially failure to assess needs and develop an after-care plan)
Poor liaison with police and probation services
Confidentiality and professional ethics (especially as barriers between health and social services, and between mental health services and the police)

Source: Lelliot et al., 1997

effectiveness of mental illness policies at the national level. In practice, however, we are not aware of any such studies at this level, and most such data are relevant to the local level (Bachrach, 1984; Scott, 1988). Third, the same applies to the inappropriate placement in *prison* of those who would be better treated in mental health facilities (Gunn *et al.*, 1991; Maden *et al.*, 1995).

The fourth possible outcome measure relevant to the national level is the use of *special enquiries*, especially those into extreme adverse events, such as homicides by patients. The results of the enquiries made in the UK have been analysed by Lelliot *et al.* (1997), who have summarised the most frequently recurring major themes emerging from these special reports on mental health services, and from five of the enquiries relating to homicides in London. These themes are shown in Table 9.4.

The fact that such meaningful outcome variables are usually missing is a reflection of the fact that mental health services are seen to be a relatively low priority in many countries. Although, as we have discussed in section 2.4, mental illnesses make a major contribution to total mortality and morbidity at the national level, nevertheless it is common for governments to see mental illnesses as of lesser importance than most other conditions. This, combined with a tendency to collect process variables that are relatively easy to collate (rather than those which are important), such as hospital admission rates, means that we are almost totally uninformed at the country/regional level about how far mental health services achieve their goals.

9.3 **Outcome at the local level**

At the local level outcome indicators can be used in three ways: (i) by interpolating from national / country data, (ii) by measuring directly at the local level, and (iii) by aggregating up to the local level information which has been collected for individuals at the patient level (the latter are described in more detail in section 9.4). For example, rates of suicide, unemployment, imprisonment and homelessness can be estimated using the first method, or directly measured using the second method if the appropriate information and resources exist. The second approach will provide more accurate and up-to-date information. At the same time, individual patient data on, for example, symptom reduction, satisfaction with services, and quality of life can be easily collapsed to relate to a particular geographical level, if institutions providing care to those local patients are willing to co-operate in data collection and collation.

An example of the application of national data to a local area is the use of national suicide data. In many countries information is not routinely available for local levels, but is collected at the country/regional level. Such information can be used directly as if such rates applied equally to the local catchment area, or can be standardised for the particular socio-demographic characteristics of the local population. This is applicable if it is meaningful and possible to measure a particular outcome for patients in a local catchment area. Unemployment rate among patients suffering from psychotic disorders, for example, are often high and such outcome data may be useful for the planning of day care and occupational rehabilitation services. Data from the PRiSM Psychosis Study of prevalent cases of functional psychosis in South London found, for example, that 81% of all patients were unemployed and a further 5% had part-time work (Thornicroft *et al.*, 1999) The implications of such structural unemployment for patients with psychotic disorders are not well researched (Warner, 1994). However, the adverse effects of unemployment on mental health more generally are now well understood (Warr, 1987), and may compound the multiple difficulties faced by such patients (Sartorius *et al.*, 1986).

The third approach is to aggregate up to the local level information gathered from individual patients. This applies largely to clinical data (defined widely as the range of outcome measures discussed below in section 9.4) and one example is the measurement of patients' needs. In the PRiSM Psychosis Study referred to earlier, the assessment of individual need was made using the Camberwell Assessment of Need (CAN), and we summarise in Table 9.5 the overall results of the service user (patient)

Table 9.5. *Met and unmet needs: changes for Camberwell psychotic patients*

Sector	Need Status	Time 1 mean (max 22)	Time 2 mean (max 22)	Change (time 2– time 1)	95% CI	p^1
Nunhead	Met needs	4.05	4.45	0.40	−0.31 to 1.10	0.26
(Intensive $n=62$)	Unmet needs	1.23	1.90	0.68	0.20 to 1.15	0.006
Norwood	Met needs	4.51	3.73	−0.78	−0.17 to -1.39	0.01
(Standard $n=63$)	Unmet needs	1.57	1.86	0.29	−0.25 to 0.83	0.29

Note:
[1] Paired *t*-test.

ratings of need from the 22 CAN domains (Phelan *et al.*, 1995). The results show that epidemiologically representative psychotic individuals, half of whom are schizophrenic, have on average about seven major needs, that about three-quarters of these are met and one-quarter unmet.

Another example of the use of individual outcomes measures at the local level is the assessment of *global function* (Phelan *et al.*, 1996). Functioning is an abstract concept which summarises the whole range of activities of a particular patient group. Various scales have been developed which attempt to provide reliable measures of a person's level of functioning in all, or nearly all areas of life. The scales vary in their construction and degree of simplicity. Perhaps the most widely used is the Global Assessment of Function Scale (GAF) (Endicott *et al.*, 1976), which has the advantage of brevity, which combines symptoms and disability in a single scale, and has been shown to be usable with reasonable reliability in ordinary clinical conditions (Jones *et al.*, 1995).

The use of outcomes measures at the level of local services is still uncommon. Yet the tools, such as the GAF scale, or the Health of the Nation Outcome Scale (HoNOS) (Wing *et al.*, 1998) and the methodologies for their application are now available. In the future, the application of evidence-based medicine to routine clinical settings will be increasingly likely to encourage the use of standardised outcome measures in everyday clinical practice.

9.4 **Outcome at the patient level**

The primary purpose of mental health services is to optimise outcomes for individual patients (cell 3C in the matrix model). Prior inputs and processes should therefore be concentrated upon their effectiveness in

Table 9.6. *Common outcome domains at the patient level*

Symptom severity
Impact of caring
Patients' satisfaction with services
Quality of life
Disabilities
Needs

terms of patient level outcomes. This is not only a technical question. Such an approach implies a whole culture change to a mental health service system that emphasises at every stage both a patient-orientation, and a specific capability to measuring health status that can be aggregated to higher service levels. If successful, such an approach will be palpable to patients themselves and to their carers. It will also be subject to systematic documentation by clinicians so that feedback can be given to patients about their clinical progress.

In this section we shall discuss the range of most commonly used domains of outcome measurement (which are summarised in Table 9.6). It is noteworthy that health service research in this field is increasingly acknowledging the importance of other outcomes apart from symptom severity.

Traditionally *symptom severity measures* have been used most often to assess the effectiveness of mental health treatments. Psychiatrists and psychologists have contributed to the early development of such assessment scales to allow this research to take place (Wetzler, 1989; Thompson, 1989; Thornicroft & Tansella, 1996). Excellent recent reviews of scales suitable for this purpose have been published (Wing, 1996; Wittchen & Nelson, 1996; Sartorius & Janca, 1996). While the primary symptoms are clearly important, for most chronic mental disorders there is symptom persistence, and it is unrealistic at present to see symptom eradication as the sole aim of treatment. Very often, after the point of maximum symptom relief, the clinical task becomes one of attempting to minimise the disability and handicaps consequent upon the primary impairment (WHO, 1980).

The importance of the *impact of caring* for those with mental illnesses upon family members and others who provide informal care has long been recognised (Creer & Wing, 1974), but has only been subjected to concerted research in relatively recent years (Schene *et al.*, 1994). Such research has shown that it is common for carers themselves to suffer from mental illnesses (most commonly depression and anxiety), and to worry about the future and how their relative will cope when the carer can no longer provide care. Many family members are distressed by the perceived underactivity of the patient, and they are often poorly informed about the clinical condition, its treatment and the likely prognosis. Clinical services rarely provide family members with a practical action plan of what to do in future should a crisis occur. Indeed, some services continue to convey to families the outmoded idea that carers, especially parents, are in some way to blame for the disorder or for relapses of the condition. In our view the regular provision of information sessions for family members is now a hallmark of a good practice.

Patients' *satisfaction with services* is a further domain which has recently become established as a legitimate, important and feasible area of outcome assessment at the local level. This involves a recognition of the contribution that patients and their carers can make to outcome assessment. Psychometrically adequate scales are those which adopt a multi-dimensional approach, which assess the full range of service characteristics, which are independently administered (so that patient ratings have no consequences upon their future clinical care), and which have established validity and reliability (Ruggeri & Dall'Agnola, 1993; Ruggeri, 1996).

Quality of life ratings have also become prominent during the last decade, and several instruments have been constructed which reflect varying basic approaches to the topic. The first distinction is between schedules which address subjective well-being only, compared with those which also measure objective elements of quality of life. The second main point of differentiation is between scales constructed for the general population, or designed for those suffering from specific disorders, including the more severe mental illnesses (Lehman, 1996). One advantage of quality of life data is that they tend to be popular with politicians, who find the concept has a powerful face validity!

After symptom treatment has been optimised, usually by treatment with medication for psychotic disorders, for example, the residual *disabilities* may need quite different types of intervention (Wiersma, 1996). Separate measurements of cognitive and social abilities, which are essential for an independent life, are therefore justified. Indeed, in a longitudinal perspective, social disability tends to have a less favourable course than psycho-pathology.

Increasing importance is being attached to the *needs* of those who suffer from mental illnesses. This new orientation marks a wider public mood that emphasises the active role of the recipients of health services as consumers,

Table 9.7. *Definitions of need, demand and supply*

Need	=	What people benefit from
Demand	=	What people ask for
Supply	=	What is provided

Source: adapted from Stevens & Gabbay, 1991.

and also raises a series of important consequent questions. How can needs be defined and by whom? (see Table 9.7). How can they be measured and compared? What importance should be accorded to both met and unmet needs in the assessment of individual patients and in the planning and evaluation of mental services as a whole? How should the needs of those suffering from schizophrenia be prioritised in relation to the needs of other diagnostic groups?

9.5 **Psychometric properties of outcome measures**

The process of establishing the psychometric qualities of new scales is detailed and time consuming. Although we would never use uncalibrated measures for height, weight or temperature, many scales used for mental health service evaluation are unfortunately of unknown validity and reliability (Hall, 1979, 1980; Salvador-Carulla, 1996). In this section we will consider scales used for adult psychiatric patients and services in the community, and we have not included reference to other important specialist areas, such as assessment of cognitive impairment, and abnormal movements, which are covered elsewhere in more detailed texts (Freeman & Tyrer, 1989; Parry & Watts, 1989; Thompson, 1989; Wetzler, 1989; Israel *et al.*, 1990).

A research instrument should first of all actually measure what it is intended to measure – it should be valid (in Latin *validus* meaning 'strong'). A single scale may be reliable and invalid or may be valid and unreliable. We therefore seek scales that exhibit both properties.

Validity poses special difficulties in the area of psychological and psychiatric assessment as the criteria against which to rate validity may themselves be indirect or imprecise. The types of validity are:

(i) *Face validity* is the subjective judgement made by the user of the instrument about whether the individual items cover the appropriate range of problems relevant to the measure as a whole. This is not a statistical yardstick of validity so much as an initial impression about the degree to which the scale correctly includes relevant items.

(ii) **Content validity** describes whether a test samples from the entire domain of that which is to be measured. Again this is rather an issue of personal judgement than a statistical measure of validity.

(iii) More widely, the opinions of experts in the field may be taken about a new measure to provide an estimate of **consensual validity**.

(iv) **Criterion-related validity** is acceptable when a new measure produces the same result as another instrument whose validity has already been established, where the latter is called the criterion measure. There are two types of criterion-related validity. *Concurrent* validity is used when the results of the two tests being compared are available simultaneously, while *predictive* validity is applicable where scores on the new test are used to predict subsequent scores on a proven test.

(v) Finally, **construct validity** addresses the psychological meaning of the test scores. It has been clearly described by NIMH (1985): 'The construct validity of a test is not established by one successful prediction: it consists of the slow, laborious process of gathering evidence from many experiments and observations on how the test is functioning'. Among these observations will be correlation coefficients with other measures of the construct under consideration, and the successful prediction of functional outcomes where these are known to be associated with the construct (Streiner & Norman, 1989).

In addition, a rating scale must give repeatable results for the same patient when used under different conditions, that is it must be *reliable*. There are four widely used methods to gauge reliability.

(i) **Inter-rater reliability** refers to two or more independent raters to agree when using the measure with the same subject. It is therefore applicable only to interviewer rated scales. In practice, this is best measured by the raters being present at the same live or recorded interview. The degree of agreement between raters may be calculated either for a total scale score, or for the ratings on individual items. A widely used measure of agreement is Cohen's kappa, which takes into account the likelihood of the raters agreeing by chance alone (Cohen, 1960). Usually kappa values of less than 40% indicate a poor level of agreement, and over 75% show very good agreement.

(ii) **Test–retest reliability** describes how far the score of a rating scale remains constant when used by the same rater with the same subject at two or more points in time. If the scores are identical from the two rating occasions the correlation would be 1.0. This does not occur in practice, because the condition of the subject may have changed, there may be a practice effect for the rater in becoming more familiar with the instrument, or because if the interval between the two interviews is sufficiently long, a child subject may have matured. Further, the original assessment may have produced a reaction for the subject which influences the second occasion, for example, subjects may be more or less willing to disclose confidential information based upon their experience of the first interview. Also, cyclical changes in what is being measured, for example, in diurnal mood variation, mean that the second test may need to be conducted in circumstances as similar as possible to the first.

(iii) *Parallel form reliability* is measured by having two different but equivalent versions of the rating instrument which are used on the same occasion, in an attempt to eliminate the change in rating scores in the test–retest situation that is attributable to actual changes in the subject's condition. Often the order in which the instruments are administered is alternated between the subjects.

(iv) *Split-half reliability* is a measure of the associations between the halves of the same test, for example between odd and even numbered items. This may be feasible even when subjects cannot complete more than one instrument (for parallel form reliability) or cannot attend on more than one occasion (for test–retest reliability). A Spearman–Brown correction is usually made to the result to account for the fact that the smaller number of items from each half produces a less reliable estimate. The measure is usually expressed in terms of Cronbach's alpha. Both parallel and split-half types of reliability are based upon the assumption of equivalence, the difference being that in the latter equivalence is assumed to apply to alternating items.

It needs to be emphasised again that there is no necessary association between the reliability and the validity of a measure: it may be highly valid but poorly reliable, or vice versa. In practice, when selecting a measure for a study of community psychiatry a number of issues must be addressed. Does the scale being considered have published validity and reliability scores available, and how strong are these results? Do the age, sex, ethnic, diagnostic and functional characteristics of the test population resemble the study population? If any doubt remains after addressing these questions, then your study may require a pilot stage to establish the psychometric properties of the selected measures under your local conditions.

9.6 Methodologies for assessing outcomes

We have previously emphasised the importance of using the best possible research design to evaluate mental health treatments and services. The best possible method may be a randomised controlled trial (RCT) or a

Table 9.8. *A hierarchy of evidence for therapy*

1a	Evidence from a meta-analysis of RCTs
1b	Evidence from at least one RCT
2a	Evidence from at least one controlled study without randomisation
2b	Evidence from at least one other type of quasi-experimental study
3	Evidence from non-experimental descriptive studies, such as comparative studies, correlation studies and case-control studies
4	Evidence from expert committee reports or opinions and / or clinical experience of respected authorities.

Source: Geddes & Harrison, 1997

less powerful design, depending upon the question to be answered and the practical constraints of the clinical setting. To suggest that the RCT design is not the only valid design is not to advocate a return to the pre-scientific era of psychiatric practice, but rather to set out the relative strengths and weaknesses of methods at each of the different levels of the model (Taylor & Thornicroft, 1996).

The matrix model offers a context in which some value can be attached to results from a range of types of research study. These can be conceptualised along a gradient of scientific power that moves from meta-analysis of RCTs, to individual RCTs, to non-randomised clinical trials, which are sometimes called quasi-experimental studies (NRCT), to structured clinical practice (SCP), and to the everyday unstructured clinical practice (UCP). Non-RCT designs may be especially appropriate to address questions for which an RCT would be too costly or too premature. A hierarchy of types of research design has recently been proposed by Geddes & Harrison (1997), as shown in Table 9.8. The particular strengths and weaknesses of these four types of study design are displayed in Table 9.9.

At the *patient level* (or for a group of similarly affected patients) the preferred direction in research design for therapeutic interventions must be from Unstructured Clinical Practice (UCP) to Randomised Clinical Trials (RCT), and may pass through the intermediate stages of Structured Clinical Practice (SCP) and Non-Randomised Clinical Trials (NRCT). At the *local level*, however, the final step of this sequence to RCT designs may either be impossible or too costly, and less technically rigorous designs may still provide valuable scientific evidence. Further, at the *country level*, a significant achievement is to take the step from UCP to SCP, for example, by promoting the widespread use of treatment protocols and clinical guidelines, by using

Table 9.9. *Comparison of the characteristics of four types of clinical research design*

Study characteristic	Randomised Clinical Trials (RCT)	Non-Randomised Clinical Trials (quasi-experimental studies) (NRCT)	Structured Clinical Practice (routine outcome studies) (SCP)	Unstructured Clinical Practice (UCP)
Defined acceptance/ exclusion criteria	√	?		
Inclusion of whole patient populations			√	√
Adequate sample size	√	√	√	√
Clear controlled conditions	√	√		
Bias reduction by double blindness	√			
Bias reduction by randomisation	√			
Standardised measures	√	√	√	
Regularly repeated outcome measurements	?	?	√	
Long-term follow-up		?	√	?
Power of statistical analysis	?	?	?	
Hypothesis generation	√	√	√	√
Generalisation	?	?	?	
Lack of constraint by ethical committee			√	√
Explicit patient consent unnecessary			√	√
Low cost for data collection			√	√

simple clinical outcome measures, or by setting explicit service targets (Department of Health, 1994). Indeed it is remarkable that clear treatment and service targets for inputs, processes and outcomes are rare in the extreme at all three geographical levels.

The further one moves down the gradient of scientific power in the research design, the greater is the possibility that research results are biased. Such biases make the interpretation of results more difficult, and in partic-ular the question of whether the clinical outcome is caused by the treatment input or is attributable to other causes. The concept of causality has been

Table 9.10. *Bradford Hill's epidemiological criteria for causality*

Strength of the association
Consistency
Specificity
Temporality
Biological gradient
Plausibility
Coherence
Experimental evidence

Source: Hill, 1965

clearly dissected by Sir Austin Bradford Hill, who has proposed eight criteria by which it can be judged (see Table 9.10), and which have also been discussed in detail by Susser (1973) and Cooper (1979).

By *strength of the association*, Bradford Hill meant whether the correlation between two variable was high. Such associations may be measured by correlations or by odds ratios (rate ratios). These measures are not the same as the statistical significance levels, which may be high when the values of the measures of association are low.

Consistency refers to an association that has been 'repeatedly observed by different persons, in different places, circumstances and times'. This depends upon the replication of research findings in different studies. As Cooper (1979) has indicated, the presence of consistency does not necessarily imply a causal effect, but the lack of consistency does argue against such an effect.

Specificity means whether a particular consequence follows *only* from a specific intervention – that is a single, necessary and sufficient cause. When it is present it does present strong support for a causal significance.

By *temporality* Hill means 'which is the cart and which the horse?' This means that a change in the independent variable occurs before a change in the dependent variable. This implies that the timing of both factors can be established with precision, a condition not always easily fulfilled within psychiatry, for example in terms of the first manifestation of onset symptoms.

Biological gradient refers to whether a dose–response relationship can be identified, so that greater exposure to the presumed risk factor does repeatably produce a greater consequent effect.

Plausibility was used by Hill to mean whether a specific statistical association was acceptable in the context of the wider scientific paradigm of the time. In other words, does the observed evidence fit what is known of the assumed pathogenesis of the disorder, and a broader underlying theoretical model? The accumulation of research findings indicating an agreed direction of causality additionally adds to the *coherence* of the findings.

Finally the importance of *experimental evidence* reinforces our earlier comments about the particular value of information from clinical trials which will usually be less contaminated by bias than the results of other types of study design. Finding an outcome which changes in the expected direction after a specific clinical intervention therefore supports the hypothesis that the association is causal.

Several of these criteria, most notably, the strength of the association, consistency, temporality, plausibility and coherence, can be used by clinicians in their everyday practice to interpret the outcomes of their treatments to patients. In the longer-term perspective, progress will be made through a chain of reasoning that starts with clinicians who treat individual patients and who generate hypotheses from their clinical reflections and systematic observations. If hypotheses survive further scrutiny they will be subjected to increasingly stringent testing by more powerful forms of verification. The life cycle of information produced in this way can then progress when research evidence is hard enough to justify changes in clinical practice, which will then be subject to further hypothesis generation.

The matrix model, which we have described here in Part III, in relation to the temporal phases, may help to encourage precisely these trends to occur also at the local and country levels, and so contribute towards making mental health services more rational as they become increasingly evidence-based (Tansella, 1997).

PART IV **Re-forming community-based mental health services**

10

The evidence base for mental health services

The aim of this chapter is to describe a stepwise approach toward an evidence base for planning or re-forming mental health services. In section 10.1 we describe this pathway in terms of the background epidemiological information which can support service development. In section 10.2 we discuss the different components of a mental health system of care, both with respect to their categories and their capacities. In section 10.3, we discuss how local service utilisation data can contribute to the evidence base that should inform planning decisions.

Although we present in this section an approach to assessing the need for mental health services, these estimates cannot be properly interpreted without first considering overall health and social care needs of the population in question. This is because it is misleading to discuss mental health needs without consideration of wider family and other social networks. Further, the specialist mental health services do not operate alone, but rather function at a whole series of interfaces with other social and health care agencies, all of which are under the influence of the wider social, political and cultural climate.

To illustrate this point, we shall refer to a enquiry carried out by Mueller (1973) in which he contacted 18 leading social psychiatrists in six countries asking for their views on the ideal psychiatric service for a population of 100000. However, reflecting the socio-political climate of the time, Franco Basaglia, in reply, refused to give figures on that basis. He criticised the way the question was put, and underlined the need for extensive background information about each particular area before any estimate of local service needs can be made. His objection would be seen as self-evident now.

In terms of assessing the needs of a population for mental health services we would also make the following preliminary remarks. *First*, there is no 'best' pattern of desired services, rather a reasonable balance of service components, which have a high 'degree-of-fit' to local circumstances. *Second*,

A **Epidemiologically based Data**

– *Population characteristics:* factors associated with psychiatric morbidity

– *Epidemiological data:* morbidity and disability for the particular area by age, sex and social status

– *Treated individuals:* appropriately/inappropriately

– *Place and type of treatment*

– *Untreated individual:* those in need of treatment

B **Services Provision Data**

–*Define categories* of service components for primary, secondary and tertiary levels of care

– *Quantify the capacities* of the service components

– *Quality of care* of the service sites

– *Quantitative and qualitative* information on staff

– *Integration and co-ordination* of components into a service system

D **Planning Process**

– *Constitution of a planning group* representing a wide range of local interest groups, including expert advisors

– *Selective assessment* of all data from, A, B and C relevant for service planning

– Setting a *medium-term time scale* for service plans (3–5 years)

– *Identify highest priority* service needs (both met and unmet)

– Identification of highest priority *unmet social needs* and information from relevant authorities

–*Plan:*

(i)   new service functions and necessary facilities
(ii) extension of capacity of current services
(iii) disinvestment from lower priority services
(iv) propose collection of new data necessary for the next planning cycle

C **Service Utilisation Data**

– *Event-based data* on clinical contacts by levels of care [in-patient, out-patient etc], number of events and rates per 10 000 population per year

– *Individual-based data* on both clinical contacts (as above) and on treatment episodes across different levels of care per year

– *Data on outcomes and costs* of different clinical contacts (disaggregated for sub-groups of patients) with which to establish substitutability and complementarity of service components in terms of cost-effectiveness

Figure 10.1 Proposed information pathway for planning or re-forming mental health services.

in any local setting there will exist no 'correct' scale of provision, only reasonable estimates based on the best available data.

In practice we propose a pragmatic strategy for the assessment of need which consists of using the best information available in each particular area. As correctly indicated by Wing (1986), this process is not linear but should be viewed as a circular pathway which can be followed more than once, as indicated in Figure 10.1. The information used in any particular cycle can therefore be influenced by the results of an earlier cycle if on that occasion a specific information deficit was identified and redressed.

10.1 **Epidemiologically based measures or estimates of local needs**

The pathway shown in Figure 10.2 can be used in areas which have both detailed recent epidemiological data on psychiatric morbidity for the local population, and a well developed information system. It is also relevant to other areas in which very little usable local information may be available.

As Figure 10.2 shows, as a first stage in this pathway we consider that the best possible information would be local epidemiological data on the occurrence of various psychiatric disorders, using a standard system of classification, and an agreed measure of needs for treatment, either by specialist or by primary care staff (A1 in Figure 10.2). Since such survey studies are expensive and time consuming, most sites will not have access to such recent local survey data.

If A1 data are not available, as is usually the case, then we suggest that country/regional epidemiological data (A2) are used instead, and are then weighted for local socio-demographic characteristics, as discussed below.

If such larger-scale epidemiological data are not available, then as a third option it is possible to use international data from 'comparator' countries or regions, weighted for local socio-demographic characteristics (A3). The results in this case will be less reliable and accurate because they are based on the additional assumption that the country/regional data can be transferred between countries.

In some cases, the data available in A1, A2 or A3 will be incomplete or insufficient, and therefore a fourth option (A4) is to use a number of experts, some of whom may be from the local area, to produce a consensus statement on levels of local morbidity, based on the best available views, taking into account specific local factors (e.g. levels of non health service provision, family support, local traditions, migration).

The final stage (A5) in our schema for estimating population-level needs is the process of producing an expert synthesis of the data arising from A1, A2, A3, and A4.

In everyday practice it will often be the case that no local epidemiological data are available, and the only feasible strategy is to make rough approximations by using the results of national (A2) or international (A3) epidemiological studies, and applying these overall, or diagnosis-specific, rates to the local area.

In carrying out the exercise shown in schematic form in Figure 10.2, two important considerations need to be kept in mind. First, the comparative

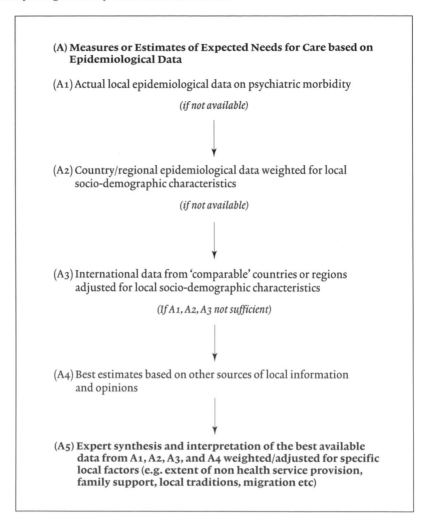

(A) Measures or Estimates of Expected Needs for Care based on Epidemiological Data

(A1) Actual local epidemiological data on psychiatric morbidity

(if not available)

(A2) Country/regional epidemiological data weighted for local socio-demographic characteristics

(if not available)

(A3) International data from 'comparable' countries or regions adjusted for local socio-demographic characteristics

(If A1, A2, A3 not sufficient)

(A4) Best estimates based on other sources of local information and opinions

(A5) Expert synthesis and interpretation of the best available data from A1, A2, A3, and A4 weighted/adjusted for specific local factors (e.g. extent of non health service provision, family support, local traditions, migration etc)

Figure 10.2 Strategies to estimate local population mental health service needs.

populations used for different geographical areas, and for the comparisons of actual and estimated needs, should be made quite clear. It may be a local total population of 100 000, for example, or the population aged 18–65. In either case the denominator being used must be precisely specified. Secondly, the 'currency', or units of service provision, must be described in unambiguous terms. For instance, the numbers of psychiatric beds needed or provided per 100 000 populations may mean adult acute beds, with or without beds intended for patients aged over 65, or for people who are demented, or the total may include intensive care or forensic beds. Again the unit of service must be stated in clear terms. Within these constraints the stepwise procedure described in Figure 10.2 can be a useful tool to give an overall assessment of how far actual provision in defined service categories matches best estimates of need.

10.1.1 The use of weighting factors derived from data collected elsewhere

Weighting can be made on the basis of two types of data collected elsewhere. First, psychiatric morbidity data, disaggregated by sex, age, marital status and other socio-demographic characteristics, which may include information on needs for treatment referring to a proportion of those who are defined as 'cases'. In this method, weighting is simply a process of standardisation which takes into account the local population, usually stratified by sex, age, and marital status. The more that local population information is available (both from the psychiatric morbidity survey and from the local population involved) the more accurate the standardisation can be. Prediction of future trends in the composition of the population (for instance expected proportion of elderly, of separated and divorced) can also be used for predicting needs for services for a limited future period of time (Kramer, 1987).

A second weighting method also uses census variables, collected in areas where some service use data (usually hospital admissions) were available at the same time. Statistical models produced from those particular areas can be used to predict rates of actual service use. The rationale for attempting to build a statistical model is that a substantial body of research has proved the associations between the rates of service use, on one hand, and particular socio-demographic (census) variables on the other hand, especially indicators of social deprivation (Shapiro *et al.*, 1985; Thornicroft, 1991).

It should be emphasised that this second weighting method assumes that use of services is a reliable proxy for psychiatric morbidity (and therefore of actual need for services), not only in the area where the model was derived, but also in the other areas to which the model is applied. Since the generation and the applications of these models occur at different times, a further assumption is that these models are stable over time. Such assumptions have rarely been tested, but are usually seen as reasonable in practice.

The latter weighting approach has been applied in Southern England (Jarman, 1983; Thornicroft, 1991; Jarman & Hirsch, 1992) and in Northern

Italy, where other types of service activity data, such as day-care contact rates, were also entered as dependent variables into the model (Thornicroft *et al.*, 1993). Another example of this method, applied at the country level in England and Wales, is the Mental Illness Needs Index (MINI, Glover, 1996). The MINI is a composite weighting score which combines six census variables, and which has been used to estimate expected capacities for in-patient and residential care services (see Table 10.4).

Table 10.1 shows census (predictor) variables which have been found to be significantly correlated with psychiatric service utilisation, most often hospital in-patient admission rates (outcome variables), in five different studies.

10.2 **Actual service provision data as information for planning**

Having examined local population needs for mental health care, we need to move now to address existing services. Two separate exercises are necessary: *first*, the best possible description of available services (structure), which will need to allow for the fact that the definitions or categories applied to services may not be consistent between sites. These structural characteristics have been described in more detail previously in Chapter 7 (inputs). *Second*, the use of these resources needs to be described, as discussed in Chapter 8 (process). The key point here is that over time both the structure and the functioning of the service will change in relation to each other.

10.2.1 **Conceptual approaches to mental health service description**

Before categorising services components, the first step is to establish an overall conceptual approach. This task can be accomplished in two main ways: as a detailed description of all the facilities (often described as programmes in North America) which have been developed, or by referring to the system of care as a whole. The first view, *the segmental approach*, considers each treatment facility or programme as essentially a separate functioning entity, with specific aims, operational policies, funding sources and selection criteria (for example in terms of patient age, diagnoses or disability). The second view, *the system approach*, sees each individual facility or programme as a part of the wider system of care, and explicitly takes account of the inter-relationships between the constituent parts.

It is important to understand that these facilities or programmes do have important effects upon each other in any local area, whether or not they are conceptualised as having such effects. The weakness of the segmental

Table 10.1. *Recent examples of statistically significant socio-demographic predictors of mental health services use*

	Jarman, 1983	Thornicroft 1991[1]	Jarman & Hirsch, 1992[2]	Thornicroft et al., 1993	Glover, 1996
Ethnic minorities	√	√			
Elderly living alone	√		√		
Children aged < 5	√				
Single parents families	√	√			
Unskilled workers	√				
Unemployed	√			√	√
Changed address	√	√			
Overcrowded	√			√	
Lack of internal amenities		√		√	
No car		√	√		√
Living in one room		√			
Population density		√		√	
Availability of general beds		√			
Household in single occupation			√	√	
Single, widowed or divorced			√	√	√
Illegitimacy index			√		
Private household with no car			√		
Dependency ratio[3]				√	
Registered as permanently disabled					√
Household not self-contained					√
Non-permanent accommodation[4]					√

Notes:

[1] Correlation coefficient of over 0.55 with standardised admission rate before principal components analysis.

[2] Six highest Pearson correlation coefficients of 169 variables entered into the model to predict standardised admission ratios based on district size and national overall rate.

[3] Percent of persons aged < 15 and aged 65 and over in relation to the population aged 15–64.

[4] Proportion of population resident in hostels, common lodging houses, miscellaneous establishments or sleeping rough.

In any particular local area many of these possible sources of data may be of poor quality or may be entirely missing. We would suggest that the available data be selected in terms of their relevance.

view in service description is that it does not provide a framework with which to understand these interactions. It cannot explain, for example, how the lack of provision of long-term residential care can mean that acute beds are inappropriately used for new long-term patients, leaving no capacity for acute crisis care. The strength of the segmental approach is that it is more specific and detailed, but this specificity is acquired at the expense of a more comprehensive and inclusive perspective.

When describing a group of services which are located in a given area, the first decision is which conceptual approach to adopt: the segmental or the system. The selection of the conceptual approach will be closely related to the actual organisation of services in each particular site. Even though it is theoretically possible to describe a fragmented service using a system approach, it is in fact easier to use a segmental conceptual approach for this purpose.

The second decision is whether to approach the question from a *service-based* or a *population-based* direction. The former requires the assembly of the best available information on the services which exist in that geographical area, and on their activities. The latter, the population-based approach, is a quite different exercise, and will be relatively straightforward where services have been intentionally organised to provide for a local reference catchment area population. Where, however, they are organised in other ways, then the population-based approach can be much more complex, since it is necessary to partition out those activities in services in local sites which are dedicated to the local population, and also to include services located elsewhere which provide care to patients from the reference catchment population. In practice this is very difficult to complete unless a case register or similar data monitoring system is already in place.

10.2.2 Categorising mental health services

Many excellent instruments have been established to measure individual psychiatric pathology. George (1989) has succinctly reported that the amount spent on such scales 'far exceeds the investment that has been made in the development and validation of measures of mental health services'.

In fact, there is no accepted standard classification of mental health service components. An ambitious approach has been taken by de Jong *et al.* (WHO, 1990) who under the aegis of WHO developed the *International Classification of Mental Health Care* (WHO-ICMHC). This is a tool for the classification of services providing mental health care, which is based upon what are called the 'modules' of care. A module of care is defined as a type of care made available to patients with comparable histories of psychopathological and social problems. The use of the scale takes place in three steps: (i) identifying the module of care to be classified, for example the departments or units of a hospital, (ii) classifying the modules of care according to qualitative aspects, and (iii) rating the extent of provision for each of the modules. There are now two editions of this schedule, and the first edition has been used in a comparison of mental health services in South Manchester and South Verona (Amaddeo *et al.*, 1995)

A second scheme for classifying types of service, proposed by the Department of Health in Britain, is called the *Spectrum of Care* (Table 10.2). It uses three main categories for services according to their functions, namely home-based care, day and out-patient care, and residential (in-patient and non-in-patient) services. Each of these main headings also allows for further specific sub-types to be defined. These services types are then further divided into 'acute' and 'long-term', and examples are shown in Table 10.2.

A third approach, is the *European Service Mapping Schedule* (Johnson *et al.*, 1997), which is being developed to allow international comparisons to be made. The ESMS allows the following tasks to be carried out in a standardised way. *First*, compiling an inventory of the mental health services serving the adult mentally ill population in a particular catchment area, with descriptions of their major characteristics. *Second*, listing the provision of health, social services, voluntary and private sectors services. *Third*, recording changes over time in the services of a particular catchment area. *Fourth*, delineating and comparing between catchment areas the structure and range of services. *Fifth*, measuring and comparing between catchment areas the levels of provision of the major types of mental health service. After an initial section which deals with overall area characteristics, this instrument allows the completion of a service mapping tree, and then a service counting tree. Although still at the pilot stage, and still to be fully standardised, it offers considerable promise for mental health service description in the future.

In comparing these three systems of classification, it is important to note that the WHO and the ESMS may be complementary in that they record different aspects of the service system, but both are relatively complex, with the most recent versions not yet fully tested in practice. We therefore consider that the 'Spectrum of Care' classification is best for those who seek a clear and simple structure for clinical and planning purposes. But for international purposes the Spectrum of Care system does not take account

Table 10.2. *Main categories of mental health service likely to be required (Spectrum of Care, Department of Health, 1996)*

	Acute / Emergency	Long-term / Continuing Care
Home-based services	Crisis intervention for assessment & treatment Intensive home support	Case management Domiciliary support services
Day care & out-patient (ambulatory) services	Acute day hospitals Hospital casualty departments Consultation / liaison services Acute / unplanned out-patient consultations	Planned out-patient consultations Drop-in centres Support groups Employment / rehabilitation workshops Day centres
Residential services **(a) hospital**	Acute in-patient units	Long-term hospital wards Medium secure units High security hospitals
(b) non-hospital	Crisis accommodation	Ordinary housing Unstaffed group homes Adult placement schemes Residential care schemes 24-hour nursed homes

Table 10.3. *The basic service profile*

Basic component	Variations

1 Out-patient and community services
  (a) home visits
  (b) out-patient services
  (c) consultation in general hospitals
	Mobile services for crisis assessment and treatment (including evening and weekend services)
	Out-patient services for specific disorders or for specialised treatments

2 Day services (including occupational / vocational rehabilitation)	Sheltered workshops Supervised work placements Co-operative work schemes Self-help and user groups Advocacy services Training courses Club houses / transitional employment programmes

Table 10.3. *(cont.)*

Basic component	Variations
3 Acute in-patient services	Specialised units for specific disorders (e.g. intensive care and forensic) Acute day hospitals Crisis houses
4 Longer-term residential services	Unsupervised housing with administrative protection Supervised housing (boarding out schemes) Unstaffed group homes Group homes with some residential or visiting staff Hostels with day staff Hostels with day and night staff Hostels and homes with 24 hour nursing staff
5 Interfaces with other services (e.g. health, social and non-governmental agencies)	*Health Services* Forensic services Old age services Learning disability/ mental handicap services/ mental retardation Specialised psychotherapies General physical and dental health Consultation to primary care / GPs *Social Services / Welfare Benefits* Income support Domiciliary care (e.g. cleaning) Holiday / respite care *Housing Agencies* Unsupervised housing / apartments *Other Government Agencies* Police Prison Probation *Non-Governmental Agencies* Religious organisation Voluntary groups For-profit private organisations

of the variety of resources in different areas, or differentiate between core 'essential' components and variations. Secondly, it does not sufficiently reflect our view that health services can only operate effectively as a part of a much wider network of care, with multiple interfaces between all the key agencies. We therefore summarise in Table 10.3 our proposed scheme for a *Basic Services Profile* (BSP), which shows the basic services we consider to be the essential elements in any system of care, along with examples of the variations which may supplement or substitute for each basic component, according to the available local assessments of need, resources, and preferred service configurations. The BSP is intended to be usable in a wide range of service patterns at different stages of development.

10.2.3 The capacities of service components

There is considerable debate about the numbers of psychiatric treatment and care places that are necessary (Wing, 1971, 1989; Thornicroft & Strathdee, 1994). The 1975 British White Paper suggests targets of 50 District General Hospital beds per 100 000 of the population, together with 35 for the elderly severely mentally infirm and 17 for the 'new' long-stay patients. More recently, the House of Commons Social Services Committee report on Community Care (1985) noted that 'a smaller number of in-patients beds is now thought necessary for general psychiatric services', and a Royal College of Psychiatrists working party has specified this as 44 acute beds for a population of 100 000 (Hirsch, 1988).

Strathdee & Thornicroft (1992) have set out targets for service provision based on likely prevalences of mental illness nationally. These targets assume that services should as far as possible be community-based rather than hospital-based, with community residential places and day care taking the place of institutional care. Wing (1992) provides some figures for targets for day provision by mental health services, which again take account of the prevalence of severe mental illness in the community. The capacities given in Table 10.4, for example, are intended to apply to a whole service where each of the other service components are present in the required capacities. The table also shows the results of a revised version of these service capacity estimates (Ramsay, 1997), which has been used in London as a basis for comparison with the actual provision of services to allow estimates of over and under provision.

Recent experience suggests that figures of this sort may be of only limited use. They can be used for local comparisons between similar areas, but they become progressively less useful at the higher geographical levels of the matrix model. They are also open to misunderstanding or to misuse.

Table 10.4. *Estimated need and actual provision of general adult mental health services (aged 15–64 only), in-patient and residential care, places per 250 000 population, estimated for England in 1992–1996*

Category of service	Range			Actual level of provision per 250 000		
	Wing 1992[a]	Strathdee & Thornicroft 1992	PRiSM 1996[b]	Outer London (overall)	Inner London (overall)	Range in London
1. Medium secure unit	1–10	1–10	5–30	8	27	0–58
2 Intensive care unit / local secure unit	5–15	5–10	5–20	8	16	0–41
3 Acute ward	50–150	50–150	50–175	73	110	48–165
4. 24 h nurse staffed units/ hostel wards/ staff awake at night	25–75	40–150 for categories 4 & 5 together	12–50	55	35	0–164
5. 24 hour non-nurse staffed hostels/ night staff sleep-in	40–110		50–300	99	162	28–330
6. Day staffed hostels	25–75	30–120	15–60	17	43	14–292 for categories 6 & 7 together
7. Lower support accommodation	n/a	48–100	30–120	55	95	

Notes:

[a] Wing (1992) estimates include old age assessment places, and the Strathdee & Thornicroft figures apply only to general adult services for those aged 16–65.

[b] PRiSM 1996 estimated need levels based upon: London actual values, and an expected 4 fold variation of need from least to most deprived parts of England, for most categories of service, with a far greater variation in medium secure beds, and NHS Executive (1996) guidance for an average of 25 places in 24-hour nurse staffed accommodation per 250 000.

[c] All estimates given assume that each category of service exists in the given appropriate range of volume.

[d] Includes respite beds and supported self-contained flats. As not all agencies gave information on these categories, these estimates should be regarded as conservative.

Source: Ramsay *et al.* (1997).

If this approach is misapplied, for example by being used to calculate in-patient bed numbers alone in the absence of other related categories, then it will produce misleading results. The reader will by now understand that our own approach is more to consider the resources of the service as a whole, than to focus on counts of service capacities of each service segment.

10.3 **Actual service utilisation data as information for planning**

Data on local service use may refer either to clinical events or to individuals. Such data can be described under four categories:

(i) *event-based information for a given service component* (e.g. annual number, or rate, of admissions)

(ii) *individual-based information for a given service component* (e.g. annual number, or rate, of separate individual patients who receive out-patient services)

(iii) *individual-based information on episodes of illness,* from onset to recovery (e.g. annual number, or rate, of episodes of depression treated by a given service)

(iv) *individual-based information on episodes of care* (e.g. annual number, or rate, of episodes of treatment for anorexia). Tansella *et al.* (1995), on the basis of data collected with the South Verona Psychiatric Case Register, suggested that a period of three months without care is a fair indicator of the end of an individual episode.

Data on individual patient contacts may be aggregated in several ways. Potentially useful methods of aggregation include: visits or admissions per year, by source or setting of service, e.g. visits to a community mental health centre, or out-patients department, by type of care provided (e.g. visits made by psychiatrists), or by episodes. It is useful to distinguish an *illness episode* (number of events in the time between the onset or recurrence of the mental health problem, and its resolution or remission), for example, contacts with psychiatric facilities during an acute episode of depression, and an *episode of care* (number of events in a specified period of time, usually one year), for example, contacts made with a series of services involved in the diagnosis and treatment of a mental heath problem (George, 1989). This distinction between an illness episode and an episode of care is important because an illness episode is based on the mental health status of the individual, whereas an episode of care is based on patterns of service use (Kessler *et al.*, 1980).

While data types (i), (ii), and (iii), as described above, can be collected in many routine information systems, data type (iv) requires a more sophisticated data management system, such as a case register. Case registers can be defined as health information systems of a geographically delimited area that record the contacts with designated medical and social services of patients or clients from the area, including in-patients, out-patients and community contacts (Wing, 1989). A WHO Working Group held in Mannheim provided an agreed definition of a Psychiatric Case Register (PCR) which resulted in the following: 'a Psychiatric Case Register is a patient-centred longitudinal record of contacts with a defined set of psychiatric services, originating from a defined population' (WHO, 1983).

Case registers represent the evolution of older systems for recording data of clinical relevance, such as *disease registers* to which hospitals and physicians used to report all cases of a certain diagnosis and *hospital-based registers*, which in general are based on aggregate data concerning patients who received care by a particular hospital or clinic (Haefner & an der Heiden, 1986).

Compared with institutionally based data collection, case registers have the advantages of avoiding selection biases and duplicated counts, and of being cumulative over time. Moreover, being patient-based (rather than contact-or episode-based) they can be used to describe the pathways to care through contacts with many agencies and they allow the calculation of number of contacts as well as rates (Wing, 1972).

Gibbons *et al.* (1984) showed that for eight British psychiatric case registers between 1.5% and 1.8% of the population were known to psychiatric services, and the rates were remarkably stable between 1976 and 1981. However by 1989, the treated prevalence rate for Salford had increased to 2.35%, due to an increase in the provision of psycho-geriatric services and the activities of mental health professionals in primary care clinics. By comparison, five case register areas in Italy showed a mean treated annual prevalence rate in 1987–1990 for all psychiatric disorders of 0.97%, probably due to the lesser availability of all services than in Britain.

If they are well designed and accurately maintained, case registers can provide a sharp photograph of their specific local areas. Case register data, however, should not be directly used to extrapolate service use over time, and they may also be poorly exportable to other areas which have considerably different populations and services (ten Horn *et al.*, 1986). Other limitations of using case registers are: geographical mobility among the population of interest and the number of mentally ill individuals who are unknown to services, and those with less severely disabling conditions may not require specialist, or indeed any, treatment. For example, the case register in South Verona was used for monitoring service utilisation over nearly 20 years to compare patterns of care in different sub-catchment areas, to study factors associated with these patterns, and to study service costs (Ammadeo *et al.*, 1997).

10.4 **The relationships between service provision and use**

It has long been recognised that there is a relationship between service provision (including the whole range of service inputs as described in Chapter 7), and service use which is similar to the economic relation between supply and demand. It appears, *first*, that where psychiatric beds are available then they are filled, whatever the quantity of provision (Hansson, 1989). *Second*, the categories of service used are usually entirely governed by the types of service available locally. If, for example, home treatment services are not provided in a given area, then the options available to staff when assessing a patient in crisis are normally restricted to in-patient or day-hospital admission. In this way supply in turn also shapes demand in that the family of a patient in crisis may demand an admission, since in their experience this is the only option which can help. *Third*, the use of the services provided depends to a large extent upon the system turnover, or, in the case of beds for example, the average length of stay. In other words, both structural and dynamic aspects need to be considered simultaneously, and we say more about this in Chapter 13.

11

The ethical base for mental health services: 'the three ACEs'

11.1 Guiding principles at the international level

We argue in this book that the twin foundations for planning community mental health services are the evidence base and the ethical base. In Chapter 10 we discussed one side of the coin, the evidence base for such planning. The aim of this chapter is to discuss the main *principles* which should form the *ethical base* of mental health services. Principles are important because they necessarily guide and shape both aspects of the general organisation and specific daily service activities. Even if these ethical issues are not made explicit in planning and service delivery, they will exert a profound influence on clinical practice. We believe that good clinical practice will be the manifestation of a sound ethical base. Indeed it is good practice to make this ethical framework explicit early in a planning cycle, so that the infrastructure of values that underpins any project can be debated by the relevant constituent interest groups at an early stage. It is our experience that if this is not done, then value conflicts will occur later, and may slow, limit or even undermine the viability of the work.

In relation to the matrix model, we shall suggest in this chapter, that each service should produce a written statement of the principles which are meant to guide the clinical activities of all staff. This process will often mean the adaptation and reconfirmation of previously produced declarations at the national or international levels for local use. This may be useful *first* because it can re-activate at local level work undertaken at higher levels. *Second*, such a statement will call the attention of staff to these values, and stimulate staff to make a commitment to act in accordance with them. *Third*, the system of values also creates a framework for the boundaries of

Table 11.1. *Summary of the declaration of Madrid*

1 Psychiatry is concerned with the provision of the best treatment for mental disorders, with rehabilitation and the promotion of mental health.
2 It is the duty of psychiatrists to keep abreast of scientific developments of the speciality.
3 The patient should be accepted as a partner by right in the therapeutic process.
4 When the patient is incapacitated and unable to exercise proper judgement because of a mental disorder, the psychiatrist should consult with the family, and, if appropriate, seek legal counsel to safeguard human dignity and the legal rights of the patient. Treatment must always be in the best interest of the patient
5 When psychiatrists are requested to assess a person, it is their duty to inform the person being assessed about the purpose of the intervention, about the use of the findings, and about the possible repercussions of the assessment.
6 Information obtained in the therapeutic relationship should be kept in confidence and used only for the purpose for improving the mental health of the patient.
7 Research which is not conducted with the canons of science is unethical. Only individuals properly trained in research should undertake or direct it. Because psychiatric patients are particularly vulnerable research subjects, extra caution should be taken to safeguard their autonomy as well as their mental and physical integrity.

Source: World Psychiatric Association (Revised at the General Assembly of Madrid in 1996).

acceptable behaviour of staff. Service users and their carers, who should be included in the initial formulation of the agreed guiding principles, may therefore later challenge unacceptable staff behaviour in relation to the agreed principles. *Fourth*, the statement of values should be seen as a dynamic rather than as a static document, and periodic revisions will be necessary to maintain a balance between ambitious aspirations and achievable goals.

Principles also contribute to building up a tradition in the style of working for a particular service. We consider that what is important in community services is not only the number and characteristics of the constituent services, but also the ways in which they are arranged as well as the style of working of the staff. This style will include the ways in which patients and their carers are included in discussions about their treatment and care, and will reflect a number of the values that we discuss in more detail in this chapter. These values will include an emphasis upon the accessibility of the services to patients when in need, and the ways in which the services attempt to co-ordinate their contributions, so as to enhance the continuity of treatment of care where this is necessary.

Table 11.2. *WHO Mental health care law: ten basic principles*

Geographical Level	WHO basic principle
Country /Regional	Promotion of mental health and prevention of mental disorders Respect for the rule of law
Local	Access to basic mental health care Availability of review procedures Automatic periodical review mechanism Qualified decision maker
Patient	Mental health assessment in accordance with internationally accepted principles Provision of least restrictive alternative Self-determination Right to be assisted in exercise of self-determination

One example of a statement of principles produced at the international level is the 'Declaration of Madrid' of 1996. In 1978 the General Assembly of the World Psychiatric Association met in Hawaii and agreed the ten ethical guidelines contained in a declaration for psychiatrists all over the world (WPA, 1978). These guidelines were intended to be minimal requirements for ethical standards of the psychiatric profession, and they were revised by the WPA General Assembly at Vienna in 1983 to increase their applicability to the wide variety of cultural, legal, social and economic conditions which exist throughout the world (referred to as the 'Declaration of Hawaii II', WPA, 1983). These principles were further revised in 1996 and the Madrid revision is summarised in Table 11.1.

Another example of an international initiative is the statement officially approved by the General Assembly of the United Nations in 1991 which deals with the protection of people suffering from mental illnesses. These 25 principles cover, for example, procedures for assessment and treatment, confidentiality, and informed consent (United Nations, 1992).

A third example of an international contribution is the document recently produced by the Division of Mental Health and Prevention of Substance Abuse (WHO, 1996a) which contains ten basic principles with annotations suggesting selected actions to promote their implementation. These principles are reported in Table 11.2.

A further WHO contribution is a document called 'Public Mental Health: Guidelines for the Elaboration and Management of National Mental Health Programmes', which is a written practical tool for decision-makers, which identifies eight main elements of mental health policy at the national level including decentralisation, inter-sectoral action, comprehensiveness, equity, continuity, community participation, mechanisms for policy formulation and implementation and selection of priorities (WHO, 1996b)

11.2 Guiding principles at the local level

The principles described above which are formulated at the international level, while useful, tend toward the abstract as they need to apply to a very wide range of circumstances. In this section we shall elaborate upon these principles in more detail in relation to the local level of the matrix model. We can draw a parallel between the statement of principles as a *compass* on the one hand. On the other hand, we see the detailed information which is available about the local area and about the local services as a *map*. The application of principles to the development or the reform of local services is an act of navigation, in which both the compass and the map are essential.

One approach to the issues at the local level is that of the British user advocacy group the National Association for Mental Health (MIND), who have set out ten principles to inform the development of community mental health services, shown in Table 11.3 (MIND, 1983)

There are also other similar lists of principles which have been proposed, and to avoid repetition we have selected the nine which we consider the most important and produced a simple scheme as the 'three ACEs'! As Table 11.4 shows, these principles are most relevant at different levels of the matrix model. While the first ACE (Autonomy Continuity and Effectiveness) applies to the patient levels, by comparison, the second and third ACEs apply only at higher levels.

We shall now define and discuss each of these principles in turn, stressing for each the advantages and disadvantages of its application. In mental health care, as in a cocktail, the final result will depend as much upon the blend as upon the ingredients. Indeed we shall argue that some of the principles should not be taken in too high a 'dose', because of adverse side-effects and interactions!

11.2.1 Autonomy

The *Shorter Oxford Dictionary* defines autonomy as 'personal freedom', 'independent', or the 'doctrine of the self-determination of the will'. This is therefore not a characteristic of the service, but rather of what the service does. It refers to the capability of the service to preserve and promote independence by positive experiences, and to reinforce the strengths or healthy

Table 11.3. *Principles to inform the development of community mental health services (MIND, 1983)*

1. **Services should be local and accessible** and to the greatest extent possible delivered in the individual's usual environment.

2. **Services should be comprehensive** and address the diversity of needs of the individual.

3. **Services should be flexible** by being available whenever and for whatever duration. There should be a range of complementary models which provide individuals with choice.

4. **Services should be consumer-orientated** that is based on the needs of the user rather than those of providers.

5. **Services should empower clients** by using and adapting treatment techniques which enable clients to enhance their self-help skills and retain the fullest possible control over their own lives.

6. **Services should be racially and culturally appropriate** and include use of culturally appropriate needs assessment tools, representation on planning groups, cross-cultural training for staff, use of indigenous workers and bilingual staff, identification and provision of alternative basic facilities.

7. **Services should focus on strengths,** and should be built on the skills and strengths of clients and help them maintain a sense of identity, dignity and self-esteem. Patients should be discouraged from adopting the sick-role and the service from developing an environment organised around permanent illness with lowered expectations.

8. **Services should be normalised and incorporate natural supports** by being in the least restrictive, most natural setting possible. The usual work, education, leisure and support facilities in the community should be used in preference to specialised developments.

9. **Services should meet special needs** with particular attention being paid to those with physical disabilities, mental retardation, the homeless or imprisoned.

10. **Services should be accountable** to the consumers and carers and evaluated to ensure their continuing appropriateness, acceptability and effectiveness on agreed parameters.

aspects of each patient, especially the most severely disabled, while controlling symptoms. There is a balance between this principle and continuity of care, such that over-intrusive or over-frequent follow-up can effectively interrupt the processes of recovery and rehabilitation. In each clinical case this balance will be a critical issue, and one that will vary over time – what is important is that a service is flexible enough to decide action (or lack of action), and does not adopt a fixed view of how and when to offer clinical contacts.

Table 11.4. *Principles for community mental health services: 'The 3 Aces' in relation to the three geographical levels of the matrix model*

	Principle	Geog. level of the matrix model		
		Patient	Local	Country
1st ACE	1 Autonomy	√		
	2 Continuity	√	√	
	3 Effectiveness	√	√	
2nd ACE	4 Accessibility		√	
	5 Comprehensiveness		√	
	6 Equity		√	√
3rd ACE	7 Accountability		√	√
	8 Co-ordination		√	√
	9 Efficiency		√	√

Autonomy is closely associated with another of our key principles: accessibility. The ability to choose is relatively unimportant unless a real choice is possible between actual alternatives that are both available and seen to be relevant by patients.

Autonomy can be defined as 'a patient characteristic consisting of the ability to make independent decisions and choices, despite the presence of symptoms or disabilities. Autonomy should be promoted by effective treatment and care'.

11.2.2 Continuity

The *Shorter Oxford Dictionary* defines continue as 'to cause to last or endure' 'to prolong, to persevere, to keep on, retain', and it defines continuity as 'a continuous or connected whole', 'an uninterrupted connection or succession', 'coherence' or 'unbrokenness'. These definitions are pertinent to our purpose here in that they stress the ongoing need by many patients for reliable sources of treatment and social support. To the extent that this can be achieved also reflects in part the degree of co-ordination between services and the extent to which the various services in any local area together act in concert.

This principle is over-used, both because it has powerful face validity and has immediate appeal, and because it has been poorly defined, often overlapping with other principles, which are shown in Table 11.4. Johnson *et al.* (1997) distinguished between longitudinal and cross-sectional dimensions of continuity of care. *Longitudinal continuity* refers to the ability of services to offer an uninterrupted series of contacts over a period of time. This implies either continuity of the same staff group, even if the individual staff members change, or to provide a line of continuity across episodes of care, for example between in-patient and community treatment. An important second meaning of longitudinal continuity is to ensure a planned transfer of care between services when the patient moves home.

Cross-sectional continuity includes continuity between different service providers, which in practice means between different mental health teams or programmes. This refers especially to fragmented types of service, since the system types usually specifically highlight this form of continuity. The second type of cross-sectional continuity applies within teams. This refers to how far team members communicate with each other about their direct clinical work, and about their strategic therapeutic goals.

The advantages of placing an emphasis on continuity are that it is easier to give consistent treatment and care, and to avoid contradictory interventions which the patients' behaviour may provoke through the splitting of staff. It may also be easier to predict relapses and remissions, to intervene early, and so to effect secondary prevention. Further, an emphasis on continuity can develop a stronger trusting relationship between staff and patients, which is both desirable in itself and can be especially invaluable in crises. The implementation of this principle may also be a way of increasing efficiency, for example the avoidance of multiple or overlapping interventions can reduce both costs and any adverse effects.

It may also increase effectiveness, not just efficiency, since it reduces risk of 'falling through the cracks' between services, which is particularly hazardous for severely mentally ill individuals, who may be poor advocates for their own interests. Continuity can improve staff morale by keeping contact with the same group of patients over a long enough time period to see improvement. It also provides a continuing service while individual members of staff are away on leave. Continuity of communication within the team also improves communication between the team and those outside, including the patient's family, who will receive a more consistent message. This principle will also lead to a more unitary way of dealing with problems, including physical problems, and so encourages access to other specialists. Finally, continuity can also increase the possibility of helping patients to solve practical problems, e.g. application for welfare benefits.

At the same time there are disadvantages from too compulsive a stress upon continuity. It can provide too rigid a framework, leaving the patient feeling trapped and making the situation unbalanced, and not retain the correct professional/emotional distance. A patient can develop an unhealthy degree of dependency on a particular clinician. It may reduce choice for patients, therapists and referrers. Continuity can also mean a slow rate of turnover of cases and this contains the possibility of producing staff disillusionment with longer-term patients who deteriorate or who do not improve, and with those who are extremely demanding in the long term.

From the patient's perspective, services organised to maximise continuity may limit access to a particular treatment if the patient has a case manager not trained in the intervention. The greatest risk, however, is that a dependence on the service will be fostered, which encourages a chronically sick role. For example, a high degree of continuity was offered in traditional mental hospitals, alongside a high degree of dependence. For these reasons we consider that a proper balance is needed so provide *variable continuity*. We would draw a parallel here with the use of medication. In the same way that we would sometimes encourage patients to use intermittent medication, or to vary the dose within an agreed range, so we would suggest that the intensity with which continuity of care is provided should be varied so as to maintain and extend autonomy for each patient.

We define *continuity* as the ability of the relevant services to offer interventions, at the patient or at the local level, (i) which refers to the coherence of interventions over a shorter time period, both within and between teams (*cross-sectional continuity*) or (ii) which are an uninterrupted series of contacts over a longer time period (*longitudinal continuity*).

11.2.3 Effectiveness

The *Shorter Oxford Dictionary* defines effectiveness as 'that which has an effect', or 'fit for work or service'. More recently the Cochrane database defines effectiveness at 'The extent to which a specific intervention, when used under ordinary clinical circumstances, does what it is intended to do'. In this sense effectiveness applies to routine clinical settings, as compared with 'efficacy'. which means how far a specific intervention achieves its intentions under ideal, experimental conditions such as those which are required for randomised controlled trials. In terms of the matrix model, effectiveness is an outcome category which is usually applied at the patient level. At this level, increasing numbers of systematic reviews are becoming available (Adams *et al.*, 1996).

As one moves from the patient to higher levels in the matrix model, so the amount of evidence from controlled studies decreases rapidly, as does its quality, and the primary issue becomes one of effectiveness rather than efficacy. To make research useful in practice we need to move from efficacy to effectiveness, that is to extend the research from selected patient groups to more representative patient samples taken from ordinary clinical settings.

Table 11.5. *Cochrane's Test (Light, 1991)*

1 Consider anything that works
2 Make effective treatments available to all
3 Minimise ill-timed interventions
4 Treat patients in the most effective place
5 Prevent only what is preventable
6 Diagnose only if treatable

At the local and country /regional levels the chance for an efficacious treatment to be proven as effectiveness depends upon the choice of patients, the skill of the therapist, patients' compliance with treatment and other factors.

At the patient level we define *effectiveness* **as 'the proven, intended benefits of treatments provided in real life situations'.**

At the local level we define *effectiveness* **as 'the proven, intended benefits of services provided in real life situations'.**

Although for the sake of clarity we discuss in this chapter each key principle separately, in fact they are intimately interlinked and they have a variable geometry in different clinical situations. Effectiveness, for example, is often related to efficiency, and Cochrane (1971) stressed the primacy of effectiveness for attaining efficiency. As Light (1991) has put it, 'can one increase efficiency through competitive contracts if the contractors do not know what is effective?' Indeed, Light has re-interpreted Cochrane's classic work to produce what he calls the 'Cochrane test' (Table 11.5). How many mental health services can pass these six central effectiveness questions?

11.2.4 Accessibility

Accessibility is defined in the *Shorter Oxford Dictionary* as 'capable of being entered or reached' or 'get-at-able'. This relates directly to the central point, which is that patients should be able to reach and 'get at' services where and when they are needed. The *Concise Oxford Dictionary* adds a further important meaning, namely '(in a form) easy to understand', which usefully refers to the need for services to make comprehensible to their users what they offer.

Accessibility remains a complex concept. It is used in relation *to geographical distance* or to *travel times* from patients' homes to mental health services sites, to *delays* in how long it takes for patients to be assessed or treated, and to *selective barriers* or filters which reduce the uptake of services by all patients (such as stigma), or for some sub-groups of the population (such as ethnic minorities). In addition accessibility can refer to the openness of the service to patients outside office hours, at night and at weekends, or to the public visibility of the service, as opposed to the remote institutions which were 'out-of-sight' and associated with shame.

There may be disadvantages associated with too much accessibility. *First*, if services are too available, then patients may have a low threshold to consult when in difficulty, may bypass primary care services where these exist, and may expect specialist attention when suffering from relatively minor, brief, and self-remitting conditions. Such contacts may divert time and resources away from more severely disabled patients, and access may be delivered at the expense of equity. *Second*, a highly accessible service may conform to Jarvis's Law, who wrote in 1850 a paper on 'The influence of distance from and proximity to an insane hospital on its use by any people'. By this he meant that the amount of use made of an unrestricted service by patients is inversely proportional to the distance that they live from that service. *Third*, if accessibility is too high, then efficiency may reduce as minor disorders are seen in the more expensive specialist services. Accessibility therefore cannot be unlimited, and in part services may need to encourage self-limited use by patients, for example, in relation to night-time emergency services.

We define *accessibility* as 'a service characteristic, experienced by users and their carers, which enables them to receive care where and when it is needed'.

11.2.5 Comprehensiveness

The *Shorter Oxford Dictionary* defines comprehensive as 'comprising much', or 'of large content or scope'. The *Concise Oxford Dictionary* adds an intriguing qualifier, 'complete; including all or nearly all elements', and so suggests that a comprehensive service may offer an almost full range of components. This addresses the central dilemma of the balance between offering all the care to all those suffering from mental disorders, and being selective according to the available budget, both in terms of the sub-groups of patients to be prioritised, and the types and duration of treatment and care which can be afforded. In our view a comprehensive service is one that has all the basic components, which were detailed in Chapter 10, with some degree of variation.

The degree of comprehensiveness of a service raises the key question: comprehensive for whom? Since mental health problems will affect about a third of the general adult population in any year, and since the capacity of the mental health services, even in the most economically developed countries, means that they can provide a service usually to about 2% or 3% of the adult population, these services will *necessarily* be limited to only a minority of those suffering from mental illnesses. The question then becomes one of quality *or* quantity. Services which selectively treat first the more severely mentally ill, such as in Britain, will provide a relatively poor service for the majority of patients who have neurotic illnesses. Many of these cases remain untreated if they are not recognised by primary care staff. This lack of treatment in turn may increase the risk of chronicity and the risk of developing subsequent disabilities and handicaps. In some countries, such as Italy, it is not mandatory for referrals to specialist care to come from primary health care staff. More open access is therefore offered, for example by self-referral, in the name of a comprehensive service. The advantages of this system are that it may avoid delays and it may decrease the stigma associated with mental health service use, by making the service routinely available. The disadvantages of this arrangement are that since comprehensiveness is limited by the capacity of the service, it may develop in the 'wrong' direction. By this we mean that services given to people with lesser degrees of disability may replace those given with more severe forms of mental illness.

This 'offset' means, in broad terms, that people with neurotic disorders are treated at the expense of those with psychotic disorders. This produces four problems. *First*, patients with these more severe disorders tend to present themselves to services less often and, in our view, require a pattern of services which can include substantial contact at home. *Second*, those with psychotic disorders, who accumulate in the lowest social class group, tend to have fewer choices than other patients, they are often ineffective advocates for their own interests and needs, and they exercise relatively little political and financial market power. *Third*, over-provision of services can produce an 'induction effect' whereby patients become used to receiving multiple types of service where only one specific type of treatment is justified on grounds of evidence. *Fourth*, setting comprehensiveness as a service goal, in an undefined way, can produce a gap for staff between expectations and clinical reality which become a potent source of stress and burnout.

In our view it is important to distinguish horizontal from vertical comprehensiveness, as described in the definition box below.

We define *comprehensiveness* as 'a service characteristic with two dimensions'.

By *horizontal comprehensiveness* we mean how far a service extends across the whole range of severity of mental illnesses, and across a wide range of patient characteristics (gender, age, ethnic group, diagnosis).

By *vertical comprehensiveness* we mean the availability of the basic components of care (out-patient and community care; day care; acute in-patient and longer-term residential care; interfaces with other services), and their use by prioritised groups of patients'.

11.2.6 Equity

The *Concise Oxford Dictionary* defines equity as 'fairness', while the *Shorter Oxford Dictionary* expands upon this by saying 'that which is fair and right', or the 'recourse to general principles of justice'. At the country/regional level, the application of this principle implies that the distribution of money should be made according to criteria which are specified, transparent, and which have widespread acceptance as being fair. We describe in detail in Chapter 10 some of the methods, such as the Mental Illness Needs Index (MINI), which have been used so far in Britain for allocating resources for mental health care to the local level. There is a clear need to adapt and apply such rational and explicit approaches to equitable resource allocation in other settings where historical patterns may predominate.

At the local level, there are two kinds of distribution of resources which should be made according to the principle of equity: firstly between health and social services, and secondly between different programmes or facilities within each mental health agency.

Finally, at the patient level the degree of discretion for funding decisions are even greater since no agreed standardised criteria exist to guide these decisions. Indeed resources are usually distributed in relation to widely differing priorities, each of which may claim to be most equitable. For example, funding distributions based upon health-gain values may lead most resources to be spent on treatment for depressed patients (usually in primary care), while those based upon the prioritisation of the most disabled, may lead to most investment in specialist services for people with severe mental illness, many of whom have limited personal resources. These two approaches would produce quite different patterns of expenditure: the former leads to relatively inexpensive treatment being given to larger numbers of patients (such as good prognosis cases of depression), and the latter to the opposite. This dilemma is universal since we know of no sites which can adequately provide services for the whole range of mental disorders. It is therefore precisely at this point that value judgements must be brought to bear, so that mental health services are based both on an evidence base and on an ethical base.

In our view there is a useful distinction between explicit and implicit equity in allocating resources to mental health services. *Implicit methods* are often based on decisions taken by restricted groups of people which are not transparent since the criteria used are not put into the public domain. These decisions may be defined as equitable by using post hoc independent procedures. Whatever the criteria used to put equity into practice, the advantage of the *explicit method* is that it can be critically tested and challenged. In the context of the public health approach which we discussed in Chapter 2, we believe that the basis upon which resources are allocated should be made explicit and should be based upon a process of needs assessment.

We define *equity* as 'the fair distribution of resources. The rationale used to prioritise between competing needs, and the methods used to calculate the allocation of resources, should be made explicit'.

11.2.7 Accountability

The *Concise Oxford Dictionary* defines accountability as 'required to account for one's conduct (accountable for one's actions)' or 'responsible'. This directs us to the central issue, namely that one of the distinct features of a community-based service, as opposed to the traditional mental hospital, is to act with a wider sense of responsibility than the purely custodial. This responsibility should apply, in our view, to a whole catchment area population. This wider boundary of responsibility includes those who may require treatment but who are not contained within the physical walls of the hospital, and this more inclusive view is, in our experience, a more optimistic perspective in that it sees patients in terms of their abilities to recover or to cope with the demands of life in spite of their symptoms.

In terms of the matrix model, at the patient level the principle of accountability refers to the relationship between staff and individual services users, a relationship that needs to be based upon confidence and trust. At this level, each patient has a legitimate expectation that the clinician will offer treatment based upon a 'duty of care', and will do this in accordance with accepted standards of professional practice. For example, one aspect of direct accountability to the patient is that clinical information remains confidential. This type of direct patient accountability may be challenged by requests from family members (or others), who express the need for services also to be accountable to them. In clinical practice these issues are common and often absorb our time and attention, as ethical dilemmas are balanced with individual circumstances.

At the local level, a wider set of considerations apply. Mental health services, to a far greater extent than other types of clinical practice, operate in a way which offers *dual accountability*: both to the patient and to the wider society. We have already discussed individual outcomes in Chapter 9. At the same time, in practice, mental health services are held accountable by the public to act in a way that maintains public confidence in their viability. In this larger sense of public accountability, mental health services are legitimated by the degree of confidence given to them by the public.

In reality the issue is even more complex in that lines of accountability operate simultaneously at all three geographical levels of the matrix model. At the country/regional level, for example, whether or not mental health services are directly provided by state agencies, in our view there remains with the state a 'duty of care' to arrange inspectorate or accreditation bodies, for example comparing services to nationally agreed minimum standards, through which services can be held to account. This is therefore a sensitive issue, and it is no coincidence that psychiatrists have been closely implicated in totalitarian regimes at times when accountability at the national level was held to be superordinate over the patient and local levels.

We define *accountability* as 'a function which consists of complex, dynamic relationships between mental health services and patients, their families and the wider public, who all have legitimate expectations of how the service should act responsibly'.

11.2.8 Co-ordination

'All unhappiness depends upon some kind of disintegration or lack of integration: there is disintegration within the self through lack of co-ordination between the conscious and unconscious mind; there is lack of integration between the self and society, where the two are not knit together by the force of objective interests and affections.'
BERTRAND RUSSELL

The *Shorter Oxford Dictionary* defines co-ordination as the 'harmonious combinations of agents of functions towards the production of a result', or 'to place things in proper position relatively to each other and to the system of which they form parts'. Again, this principle is linked with others in the three ACEs, in particular with continuity and with effectiveness. As we indicate in the definition box, we can distinguish between cross-sectional and longitudinal co-ordination. The first refers to the co-ordination of information and services within an episode of care (both within and between services). The latter refers to the interlinkages between staff and between agencies over a longer period of treatment, often spanning several episodes.

The communication necessary to ensure proper co-ordination can be informal or formal. In decentralised service systems, such as community mental health teams, more careful attention may need to be paid to lines of communications since staff will less often see each other on a day-to-day basis than in a traditional hospital, and this may mean that more formal systems of communications are needed, for example, daily morning hand-over meetings to inform all staff of clinical developments. The key role of the case manager is to provide co-ordination, both cross-sectional and lon-gitudinal, indeed in Italian local Departments of Mental Health the role is referred to as 'coordinatore'.

We define *co-ordination* as 'a service characteristic which is manifested by coherent treatment plans for individual patients. Each plan should have clear goals and should include interventions which are needed and effective: no more and no less'.

By *cross-sectional co-ordination* we mean the co-ordination of informa-tion and services within an episode of care (both within and between services). By *longitudinal co-ordination* we mean the interlinkages between staff and between agencies over a longer period of treat-ment, often spanning several episodes'.

11.2.9 Efficiency

The *Shorter Oxford Dictionary* defines efficiency as 'productive of effects' or 'operative'. While this rightly refers to the effects of clinical prac-tice (outcomes in the matrix model), it does not also consider the inputs needed to produce these effects. There will never be 'enough' resources allo-cated for health services in the eyes of staff or patients. If we accept scarcity as the basic condition, our starting point is therefore the narrower question of allocation. The pursuit of efficiency can mean, therefore, reducing the costs for a given level of effectiveness (outcome), or improving the level of effectiveness or the volume and quality of outcomes achieved from fixed budgets. Efficiency does not have to mean cut-backs, and a more efficient solution may cost more (Knapp, 1995).

Three types of economic efficiency have been defined by Davies & Drummond (1994). *Technical efficiency* is 'achieving maximum physical output from resource use' (without considering the costs implications). *Productive efficiency* means 'achieving maximisation of output for a given cost'. *Allocative efficiency* is defined as 'achieving maximisation of the value attached to the output for a given cost'.

In terms of the patient level, Cochrane (1971) identified two aspects of

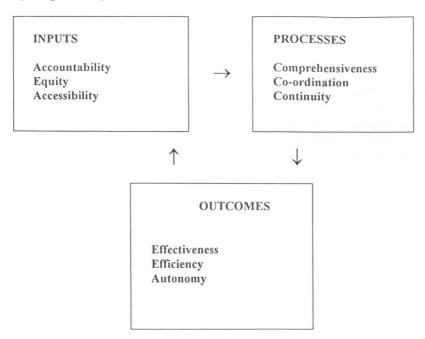

Figure 11.1 Principles for mental health services in relation to the three temporal phases of the matrix model.

inefficiency: the use of ineffective therapies and the use of effective therapies at the wrong time. Our own definition of efficiency, shown in the box below, is designed to assist the production in future of operationalised measures of this principle which can be incorporated into mental health service evaluation.

We define *efficiency* as 'a service characteristic, which minimises the inputs needed to achieve a given level of outcomes, or which maximises the outcomes for a given level of inputs'.

11.3 Clinical values as complementary to cost-effectiveness

In this chapter we have enumerated nine principles, and we have described them in relation to the patient, local and country/regional geographical levels of the matrix model. Another way to consider these principles is in terms of the other dimension of the matrix model, that is in relation to their temporal sequence after entry into the service, according to the input, process and outcome phases of the matrix model, as shown in Figure 11.1. This scheme is intended to improve clarity by emphasising the principles which apply most actively, but not exclusively, to each of the three phases. It is not necessary to consider this scheme as starting only at the input phase, since on coming into a new post, it is common that a senior member of staff will not be in a position to initiate a new cycle of planning at the input phase, and may need to begin the analysis at the process or output phases. The order in which the principles are considered and put into action is therefore often as much a tactical as a strategic question, depending upon local circumstances. Whatever the order, we believe that the use of clinical values for re-forming mental health services can be regarded as an iterative process.

Our main point in this chapter is that whatever the strength of the evidence on cost-effectiveness (which may be misused for cost-saving reasons), the technical solutions of evidence-based medicine should not be used alone to respond adequately to complex planning choices. Rather, the evidence base should be counter-balanced by a principled ethical base, and in our view the primary responsibility for introducing clinical values to these decisions lies with clinicians.

Key resources: training and morale of staff

12.1 **The central role of human resources**

This book is written for the range of people who are interested in improving mental health services, and this particular chapter will probably be of more interest to clinicians than to administrators and planners. Having already discussed in the last two chapters how to establish the overall needs for information and services, our aim here is to suggest how the staff who constitute the service can be directly involved in formulating plans and putting them into practice. Our main guiding theme is the question: how can the human resources in any existing mental health service best be deployed for the benefit of patients? We take again as our frame of reference the public health approach, which we have outlined in somewhat idealised terms in Chapter 10. In this chapter we shall concentrate upon more pragmatic and day-to-day issues, and in effect we shall base our comments upon the evidence of our experience, rather than the evidence of research. This is simply because there is a striking poverty of relevant research.

To a much greater extent than most other areas of medicine and health sciences, mental health services rely almost entirely upon human technology rather than upon instrumental technology, both for diagnosis and for therapy. For example, the best way to validate a questionnaire as a screening instrument is still by comparison with a clinical interview. In spite of the progress made recently in biological markers, none are yet available as clinical tests for the diagnosis of mental disorders. In terms of treatment, it is clear that the human factor is also central to how far, for example, patients comply with prescribed medication. Indeed it is within mental health services that the importance of the relationship between clinician and patient, which is a basic issue in all medical settings, is most accentuated.

There are important implications for this central role of the human factor. *First*, apart from capital (buildings) costs, recurrent expenditure in mental health services is almost entirely needed for the development and maintenance of human resources. *Second*, the nature of clinical contact with psychiatric patients puts demands upon staff that draw upon all their reserves, and which render staff at risk of a depletion of motivation and compassion, the so-called 'burnout syndrome'. These human resources are therefore not fixed resources, but are continually subject to deterioration or degradation unless restored and upgraded.

At the outset we want to make the distinction between *primary* and *secondary service goals*. By primary goals we refer to interventions intended to give treatment, care and assistance to patients. In our view this is the central purpose of the service and should always remain centre stage. By secondary goals we mean measures which are addressed to the needs of staff. Although in this chapter we shall argue that unless these necessary and legitimate staff needs are properly addressed, then the quality of service to patients will suffer, nevertheless our remarks are within a wider context that continues to give primacy to patients needs over those of staff. Indeed when clinical teams can select only desirable patients (and exclude patients who are less rewarding or attractive), then patients' needs may become subsidiary to those of staff. This risk is greater in more highly segmental services (see Chapter 10), which are made up of specialist treatment components. The public health approach, which we favour, counteracts these tendencies by discouraging patient selection, it tends to prevent exclusion, and emphasises the rights of all those who suffer from mental illness to treatment and care.

In this chapter we shall discuss issues in relation to two of the levels of the matrix model: the individual staff member level (corresponding to the patient level), and the clinical team (equivalent to the local level). We shall focus upon *individual members of staff* for two reasons: first, this is the basic component of the clinical team and, second, because one-to-one contact between staff and patient is the primary vehicle for the direct delivery of services. We shall then consider those issues which concern the *clinical team*, which we consider as the crux of mental health service delivery. Our reasons for this are: (i) the team allows a more complete assessment of the needs of each patient and consequently a fuller range of multi-disciplinary interventions than an individual practitioner can achieve alone, (ii) the team provides a greater degree of continuity of care, in that team members can substitute for each other during periods of planned and unplanned leave, and the use of staff rotas outside office hours can give an extended range of care, (iii) the team may offer a more sustainable model of service because staff members can exchange roles within a team, may work full time or part time depending upon their other commitments, can take periods of further training or career development breaks, and also because the key role of case manager can be rotated between staff members for the most difficult cases, or shared between more than one clinician at a time, and (iv) the team can extend to patients a greater choice between clinicians, while remaining within the service as a whole.

12.2 The renewable resources of individual staff

While there are many books on the training of the various members of the mental health team, especially in relation to specific techniques for assessment and treatment, the question of how staff can be managed in the wider perspective of a community-orientated service has received remarkably little attention. There is a need to consider *personality and attitudinal factors*, which are most important at the selection stage, followed by both the content and the form of the training. The next stage is to acquire *clinical expertise*, which has to be differentiated from *clinical experience*. Experience is simply directly proportional to the period of time spent on a particular task, without reference to quality, and derives from *experientia,* meaning to try, without necessarily succeeding. Expertise, on the other hand, is the acquisition of knowledge and skill or judgement for a given purpose. While a certain degree of experience is necessary to establish expertise, it does not necessarily follow that experience *per se* leads to expertise. Indeed some long-term staff may have accumulated many years of adverse or irrelevant experience, such as the custodial practices of some clinical staff in poor quality institutions. In other words, it is expertise rather than experience that counts.

We consider first *personality characteristics and attitudes* and we agree with the qualities which Mosher & Burti (1989) have described as desirable and undesirable for community mental health staff, and which are summarised in Table 12.1. While these characteristics sketch a desirable profile for mental health practitioners, quite often one finds staff who are unsuited to clinical work, but who nevertheless have direct care responsibilities. Although it may not be possible to reallocate these staff to non-clinical roles, it is usually feasible to find a new post in which they undertake subsidiary activities and can contribute to the service with fewer opportunities to have face-to-face contact with patients. The opposite can also occur when individuals have particular rare therapeutic skills, and so can be valued members of the team, despite demonstrating other characteristics which run counter to the

Table 12.1. *Desirable and undesirable personality characteristics for community mental health staff (after Mosher & Burti, 1994)*

Desirable characteristics
1 Strong sense of self: comfort with uncertainty
2 Open minded: accepting and non-judgmental
3 Patient and non-intrusive
4 Practical, problem-solving orientation
5 Flexible
6 Empathic
7 Optimistic and supportive
8 Gentle firmness
9 Humorous
10 Humble
11 Thinks contextually

Undesirable characteristics
1 The rescue fantasy
2 Consistent distortion of information
3 Pessimistic outlook
4 Exploit clients for own needs
5 Over controlling and needing to do for others
6 Suspicious and blaming others

service model used by the other staff. Such compromises are the stuff of everyday clinical work. These factors are best identified at the interview or selection stage because, although not entirely unmodifiable, our experience is that it is usually better not to appoint an unsuitable candidate if the local administrative arrangements allow a second recruitment process.

We shall move now to *clinical training*, and we refer here not to the content of training courses, but rather to their structure, in terms of the place of training, the types of trainer, and their quality and scope. *First*, such training is usually more effective *in situ*, namely in the whole range of community-based settings rather than in hospital, both for initial vocational courses and for continuing professional development. *Second*, it is often beneficial for students of all specialities to undergo some cross-disciplinary training by having teachers from other disciplines or teaching sessions with students of other professions. An important part of the training process is to have time to reflect upon individual cases in detail with clinical teachers. *Third*, work in community settings better allows a longitudinal rather than a cross-sectional perspective. This perspective has the important consequence that assessment, except in crises, can take place over a period of time and involve a wider set of relevant information, including family members, other key informants, and the sometimes invaluable detail available from home assessment.

Treatment, similarly, should take account of information from a wider social context, for example, the degree of sedation or other adverse effects that a patient can tolerate are related to the usual activities and preferences of that particular individual. For assessing outcome, a longitudinal perspective allows us to consider patterns of recovery or relapse over months and years, and to identify risk factors and protective factors specific to each patient. Part of the clinical training, therefore, should be dedicated to teaching the limitations and biases of clinical experience, as well as research evidence, in predicting outcome. Finally, we consider that an essential part of good clinical training is instruction on clear entries in clinical case records. This is important because clinical assessments and care plans accumulate over time to form a potentially invaluable information resource for all staff.

There is now a considerable amount of research on the relationships between clinical training, experience, techniques and outcomes, especially in relation to psychotherapy, which has been subjected to a recent thorough overview (Roth & Fonagy, 1996). First, this research has confirmed that there are wide variations in outcome, even for relatively homogeneous treatments, and these are variations which cannot be accounted for by client factors or by the type of treatment techniques, but which are associated with the individual therapist. Surprisingly, there are only modest direct associations between training and outcome, and between experience and outcome, where these may have a specific importance in preventing early attrition and in retaining more difficult patients in clinical contact.

This body of research has also convincingly shown that the capacity to develop a productive treatment alliance is the single best predictor of outcome, and accounts for 26% of the difference in rates of therapist success. This alliance, in turn, is best predicted by therapeutic expertise (rather than by clinical experience), and by the presence of clinical supervision.

The essence of such *therapeutic expertise* consists of skills and personal qualities of the therapist, and the ability to use technical skills flexibly. There may be some additional benefit if the therapist has received in-depth training in multiple treatment modalities. In terms of the factors which are associated with the success of therapeutic interventions for patients, in 1961 Jerome Frank (see Frank *et al.*, 1993) described four key predictors of improved outcome, shown in Table 12.2.

Table 12.2. *Common features and key influences of effective psychotherapy (Frank, 1993)*

Common features of the intervention
1 The patient has confidence in the therapist's competence and desire to be of help
2 The locale of psychotherapy is designated by society as a place of healing
3 The treatment is based on a rationale which includes an explanation of illness and health, and which implies an optimistic philosophy of human nature
4 The therapeutic procedure requires some effort or sacrifice by the patient

Key influences of the intervention
1 Provides new opportunities for learning
2 Enhances patient's hope of relief
3 Provision of success experiences
4 Helps patient to overcome the demoralising sense of alienation from others
5 The treatment produces emotional arousal in the patient.

12.3 **The clinical team as a therapeutic agent**

Even if the individual staff member level is of central importance in providing good quality direct treatment to patients, it is the quality of the team which makes the difference between good and bad quality mental health services. We see the staff team both as made up of individual clinicians, and as an important entity in its own right. The characteristics of a team as a whole are not simply the sum of the parts, but includes the clinical setting, the style of leadership, and the degree of co-ordination with other staff. It is therefore necessary to consider the clinical team as an agent or as a vehicle of service provision separately from the contribution of individual clinicians.

A simple and useful scheme is to think of the clinical team in four stages: new team building, major reconstruction, maintenance and minor reconstruction. In most cases, what happens is that a new team leader inherits a current staff group, so the primary questions are how far and how fast to change. Figure 12.1 shows the cyclical relationship between the phases of team maintenance and initial construction or subsequent reconstruction.

Although Stage A (*new team building*) is relatively uncommon, it occurs more often when the service is experimental, in other words when it is supported by research funds from the outset, and so has clear goals to be achieved within a limited period of time, which is defined by the research purpose, with the clinical work being purely instrumental to this aim. All biases which are known to influence the process and improve the outcome

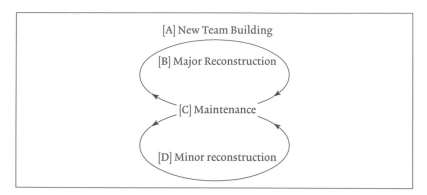

Figure 12.1 Cycles of clinical team building, maintenance and reconstruction.

of the service are in action, i.e. motivation of staff, major attention to patient conditions, introduction of new assessments of clinical status and positive expectations. Since these biases cannot be eliminated, in the research setting they can be controlled for, usually through random allocation. We therefore compare the standard treatment with the treatment and care provided in an experimental service which is set up. In routine settings, by comparison, there may be limited opportunities to establish new services, mainly for clinical purposes, but the pressures from evidence-based medicine almost always imposes a research agenda on to the clinical initiative.

Briefly, at the start of a *new clinical team*, there is the opportunity for the team leader(s) to influence powerfully the shape and style of the nascent service. Many of the routines and traditions which quickly become institutionalised within work groups are initially absent and can effectively be invented. The allocation of room space, for example, can alter patterns of behaviour in the working of the team, and also set the tone for a more or less hierarchical social relationships between team members. The name of the team can exert a strong influence upon how it is perceived by its own staff and by external agencies. The extent to which the goals of the team are jointly developed and explicitly stated may directly impinge upon the team's effectiveness. In short, the construction of new team provides an opportunity to set up a coherent pattern of service components, since there are no pre-existing barriers, but it is in itself neither necessary nor sufficient to achieve such coherence.

Stage B is that of *major team reconstruction*, which in many ways is parallel to that of establishing a new team. Major reconstruction can occur proactively or reactively. The first case, *proactive major reconstruction*, is usually associated with the arrival of a new team leader, and this may occur at the service as well as at the regional/country level, especially following the election of a new local or national government. The second case, *reactive major construction*, is most often found after and in consequence of a perceived system failure. The Italian reforms of 1978, for example, typify such reaction in that they were formulated against a background of widespread dissatisfaction with the traditional asylums. The Swedish mental health reforms of 1995, in which clinical and financial responsibility for long-term patients no longer needing acute treatment was transferred from medical to social services, is a more recent example of a major reconstruction at the country level. In both cases such reconstruction is associated with positive expectations to exceed the quality or quantity of service being provided before changes.

At the local level, substantial alterations to mental health teams can occur in response to changes in clinical leadership, changes in the local political complexion, from reactions to scandals, or from substantial staff vacancies. This stage differs from the establishment of a new team. Existing staff need to be accommodated within the new structure; current service patterns, traditions and customs may prove resistant to alteration, and there will be an already established set of expectations by patients and outside agencies of what service has been offered in the past and what should be provided in future.

Phase C, *maintenance*, is the most common and probably the most important of the four phases, as it occupies by far the longest time periods in the life of a team. It is the most difficult phase as it is routine but should not be repetitive, and because when these maintenance functions are well performed, they are almost invisible. This is exactly the paradox, since there is an absence of positive feedback about good team management, while negative feedback is instantaneous!

The first logical step in the maintenance phase, although not usually the first step in practice, is the *definition of the goals* or the *purposes of the team*. These should be based upon a consideration of the guiding principle, as we discussed in Chapter 11, and may be placed in the context of writing a team strategy as we shall go on to describe in Chapter 13.

The second key element in the maintenance phase is setting the *boundary conditions*. Setting the boundaries of the team work consists in identifying: (i) the specific goals and aims of the service in relation to the aims of other local services and agencies, (ii) the particular patient group or groups to be served, for example on the basis of diagnosis or disability, (iii) the intended duration of clinical contact, or episodes of care, which are indicated by clinical considerations and financial constraints, (iv) the limits of staff tolerance and duty, and (v) the degree to which each particular service acts as a substitute for other service components or social support networks, which may be limited, dysfunctional or wholly absent.

Such boundaries are entirely necessary for the integrity and sustainability of the work of the clinical team. They may be implicit or explicit, and this is immaterial as long as the team functions effectively. When, however, the team enters a period of relatively poor functioning, then the absence of explicit and written boundaries becomes crucial, as the boundary conditions are not immediately available for review. Without such clear and agreed boundaries, the roles expected of such teams can vary rapidly, and can cause staff anxiety, which in itself encourages destabilisation and stress. This is especially the case for teams providing general mental health services for adults, as other specialist or sub-specialist teams can, through effective boundary setting, retreat from whole categories of patients, and the 'general adult' teams are left to act as the default, to treat all those not receiving services from other teams.

A *systemic* community mental health team differs from a *fragmented* service in that the former will usually have less rigid (and robust) explicit boundary conditions. Equally, most community mental health teams have far less clear-cut boundaries than do in-patient institutional services, where the physical domain of the ward to a large extent automatically defines the proper territory for clinical duties. This is most accentuated in community mental health teams, which set a high priority upon 'comprehensiveness' and 'accessibility' (discussed in Chapter 11), and which therefore have an ideological aversion to excluding any patients. As we shall argue in Chapter 13, there is an strong case for mental health services to define their proper remit in terms of clinical case load. In many economically developed countries the capacity of the mental health services is to treat 2%–3% of the general population each year, while ten times as many people will suffer annually from some mental health problem.

If the specialist service does not target its resources it will (i) be overwhelmed by clinical cases, and (ii) fail to deliver an adequate service to people most disabled by mental illness. If such boundaries are not set proactively at the outset by the CMHT, therefore, clinical pressures are likely to be such that they will need to be asserted reactively at a later stage. This most usually follows a period in which staff feel they are working under unsustainable stress, with too great a gap between the aspirations of the service and what they can actually deliver. The advantage of having clear and realistic boundaries, stating both what the service is and is not able to provide and which are widely known from the outset, is that it helps to limit inappropriate demand, and it avoids the additional stress on staff of having to narrow the role of the team at a later stage, with the consequent disappointment of staff and of outside referral agencies.

Phase D refers to *minor reconstruction*, the episodes during which less vital 'running repairs' are conducted to improve a team's effectiveness. This phase is necessary at regular intervals in each service, to monitor the team's performance in relation to changing conditions and because a moderate degree of change is important for staff morale. This phase depends upon the ability of the team to diagnose dysfunction in their own work at an early stage, before the point at which major reconstruction becomes necessary. Common occasions for minor reconstruction are times of limited staff turnover. Such changes can also occur in reaction to the injection of ideas from visitors to the team, from visits of staff to teams elsewhere, from an appreciation of the research literature, from relatively minor budgetary changes, or from external 'diagnosticians', such as group facilitators, who are brought in temporarily to suggest minor improvements. Whatever the source of the ideas, the phase of minor reconstruction is important to fix problems early, and as an antidote to the routinisation of everyday work.

12.4 **Staff morale and burnout**

One of the characteristics of staff working in mental health services is that they frequently feel high levels of stress for several reasons. Their work sets unusual demands: they will have to deal with patients whose behaviour may be odd or bizarre, and occasionally may be disturbed, or disturbing; rarely patients are verbally or physically aggressive or threaten suicide, and because of this staff need to be continually prepared for such attacks upon their physical integrity; and indeed some patients have a powerful tendency to blame those offering help for their difficulties.

There is also a common wider tendency for the representatives of social opinion also to blame staff for the symptoms and behaviours indicative of mental illness; and patients with more severe disorders may improve to only a limited extent, depriving staff of the reward to seeing rapid clinical improvement. In addition, communication difficulties between staff are common, and are often experienced as more stressful than the clinical problems that arise in dealing with patients! One particular example, as Mosher & Burti (1989) have pointed out, is that which concerns those who are low in the organisational hierarchy. These staff have the most direct contact with patients, and they have the least power in terms of clinical and managerial decisions.

Table 12.3. *Characteristics of staff burnout (Mosher & Burti, 1989)*

Description
1 No energy
2 No interest in clients
3 Clients frustrating, hopeless, or untreatable
4 Higher absenteeism
5 High staff turnover
6 Demoralisation

Causes
1 Setting too hierarchical: staff not empowered
2 Too many externally introduced rules, no local authority and responsibility
3 Work group too large or non-cohesive
4 Too many clients, feels overwhelmed
5 Too little stimulation, routinisation

' **Stress can be good, stress can be bad.**'
CHARLES HANDY, 1976.

At the same time a limited amount of stress is necessary to increase work performance. Handy (1976) has distinguished the beneficial role of stress *(role pressure)* from the harmful role of stress *(role strain),* and pointed out that one of the major tasks of management in organisations is to control the level of stress. He described the symptoms of role strain as tension (often expressed as irritability and excessive preoccupation with trivia, great attention to precision or periods of sickness), low morale (low confidence in the organisation, expressions of dissatisfaction with the job or sense or futility), and communication difficulties (absenteeism is an extreme form of this symptom).

Burnout is a term which has come to be widely used and recognised as the consequence of prolonged and severe role strain. It has been defined by Maslach & Jackson (1979) as a dysfunctional psychological state that seems to be most common among persons working in job settings characterised by a great deal of personal interaction, under conditions of chronic stress and tension. These conditions are frequently found in community mental health teams, which we consider to be continually at risk of fostering staff burnout, and a recent study in South London has shown higher burnout levels among community than among hospital staff (Prosser *et al.*, 1996). The characteristics and causes of burnout have been summarised by Mosher & Burti (1994), and are shown in Table 12.3.

A number of strategies have been proposed for dealing with role strain

Table 12.4. *Features affecting the experience of work (Warr, 1987)*

1 Opportunities for control
2 Opportunities for skill use
3 Externally generated goals
4 Variety
5 Environmental clarity
6 Availability of money
7 Physical security
8 Opportunity for inter-personal contact
9 Valued social position

(Watts & Bennett, 1983). In relation to the matrix model, at the individual (patient) level, Handy (1976) has suggested the following strategies: repression, withdrawal and rationalisation. In *repression* the individual refuses to admit that there is any problem, in *withdrawal* the individual retreats behind a psychological barrier or leaves the organisation, and in *rationalisation* the individual decides that the conflict is inevitable and must be lived with.

The features of work within community mental health teams which are conducive to positive experiences are, we believe, the same as in other work settings. Warr (1987) has summarised these factors, which are listed in Table 12.4, and we shall highlight those which are most important to our discussion. In terms of *opportunities for control*, which have two components: the opportunity to decide and act, and to predict the consequences of one's actions. Staff need to be allowed considerable discretion in their treatment plan for patients, within a context of supervision and professional support. Such control can also be exercised through meaningful involvement of all staff in the formulation and execution of team operational policies. *Opportunities for skill use* is important for mental health teams in relation to how far members of different disciplines exercise skills specific to that discipline, or undertake generic tasks that could be carried out by staff with other types of professional training.

Variety is important to avoid repetitive or invariant actions, for example, by dealing too frequently with the same types of clinical problems. In many clinical teams there may be a positive aspect of increased variety in community services which include visits to patient's homes, counter-acted by a tendency in teams targeted to patients with more severe disabilities to narrow the spectrum of diagnoses seen to little more than those with psychotic disorders. Environmental clarity is the degree to which the work setting is clear or opaque in three senses: the availability of feedback on the consequences of one's actions, the degree to which the actions of other people are predictable, and the clarity of role expectations.

At the team level, there are a number of techniques to prevent and reverse burnout, including: didactic training exercises, regular staff-meetings for inter-personal problem resolution, routine case conferences to discuss difficult cases, and regular supervision (Mosher & Burti, 1989). In addition there are a number of features of community mental health teams which encourage functional rather than dysfunctional performance: small team size (usually 6–12), more open patterns of decision making, mutual support, and consultation between staff members.

There are also possible sources of increased staff satisfaction in adopting a community-based mental health care model. *First*, the move away from traditional roles and leadership structures may give staff from disciplines such as nursing considerably greater autonomy and responsibility, which may increase their job satisfaction and sense of mastery. *Second*, patients and relatives appear often to prefer community-based care to hospital care, and staff may feel happier about their work when the recipients are more satisfied. *Third*, staff may feel that their work is more effective when they move into the community. *Fourth*, the traditional psychiatric hospital may be experienced by staff as well as patients as a depressing and institutionalising environment, and community mental health centres, primary care health centres and patients' homes may in general be more pleasant and stimulating work settings (Prosser *et al.*, 1996).

12.5 **The clinical team as a lens**

We outlined at the beginning of this chapter why staff are important. In terms of the matrix model, staff, who are the main resource of mental health services, can act as a vehicle to deliver interventions to patients which are both evidence-based and ethically-based. Figure 12.2 gives graphical representation to our view that the clinical team should act as a lens which focuses these two types of input in the process of providing care to individual patients, so optimising their clinical and social outcomes. These outcomes for patients therefore depend both upon the extent to which staff put into practice the values which are accepted in each local area, and how far actual practice reflects the best evidence from research on clinical effectiveness. Both of these are dynamic rather than static characteristics, and they change at different rates. The guiding principles may remain

Geographical
Dimension

Temporal Dimension

	(A) Input Phase	(B) Process Phase	(C) Outcome Phase
(1) Country/Regional Level	1A PRINCIPLES (ETHICAL-BASE) ←→ RESEARCH FINDINGS (EVIDENCE-BASE)	1B	1C
(2) Local Level (catchment area)	2A	2B CLINICAL TEAM INTERVENTIONS	2C
(3) Patient Level	3A	3B	3C INDIVIDUAL PATIENT OUTCOMES

Figure 12.2   The focus of clinical team interventions on individual patient outcomes taking into account principles and evidence within the matrix model.

invisible for years, for example, and then relatively suddenly become more libertarian or custodial, depending upon the balance of forces in the wider public debate over the proper role of mental health services for the patients, directly and indirectly for the wider society.

By contrast, while researchers seek a treatment breakthrough, more often there is a slow and more prosaic accumulation of evidence of which treatments are effective. The skills required of any clinical treatment teams will therefore necessarily need to be updated on an ongoing basis, and this will apply differentially to members of different specialities according to professional developments in each field. Further, the type of evidence produced by research is also in part a product of the social and political climate of the time.

What we propose is a long-term perspective to invest in the key assets of a mental health service – the staff. This is because there will often be a considerable delay between the initial investment in staff training and the eventual improvement in patient outcomes, and also there is often a long delay between the lack of training and other investment in staff consequent upon poor clinical standards. Indeed it is common when budgets are reduced to cut the training budget first. An equivalent could be stopping all routine maintenance on a passenger aircraft: it will fly on for some time, but the need for consequent major repair, if not the risk of serious adverse outcome, increases with time. In other words, if the mental health team is seen as an asset, then investment in frequent and planned minor maintenance is likely to be cost-effective in the long term, since it keeps clinical standards high and reduces the need for unplanned and reactive major reconstructions, which are often more expensive in the long term.

If staff investment is recognised as indispensable, then it requires a reasonable budgetary allowance that is not vulnerable to short-term budgetary pressures. Staff investment goes beyond training and in this respect public services have much to learn from private enterprises who routinely invest in a wide range of non-financial staff benefits as incentives. These will include child-care services for staff, flexible working hours, high-quality supervision and career guidance, and sporting and leisure facilities.

In practice, different blends of principles and evidence will be used at the country/regional levels, and by clinical teams at the local level. The Italian reform of 1978, for example, was almost entirely based upon principles, and anything beyond face evidence for changing the backward in the institutions was considered unnecessary. The scientific foundations of psychiatric practice are only about 25 years old, and before about 1970 relevant research information was almost entirely absent. As discussed in

Table 12.5. *Traditional hospital and community-based staff orientations*

	Traditional hospital	Community-based
Staff attitudes	Short-term view	Longer-term view
	Focus on control and structure	Unplanned responses
	Routine contacts with patients	Family focus
	Use of policies and procedures	Emphasis on social disability
	Hierarchical decision making	Negotiation mode
Staff training	Biological orientation	Eclectic orientation
	Training rotates between specialist units for diagnostic groups	Community training often absent
		Problem solving approach
		Training rotates between specialist & general units
Therapeutic orientation	Emphasis on symptoms relief	Greater staff independence
	Improved facilities and expertise for physical assessment, investigation, procedures and treatment	Longer term assessment process
		More individual treatment
		May neglect physical diagnosis and treatment
	Brief assessment package	Integrated therapeutic and social interventions
	Seek decision from above in the hierarchy	
	Better control for suicidal / violent patients	
	Block treatment of patient groups	
	Regulated timetable	
	Separated short-term treatment and rehabilitation	

Chapter 11, this view, taken naively, raises the contrary risk, namely that research results alone will guide policy and clinical decisions.

In this chapter we have argued that the central resource of a mental health service is the staff who treat patients, and that this resource needs ongoing investment. If we look back at the last 25 years we can seen clear signs of a trend in staff attitudes. Table 12.5 compares some of the characteristics of what we call the 'traditional hospital' view with the 'community-based' perspective, and, for the reasons we have advanced in the two preceding chapters, we believe that investment in staff should be made to accelerate the movement from the hospital to the community perspective.

13
Planning based on evidence and on ethical principles

13.1 **Defining the planning process**

In Chapter 10 we outlined two ways of describing mental health services which are located in a particular area: the *segmental approach* (which considers separately each service component, treatment facility or programme) and the *system approach* which underlines the contribution that each programme gives to the wider system of care at the local level, and which explicitly considers the inter-relationships between the different services. We have also stressed the point that the selection of one of these two approaches for describing services is closely related to the actual organisation of services in each particular site being described.

In this chapter we shall deal with the planning of mental health services, defined in Table 13.1, using both the evidence and the ethical bases which have been discussed in the previous two chapters. It is often difficult to know whether values or evidence should be given first consideration. Here we propose to reverse the usual order (which is first evidence and later, maybe, ethics!), for the simple reason that even the choice of which evidence is to be collected and used is influenced by value judgements. We address planning for general adult services at the local level, and for simplicity we refer mainly to planning which is limited by a fixed resource input, and the task then becomes one of considering alternative ways in which to shape services for the best outcomes. We recognise that resource inputs may also vary, both to increase or decrease the total resources available.

Our discussion of the planning process will begin with a more detailed consideration of the differences between the ethical based and evidence-based approaches, and we shall then move on to offer a model of the whole mental health service system in terms of a 'hydraulic' scheme, in which we suggest that the 'pressure of morbidity' is transferred between the components of the system as a whole, and so activity within one component will have consequent reactions within other component parts of the system. We

Table 13.1. *Definition of mental health service planning*

We *define planning* as 'a linked series of actions designed to achieve a particular goal, and which requires the completion of increasingly specific tasks within a given timescale'.

In relation to the matrix model, 'planning is the process which intends to transform given inputs into optimum outputs. At the local level we distinguish mental health *service component planning* from mental health *system planning*'.

---

go on to describe the importance of clarifying the boundaries between these components, which act both to contain or to reject categories of work, and as interfaces across which patients and information flow. This leads us to consider how general adult mental heath services can prioritise the many possible demands upon their resources and to decide which groups of patients may be targeted. Finally we shall propose a straightforward method to guide the planning process, which follows seven steps.

13.2 'Service component' or 'system' planning

We can distinguish mental health *service component* planning from mental health *system planning*. The first type of planning is segmental in the sense that it takes the needs of individual institutions or particular types of patients one at a time without putting these needs in a general framework of the other services available in the same area. However, system planning is often population-based and aims to organise for defined populations a system of care which underlines the connections between different components, and even the relationships with other health as well as social and private services in the same area. In other words, the system approach to planning is the practical consequence of taking a public health approach to assessing the mental health needs of a population.

There are also other differential characteristics of the two models of service planning and delivery, which are summarised in Table 13.2 in relation to how far they reflect the nine guiding principles we introduced in Chapter 11. Autonomy and effectiveness are not differentially affected by the two approaches.

The segmental approach relies far more heavily than the system approach upon a strongly motivated patient clientele, and is far less suited to conditions in which the co-operation of patients may be, at best, equivocal, and this can adversely affect the *continuity* of treatment they receive.

Individual facilities planned using the segmental approach will often

Table 13.2. *Principles for community mental health services in relation to the strengths of segmental and system approaches to planning*

Principle	Strengths of different planning approaches at the local level	
	Segmental (service component)	System
1 Autonomy	√	√
2 Continuity		√
3 Effectiveness	√	√
4 Accessibility		√
5 Comprehensiveness		√
6 Equity		√
7 Accountability		√
8 Co-ordination		√
9 Efficiency		√

attract patients from a wider geographical reference population, and therefore will reduce the ability of the service to offer a locally *accessible* provision to people not able to travel, or not able for other reasons to gain entry to remote resources.

Comprehensiveness we defined in Chapter 11 in two ways. By *horizontal comprehensiveness* we mean how far a service extends across the whole range of severity of mental illnesses and patient personal characteristics. Similarly, we have defined *vertical comprehensiveness* to mean the availability of the basic components of care (out-patient and community care; day care; acute in-patient and longer-term residential care; interfaces with other services), and their use by prioritised groups of patients. The 'service component' approach in planning tries to limit both aspects of horizontal comprehensiveness to different degrees in different sites. The guidelines for these limitations are not always very clear-cut and they may change over time according to variations in the goals of the service. For instance, if the service is privately operated, as is often the case in segmentally organised services, this goal can be influenced by cost issues. On the contrary, the 'system approach' has a wider degree of horizontal comprehensiveness, which is mainly regulated by two boundaries, the geographical catchment area definition, and the priority treatment groups defined by policy or by practice. As far as vertical comprehensiveness is concerned, the difference between the two approaches to service planning is even more pronounced. The service component approach tends to provide one type of care only, while the system approach explicitly seeks to inter-link the different multiple types of care which are delivered at any one time.

If *equity* is defined as the fair distribution of resources, then we consider that the service component approach is a much more limited frame of reference in that it leads to staff time and expertise being distributed only between patients in contact with that particular service. The system approach, by comparison, takes as the frame of reference the whole morbid population within a given geographical area, and allows explicit consideration of how patients simultaneously use different components as part of a larger package of care. To this extent the system view seeks to be inclusive of the needs of *all* those needing care rather than only those who happen at any time to be in contact with a particular service component.

In our view the system approach also has advantages in terms of *accountability*. As we indicated in Chapter 11, accountability is a function which consists of complex dynamic relationships between mental health services and patients, their families and the wider public, who all have legitimate expectations of how the service should act responsibly. Such accountability can be enhanced in a local service over a period of time, and will be shaped by the information available to patients and their consequent expectations of the service. While both the service component and the system views can allow lines of accountability to individual patients to develop, only the latter also allows the possibility of a wider accountability to be given to a population as a whole. The question of what are legitimate expectations also needs further consideration. While in principle all opinions on how a mental health service should be planned are legitimate, in practice it is usual for a small number of the most active, rather than the most representative, local figures to shape the planning process, and we would propose a pragmatic view which again seeks to include some representation from a wide base of local interests.

Co-ordination is the primary intended advantage of the system over the service component approach. In our view, the degree to which this principle is enacted makes the biggest difference to visions of planning. Planning on the basis of service components alone always runs the risk of fixing one local difficulty at the price of displacing it to another part of the system, for example, the question of where patients with personality disorders are seen.

In parallel, there may be considerable gains for *efficiency* in that a system view can take account of any duplication between services, and so reduce redundancy, and can also seek to ensure that the most efficient service inputs are provided for patients, for example, more appropriate and less expensive supported residential care for disabled and longer-term patients rather than inefficient placements in acute in-patient units. In this case a distinction needs to be recognised between the efficiency of individual service components, for example in terms of fast patient turnover, and efficiency of the system as a whole, which may best be served by longer lengths of stay in some forms of residential care.

There is an increasing attention to the evidence-based approach for all health services. The reasons for this relate to the need to make the best use of available resources, to apply interventions precisely to conditions for which they can lead to positive outcomes, and to identify and stop interventions which are ineffective. The risk for mental health services is that the evidence-based view is taken in isolation and overshadows the ethical contribution. This would be perfectly understandable in economic terms alone, but it is not acceptable in the wider social milieu of the planning process.

A further limitation of the evidence-based approach is that the evidence available so far refers mainly to service components, and tends to be extrapolated incorrectly from one component to another or even from one country or region to another, for example, the widespread reference in European countries to studies using case management in the USA. The reason for this lack of evidence at the system-level is that it is more difficult to collect. We therefore need, first of all, to create an evidence base at the system level, without which we shall be drawn to the ecological fallacy, which is to take data gained from one level and to apply it indiscriminately to another. It may be better to admit having no relevant data for particular planning questions, than to use an inappropriate evidence-based approach.

Table 13.3 summarises the differences between the two main approaches, at the level of the local mental health service, across the three steps for collecting evidence on which to base planning: the collection of data on needs, service provision and service use (see Chapter 10 for further elaboration of these three steps).

For the reasons we have indicated in the previous section, we prefer the system to the service component approach to planning. One useful metaphor to visualise the system approach is to see a mental health service in hydraulic terms. In other words, we can conceive of how mental health services as a whole operate as, in some ways, similar to a closed system containing fluid, such as a central heating system. In these terms we can draw parallels between the fixed 'pressure of morbidity' and the water pressure, between the flows of patients between the different service components

Table 13.3. *Evidence used in planning for community mental health services in relation to the segmental and system approaches*

	Planning approach at the local level	
Evidence	Segmental (service component)	System
1. Needs assessment	For selected patient sub-groups Problem or diagnosis-specific assessments	More comprehensive assessments Population based
2. Service provision	Institution based data Service activity reported separately (e.g. beds from day centre activity)	Population-based data Attempt to consider different clinical activities in an integrated way
3. Service use	Institution-based data Service activity reported separately	Population-based data (e.g. case register data) Consider offset or substitution effects

and the flow of water between the chambers of the fluid system, and the effects in terms of back-pressure of closure or restricting access to any one key compartment.

13.3 Service components in a service system: the hydraulic model

We therefore propose that the totality of mental health service components be considered as a series of inter-related elements, in which the behaviour of each affects (directly or indirectly) all the others. Such a view allows us to speak of the volume and the capacity of components and of the whole system (both for under and over-capacity), to calculate rates of flow between components, to build in control taps and safety valves for periods of expected and unexpected excess pressure, and to make allowance for overflow capacity in times of excess volume, for the 'leakage' of some patients out of the system (when patients may be inappropriately lost to contact with services). Such a metaphor also allows us to consider the need for routine and emergency maintenance to avoid system breakdowns, and to build in sentinel events or alarm systems to warn of incipient system failures. While not wishing to overstretch this parallel, we do find that such a view helps to understand the links between service components.

'How many beds?' or 'How many day places?': these are common questions for those planning mental health services (Wing, 1971; Thornicroft & Strathdee, 1994). The system view can produce a more efficient consideration of such questions which at first sight require a component-level answer. For example, if a particular mental health service usually has all its beds fully occupied and has great difficulty identifying beds for patients needing admission, a response framed in terms of service components alone will simply point to the need for more beds or more efficient use of current beds. A system view, by comparison, would take account of flows of patients into and out of beds, and the thresholds and delays for such transitions, and may point to the need to establish more highly staffed long-term hostels for long-term disabled patients who may be inappropriately placed in acute psychiatric beds.

In situations where community services are provided in addition to more traditional services (both hospital and residential) and where the capacity of these institutions is such that they provide for the majority of people severely disabled by psychotic disorders, then the case-load of the community services will predominantly include less severe forms of mental disorder. This was the case to some extent in the first phase after the introduction of community mental health centres in the United States after 1963. Many severely mentally ill people were discharged from mental hospitals and transferred to variable quality residential institutions (Eisenberg, 1997) while the new mental health services in the community were offering their newly established resources to less severely ill individuals. If under similar circumstances the capacity of the traditional system providing long-term hospital and residential care services was limited, then community services, if operating effectively, will be likely to detect previously untreated or under-treated cases. This may produce a greater demand for in-patient treatment, producing a paradoxical simultaneous increase in expenditure on both community and hospital care (Tyrer *et al.*, 1995).

Although we recognise the existence of interactions in which, for example, the presence of acute day hospital places, substitute for acute in-patient beds, we have little information about the gearing or calibration of these offsetting effects. This is for two reasons: the absence of system-level research which takes accounts of such possible interactions, and the focus of studies which have been completed upon efficacy rather than upon effectiveness, for example, the completion of several experimental assertive outreach services as a substitute for acute beds, but few similar studies in routine clinical settings. Indeed there is a danger that efficiency judgements are made on individual service components based upon evidence of their efficacy rather than of their effectiveness. In our view, the correct sequence is: (i) adopt a system approach, (ii) assess the initial effectiveness of the system, (iii) monitor the ongoing efficiency of the system as a whole.

13.4 **Interfaces between components of the service system**

Once we have clarified that mental health services should be seen as a system, we can use this overall framework to consider three types of *interface*: (i) those *within the mental health service*, between its components, (ii) those *within the health service*, between mental health and other services (both primary and secondary care), and (iii) those *between health and other public services*, including Social Services and the Housing Department. The sheer complexity of the operation of all these simultaneous interfaces is a further basis to reinforce our view that a first requirement, before addressing links with non-mental health services, is to clarify the ways in which the separate mental health service components operate together as a system. Indeed once this is successfully achieved, then the quality of contacts with other services becomes vastly more coherent. Figure 13.1 graphically displays firstly some of the most important linkages between the core general adult mental health service system and eight other key health components, and secondly it shows the four main categories of public service with which health services connect.

The *permeability* of each interface may change over time and may differ for the direction of referral. Each facet between adjacent services can act as a filter in the same sense as that used by Goldberg & Huxley (1980, 1992) in their model of the pathways from the general population to primary and then to specialist psychiatric care. Although in clinical practice the existence of interactions between these services elements is well recognised, for example in terms of the transfer of patients from the criminal justice system to health facilities through prison or court diversion schemes, in theory such linkages are not usually described. Indeed the only interface which has been well characterised is that shown in Table 13.1 between primary care and community mental health services, known as Filter 3 in the Goldberg & Huxley scheme. As a consequence, there is little relevant research which quantifies the extent of patient flows across these interfaces. It does seem clear, however, that the ground rules of engagement for these interfaces vary enormously, even within regions. The criteria for acceptance in old age psychiatric services may be: all patients aged over 65, or those over 70, or those suffering from late onset dementing disorders, or other criteria which may or may not be known to the providers of other local services.

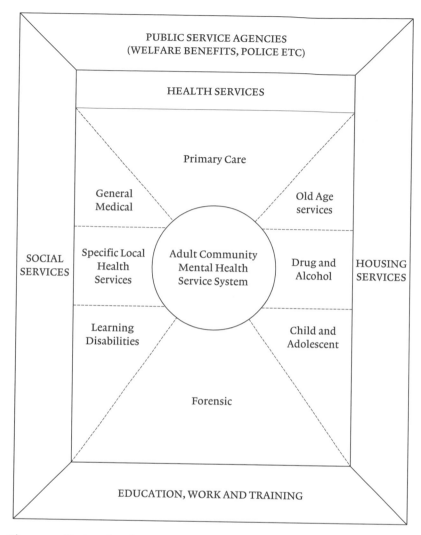

Figure 13.1 Key interfaces between the community mental health service system and (i) other health services and (ii) other public service agencies.

Just as we described the functioning of mental health services in terms of a hydraulic system, so this metaphor can be applied at a large scale to the whole nested series of interactions between the service elements shown in Table 13.1. The ways in which these semi-permeable membranes or filters act will exert a powerful influence on the required capacity of any single element. When the interfaces are seen as filters, then their properties include what types of referrals pass each stage (*selectivity*), and the rate of passage across each interface (*flow rate*).

Planning Approach	Service with a traditional mental hospital	Service without a traditional mental hospital
Segmental approach	[A] Commom starting point for local planning ↓	[C] → ↓
Systemic approach	[B] ↓ →	[D] ↓ Desired planning target

Figure 13.2 Paths from traditional and segmental services to a community-based care system.

13.5 **Planning the transition to a community-based system of care**

Turning now to the application of this conceptual approach to actual planning decisions, we shall use as an illustration the question common in many economically developed countries of how to plan the transition from a pattern of services largely dependent upon a traditional mental hospital to one which encompasses an array of more local provisions, including in-patient beds. The need to plan this transition is usually based on a mixture of political, social and clinical reasons, although the local variations on this theme and the pace of change vary a great deal. In fact, as Figure 13.2 shows, this is usually a two-fold transition: from a service component to a system approach, and from an institutional to a community orientation.

Practically speaking most organisations can manage only one major change at a time, and so a choice arises: should an organisation proceed from (A) to (C) to (D), or from (A) to (B) to (D) in the scheme shown in Figure 13.2? We suggest that the latter is preferable, and we suggest that the organisational reform is undertaken before the institutional reform. Our reasons for this are that the process of reprovision from older asylums is a complex task, and that institutional practices and facilities can more easily be reconstructed within the context of the service component approach. We do not underestimate the difficulty of this task since no country has yet fully successfully completed the transition from dependence upon older asylums.

Second, we consider that the system approach produces a higher likelihood of replacing the protective functions of the asylum by community-based alternatives which are less custodial in orientation, and probably which induce less long-term dependency upon services.

Two recent examples can be given to illustrate transition planning. In Italy the approach chosen in 1978 was 'to close the front door', so that no more patients were admitted to the asylums. The disadvantage of this approach is that it incurs double-running costs for a prolonged period. It is notable that while this decision to stop further admissions was made at the country level in a matter of weeks in 1978, the responsibility for constructing a replacement community system was left to the regional levels without sufficient policy guidance. In essence these changes were based upon a diagnosis of a dysfunctional system, the intervention was aimed only at a single, service component, and no detailed recommendations were made about how to construct an adequate alternative system, and so heterogeneous responses were produced. This process was therefore intended to proceed from (A) to (B) to (D), but has been implemented in a partial and inconsistent way across the different regions of Italy.

By comparison, England offers an example of the (A) to (C) to (D) route, in that asylums have more often completely closed, but again this has been achieved usually within a component rather than a system planning context. Service integration has most often been addressed as a subsequent issue. Two important adverse consequences have accrued from this lack of integrated planning. *First*, the planning of places for long-term patients has only been applied to previously long-term in-patients, and not to the accumulating generations of their successors. *Second*, no allowance was made in the calculations of acute bed requirements for the occasional need for re-admission to hospital of former long-term in-patients discharged to homes and hostels in the community. These two shortcomings have contributed towards the current inappropriate use of about 30% of acute in-patient beds by long-term patients in most parts of England. This is in part a consequence of the compartmentalisation of planning which reprovides for each service component one at a time, and which cannot take into account the dynamic transfer of pressure around the whole service system.

13.6 Seven steps from planning to practice

Following on from the preceding discussion, we now propose a seven-step procedure to lead from planning to practice (Table 13.4). This scheme is intended as a guide or an *aide memoire* about the key stages in the

Table 13.4. *Seven steps to reform community services*

1 Establishing the service principles
2 Setting the boundary conditions
3 Assessing population needs
4 Assessing current provision
5 Formulating a strategic plan for a local system of mental health services
6 Implementing the service components at the local level
7 Monitoring and review cycle

planning process. In real life we expect that it will be rare for these steps to be followed sequentially, and in practice the order of events can change, or several stages can occur simultaneously. Nevertheless, in our view each step is a significant contribution to a thorough planning process, and the entire absence of any step will weaken the relevance or the robustness of the services which are put into practice.

The *first step*, as we described above in Chapter 11, refers to establishing the service principles. Although we place these as the foundation stone for planning, such principles are usually excluded from the whole process. Even when values are considered, most often at an early stage of planning, they remain without consequence for three reasons. First, those involved may assume that their colleagues share common ground and that such agreement goes without saying. Second, they may tacitly acknowledge substantial differences in core values within the planning group, and reckon that better progress will be made by avoiding than by addressing these differences. Third, planners may judge that discussion about underlying values is not sufficiently important to take up scarce planning time. In our opinion all three views, although common, are mistaken and will lead to the re-emergence of disagreements later in the planning process, when value differences become displaced onto operational matters.

The *second step* in planning is to *set the boundary conditions*. This is closely related to the operation of the interfaces we have discussed in Section 13.4. In terms of the general adult service, two types of boundary are of primary concern: the 'geographical' and the 'functional'. The former is the delimitation of the area for which the service has responsibility and is closely linked to the concept of a catchment area (variously called '*district, secteur, territorio* or *bezirk*'). The size of the area is usually very informative in that the smaller the population size, the more likely it is that a single team will have generic responsibility, and by comparison, increasingly specialised services will have greater reference populations. In Victoria, Australia, for example, the

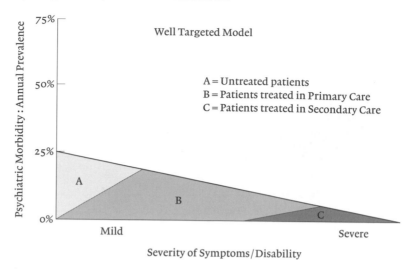

Figure 13.3 Relationship between degree of disability and treatment setting (primary or secondary care) for a well-targeted service.

basic population unit for adult services is a catchment area of about 250 000 for which separate community crisis teams and mobile continuing care teams operate. In England, however, the average sector size is 50 000, and it follows that usually a single generic team will provide all community treatment services for the resident population of a sector.

In terms of the 'functional boundaries', these apply within the adult mental health service, and across the interface with other health and social services, as illustrated in Figure 13.1. One key example of such a boundary is that between primary health services and secondary (or specialist) mental health services. Since up to 25% of all adults suffer from some mental health problem in any year and since the capacity of the specialist mental health services in most economically developed countries is that they can offer contact to 2%–3% of the population in any year, it is clear that only about a tenth of all psychiatric morbidity can receive any clinical contact from specialist services. The central question then becomes: *which* 10%?

The severity of mental health problems is in most areas poorly related to the intensity of care received (Goldberg & Gournay, 1997). As specialist services are scarce and expensive services, we believe that they should target their skilled impact upon those with the most severe symptoms and the greatest degree of disability consequent from mental illness. To achieve this

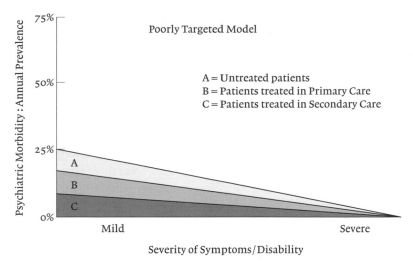

Figure 13.4 Relationship between degree of disability and treatment setting (primary or secondary care) for poorly targeted services.

consistently a service will need to set priorities for the groups of patients who should receive highest priority for contact. Figure 13.3 illustrates what we call a well-targeted service in that the secondary (specialist) services concentrate their efforts entirely upon people with the most severe degrees of symptom/disability (area C). Primary care services then provide for all other patients with lesser severity conditions (area B). Even so there is an oblique interface between C and B since some of the more severe cases will still be treated only by primary care services, towards the right side of the figure. The gradient of this interface will vary in different health systems and, for a 'perfectly' configured primary/secondary care interface, is vertical. Area A represents true cases who are not receiving treatment, that is untreated prevalence. Such cases may not have presented to services, may have presented and not been recognised, or may have been identified and no treatment was given. The extent to which such morbidity, which is usually of relatively minor severity, is treated varies considerably between sites (Robins & Regier, 1991), as does the gradient of the interface between A and B. In poorly targeted services there may be horizontally parallel layers of A, B and C so that some very minor cases are treated by specialist services, and some severe cases go untreated, as shown in extreme form in Figure 13.4.

Targeting is necessary but not sufficient. A second key element is that the capacity of the secondary (specialist) service is large enough to absorb or accommodate all the cases who fulfil the entry criteria for the priority groups of patients (assuming that such entry criteria have been defined in advance). The third central characteristic of well-functioning specialist services is that, once in contact with the target patient group, they deliver cost-effective (efficient) treatments.

The *third step* is to assess population needs. Needs assessment, like so many aspects of life, is more talked about than done. This step is closely related to targeting since the degree of stringency necessary in defining the highest priority group in any service will depend upon three factors: (i) the overall rates of psychiatric morbidity in each local population, (ii) the capacity of each local mental health service in terms of the number of cases which can be treated at any one time, and (iii) the degree to which these services effectively target the severely mentally ill. As we have discussed in Chapter 10, there are a series of methods which allow the measurement or the estimation of true (treated and untreated) prevalence, and the use of treated prevalence rates alone can produce a highly distorted picture of met and unmet need at the population level. At the same time a population-based needs assessment only has value for planning if it is more than an academic exercise, when it is an integral part of a programme of service development and reform.

Step four is the assessment of current service provision. The literature on this topic is vast but difficult to summarise because of the different methods and indices used. Service use information *per se* is of only limited importance, in that it is one type of data on process. It may be valuable to compare sites cross-sectionally which differ on key characteristics which allow us to test hypotheses, or to make comparisons within sites over time about the effect of changes in inputs. But beyond this, service utilisation data are limited to the descriptive unless they are combined with information on needs and outcomes. We argue throughout this book that the main purpose of mental health services is to improve clinical outcomes for individual patients, and therefore service utilisation data can be seen as the characteristics of the vehicle which is necessary to deliver such improved outcomes.

After such background information has been assembled, we recommend that *step five* is the formulation of a strategic plan for the local system of mental health services. Such a written plan will usually involve: the setting of short- and long-term objectives, and widespread consultation and involvement in the plan. An example of those likely to be involved in such a consultation process in Britain are shown in Table 13.5. The strategic plan will also estimate gaps in categories of services, will separately esti-

Table 13.5. *Who should be involved in writing the strategic plan?*

Group	Involved in strategy group	Involved in consultation on draft strategy	Involved in endorsement of final strategy
Health service managers	r	r	
Clinicians	r	r	r
Administrators	r		
Service users and their representatives	r	r	r
Hospital board members		r	r
Contract managers	d/s		
Social services managers	r	r	
Director of social services		r	r
Voluntary agencies	d	r	d
General practitioners	r	r	r
Housing department staff	d	r	d
Politicians		s	s
External advisers	s	s	

Key: r, required; d, desirable; s, invited for specific issues.
Source: adapted from Reynolds & Thornicroft (1999)

mate gaps in the capacities of services; will include a specific costing; and will set out a detailed project management timetable which indicates the timepoints at which each service change will take place.

The *sixth step* in planning is the implementation of the essential service components. The relevant decisions here will follow on from the previous steps, especially the identification of unmet needs at the population level. Pragmatically it will almost always be true that planners consider that several service components are absent, weak or inappropriately provided, and so the question arises of how to prioritise between competing components for the sequence of implementation. We would suggest that there should be some provision in each category of the basic service components, which are shown in Table 10.3. If any single category is totally absent in a local area, then the planning team will need to consider whether the provision of some capacity in this missing category should be one of the highest priorities. Again it will be important to use a system perspective so that priorities are conceptualised within the wider 'hydraulic' framework of the system as a whole. For example, the provision of highly staffed residential care should usually be considered for individual patients only if lesser degrees of support have proven insufficient.

Finally, the *seventh step* is that of monitoring and conducting a review cycle. This step is often forgotten, so that there is a discrepancy between the resources invested in changing and maintaining health services, and the budget dedicated to evaluate the effect of these interventions. We consider that this is wrong because sufficient attention should be paid to reveal whether the services are providing benefits to patients and, if so, how efficiently. A proper evaluation will be beneficial to improve that particular service, and will indicate how far the results could be generalised to other similar areas. The reasons why this often does not occur are twofold. First, it is not usual to find in the same location knowledge of both service re-form and service evaluation. Second, the timescales intrinsic to service planning and to service evaluation often do not coincide. Senior staff, both administrators and clinicians, who make planning decisions commonly prefer access to quick and available information and may not be able to wait for the more precise data that will result from long-term research studies. Under these circumstances the money that is needed for such research is not considered an investment but only an extra cost. Wing (1986) made clear that a continuous cycle of planning and evaluation is necessary and both parts of the cycle should have, whenever possible, an epidemiological basis. Since monitoring is a first step before more formal evaluative research we would encourage the more widespread practice of service monitoring using agreed definitions and indicators, and for both of these we hope that this book can make a contribution. In relation to the conduct of more formal research we have discussed these issues in detail in previous volumes (Knudsen & Thornicroft, 1996; Thornicroft & Tansella, 1996; Tansella, 1997).

In terms of the matrix model, in our view it is necessary to improve the extent and the quality of monitoring of routine clinical practice, and the responsibility to initiate this change lies mainly at the country/regional level. There will be occasions when a research programme, added to a routine monitoring programme, will be of special importance, most often when major service changes are anticipated. It may be necessary to import such research expertise from other regions, or even other countries, if it is not sufficiently well developed *in situ*.

PART V **International perspectives on re-forming mental health services**

14

Australia

From colonial rivalries to a national mental health strategy

ALAN ROSEN

14.1 Historical development of mental health services in Australia

This history is entwined with the impact of European (British) invasion and settlement, initially in 1788, to form penal colonies to alleviate the overcrowding of English jails. As European settlement in Australia expanded, the colonisers tried to come to terms with this remote vast landscape, and fought with the original Aboriginal inhabitants over land and resources. This resulted in fear and isolation for Europeans, and widespread, deadly epidemics and determined attempts at extermination, seriously endangering the indigenous peoples. People of European stock were, therefore, seen as vulnerable to 'bush madness', 'moral insanity', 'sunstroke' and 'intemperance', the latter being due to binge drinking and adulterated alcohol. Aboriginal peoples have been subjected to dispossession and 'spirit-breaking': largely undocumented emotional traumas through massacres, forced removal from their parents ('the lost generations'), traditional lands, culture and language, amounting to genocide (Rosen, 1994, Wilson, 1997).

Initially, people with mental illness were confined in irons on ships and in jails alongside troublesome convicts. It was some years before the first suicide was recorded: 'When life is cheap suicide is rare' (Dax, 1989). No separate provision was made until 1811, with the first small institution for the 'insane' opening in Castle Hill, New South Wales, (NSW) accommodating 20 people. Two small asylums were opened in Van Dieman's Land, now Tasmania, in 1824. The first large asylum at Tarban Creek, NSW, was opened in 1838 (later named Gladesville Hospital, which finally ceased operating as an in-patient psychiatric facility in 1997).

Gold Rushes from 1851 brought rapid population increases, 'gold mania' and the building of 10 asylums, particularly in Victoria and Queensland, between 1860 and 1890. The first private provision in hospitals and 'inebriates retreats' appeared in the 1880s. Further population expansion saw the emergence of many institutions over the next 100 years, and their story in Australia is similar to the chillingly consistent and familiar multinational experience throughout the Western world: overcrowding, loss of connection with families and the community, 'institutionalisation', oppressive practices and 'vocational ownership' (Thornicroft *et al.*, 1993) countered by earnest but often thwarted attempts to improve conditions and reform practices (Dax, 1989). The exception was the disproportionately high rate of incarceration of Aboriginal people in our mental and 'corrective' institutions, in parallel up to the 1960s with indigenous people becoming the object of fascination as psychopathological exotica, during brief psychiatric safaris to remote Australia (Hunter, 1997).

A non-systematic trend towards deinstitutionalisation picked up momentum from the 1950s or 1960s partly on the basis of renewed clinical optimism, availability of employment and changing social attitudes. But more often it appeared to be determined by economic and political imperatives, in response to scandals, inquiries, and the reluctance of governments to allocate funds to upgrade these facilities. Mental health services and resources, however, did not follow their patients into the community. In fact, by 1984, virtually 90% of people with severe mental illness in NSW were living in the community, whereas approximately 90% of public mental health staff and funding were retained in hospitals (Rosen *et al.*, 1987).

The development of local general hospital psychiatric in-patient units initially did not shift the concentration of work with in-patients with severe mental illness from the psychiatric hospitals. The general hospital units were initially highly selective, were not designated in some states to take involuntary patients and were reluctant to become so. Some of them used their resources and beds to favour academic interests and/or super-speciality tertiary referral programmes. This is similar to the UK experience, as described by Baruch & Treacher (1978).

Compounding these trends, Australia has developed a substantial private medical sector, now funded nationally by taxpayers through our Health Insurance Commission, as well as via private health insurance schemes. This has promoted a parallel growth in private psychiatrist practices and psychiatric in-patient beds, concurrently moving 'up market' to deal increasingly with less severe disorders and the demand for psychotherapy. Working with involuntary patients, those with fewer economic resources, and people not prepared to come in at convenient times to private clinics to have their crises, was left largely to the public sector.

Meanwhile from the early 1970s some community health teams were put in place nationally through the Australian Assistance Plan, but they were often idealistically focused on primary prevention, offering generic rather than specialist mental health services on a business hours, weekday basis.

In 1983 David Richmond was commissioned from outside the Mental Health field to report on these circumstances in NSW. Consulting widely, including via a publicised consumer and family phone-in, he was struck by the lack of provision of services and support for people with severe mental illness and their families in the community, and recommended a gradual shifting of resources to where most of these people now lived.

Richmond's Report (1983) endorsed the published results of a seminal randomised control study in Sydney (Hoult *et al.*, 1984) of 24-hour community-based psychiatric care as an alternative to hospital-centred acute care and office-hours only aftercare, replicating similar studies in North America (Stein & Test, 1980). From 1984 to 1987, The Richmond Implementation proceeded in NSW, demonstrating that with pump-priming funding, 24-hour mobile community mental health services in most localities could be established. These would prioritise the needs of individuals with severe mental illness and their families, and could be integrated with local general hospital psychiatric units, now increasingly under pressure to become accredited to accommodate security risk acute inpatients, on an involuntary basis if necessary.

14.2 **Recent national developments**

The National Mental Health Policy was endorsed by all Australian Health Ministers and published in 1992, generalising this policy direction to all states and providing transitional funding in the national budget through the accompanying National Mental Health Strategy to shift services from institutions to local communities. The aims of this strategy were:

- to promote the mental health of the Australian community and, where possible, prevent the development of mental health problems and mental disorders;
- to reduce the impact of mental disorders on individuals, families and the community; and
- to assure the rights of people with mental disorders.

These services were to be community based, 'mainstreamed', that is, integrated with and accessible via general health services, though remaining distinct as specialised mental health services. They were to develop strong links with groups of consumers, families, general practitioners, the non-government service organisations, and other non-health local services, like housing, general disability services, social security and employment.

The National (General) Health Strategy followed with an extensive issues paper on 'continuity of care for people with chronic mental illness' (Whiteford, 1993), supporting a similar trajectory, particularly with respect to systematised alternatives to institutionally based services, and orderly transfer of services. A subsequent report on the status of Australian indigenous mental health services (Swan & Raphael, 1995) recommended considerable changes to be applied with cultural sensitivity.

14.3 Application of the three geographic levels

14.3.1 Background

Australia essentially came together as a Federation or collection of colonies which do not quite trust each other. Consequently, we have a Commonwealth (national) government responsible for personal tax collection, unemployment and welfare benefits, and general policy directions in health, disability, education, employment, etc. The State Governments retain responsibility, through their State Health Departments, for organising all their own health services and facilities on the ground, including mental health services. Consequently, such provision is diverse, though influenced to some extent by policy directions driven by the Commonwealth Department of Health, particularly when attached to funding specifically tied to implementation of such programmes, e.g. the National Mental Health Strategy. This leverage has been enhanced in recent years by seeking consensus about such programmes among all health ministers, State and Federal, through AHMAC (The Australian Health Ministers' Conference), and by formalised agreements between Commonwealth and States (Schedule F of the Medicare Agreement) in return for transitional implementation funds derived from the Medicare Levy raised nationally with personal taxation.

14.3.2 The country/regional level

In Australia this must be divided into Federal and State responsibilities.

Federal (Commonwealth) Government
An allocation has been made in the annual Federal budget for implementing the National Mental Health Strategy, largely due to the AHMAC Consensus and Community pressures. This strategy has enjoyed bipartisan support as national government has passed from Labour to Conservative,

although the funding has been wound back in recent years. The National Strategy is responsible for:

    (a) Developing National Mental Health Standards (Gianfrancesco *et al.*, 1997), which will be implemented through independent hospital and community health national accreditation bodies.

    (b) National data sets and annual reports comparing state and regional mental health service provision, and performance.

    (c) National studies and projects, developing models and pilots for consideration and possible implementation by the states. These include: mental health treatment category classification and costing study of whole episodes of care, as an alternative or adjunct to hospital-based casemix; community epidemiological studies to ascertain prevalence and needs, evaluating outcome measures for national use, and promoting national networks and training (e.g. service development, site visiting, conference and awards programmes in the areas of local integrated services, early intervention, dual diagnoses, rural and remote services, indigenous and transcultural mental health services, consumer and carer service initiatives, etc.).

    (d) Community Awareness Media Campaign and studies in community and staff attitudes to people with mental illness.

    (e) Promoting consumer and carer participation in policy and planning at every level through the National Consumer Advisory Group (NCAG) with direct Ministerial Access relating to a network of state 'CAG's'. The present Commonwealth Government has opted to disband the National CAG, however, and put in place a National body of non-government advocacy and service organisations.

    (f) Develop some principles for workforce planning, professional competencies and university professional training, though practical provision has been left so far to the states and the professions involved.

    (g) Encouraging early prevention and improved detection, consumer access to services, and early intervention and shared mental health care with general practitioners in all age groups, but particularly for depression and psychosis in young people, and others at risk of suicide.

    (h) Improving mental health services for Aboriginal and Torres Strait Islander populations and people with non-English-speaking backgrounds.

State

At this level, there are usually explicit State Mental Health Policies, which form the blueprint for the next stage or commentary on the current stage of development. Each strategy has its own Mental Health Act and

Table 14.1. *Comparisons between states*

Australian state	Victoria	NSW
State Mental Health Directorate	Historically large	Historically small*
	Substantial control and policy direction	Little control
	Clear and accessible policy documentation	Advisory mainly
	Well defined and retained mental health budget and expenditure	Little public policy documentation since early 90s*
		Variably defined and continually eroded mental health budgets
Early consequences for services	Remained conservative and institutionally based longer.	Allowed diversity of service innovation and experimentation.
Time-frame for change training	Very short (2–3 years).	Fairly long (13 years)
	Belated but well co-ordinated training packages (1990's) for professional and non-professional staff	Pioneering training packages (1980's) long since mainly devolved to tertiary education sector
Staff response to change	Top down: (State to local level): staff felt very buffeted and imposed upon initially	Bottom up: (Local to state level): broad commitment and strong sense of ownership of changes from early 1980's, but...
	Voluntary redundancy packages accepted by some	Frustration and depletion more recently with uncertain funding, staffing and support.
	Sense of local ownership emerging recently.	
System impetus and response to change	Strong central committed leadership	Widely dispersed leadership
	Initial apparent bed crises, government inquiries, media reports playing up discordant relations with other agencies, e.g. police shootings of mentally ill individuals	Strong grass-roots movement
		Relatively uneventful transition except for sporadic media beat-ups
	Jarring transition at first	Some service shortages emerging now, due to resource erosion, maldistribution and system coordination problems

Per capita expenditure on public mental health services (1995)	Highest in Australia	Lowest in Australia (allowing for some ambiguity in attribution of overheads costs)*
Later consequences for services	Well systematised, regulated and consistent More complete deinstitutionalisation and resettlement programmes for inpatient staff and residents More orderly resource shift to local integrated services	Inconsistent patchwork and training of services, but some very experienced and evolved services, and strong ground-level movement. Incomplete patchy deinstitutionalisation and consequent limited resource transfer.
Major contributions to the national strategy	Well organised transfer of resources Consumer evaluation of services Health service contracts on price and volume of services (since 1989) Performance indicators Transparent accounting Consistency of service components in each catchment Early prevention and intervention in psychosis programmes Transcultural mental health programmes Economic models for whole episodes of care	Initial Australian controlled research into 24-hour community based services Consumer participation in service managements Very strong networking via team forums, conferences and award programmes Integrated standards and services (urban, rural and remote) Postgraduate University courses for mental health professionals with training for remote areas by interactive television Torture and trauma counselling services Youth depression guidelines

Notes:

* Though some increase recently.

Sources: National Mental Health Report 1994, 1995

Guardianship Legislation, which results in some variability in provision for medical and legal professional and lay involvement in the involuntary admission process, community orders, guardianship, forensic issues, etc. Through the National Strategy however, Model Mental Health Legislation has been developed as a suggested template for the further development of State laws.

The regional level The Mental Health Directorates in some states have a high level of top-down control and close regulation of regional services (e.g. Victoria), while in others, (e.g. NSW) only policy direction can be advised from the Directorate, as administrative control of Mental Health Services has been devolved to the Area Health Services, which act as semi-independent quasi-corporate business units managing all health services for populations up to 750000. In Australia, these differing relationships have been the subject of some instructive comparisons (see Table 14.1). At state level, the historical lack of a strong centralised mental health directorate in NSW compared to Victoria allowed a *bottom-up* movement to develop a ground-swell for innovative change at the local level.

The consequences in Victoria were that services remained institutionally based much longer, but when at last they were ready to change, it was in a fairly systematic *top-down* manner, largely retaining control of resources for mental health services. In spite of traditional rivalries between these two most populous states, they undoubtedly have needed each other as powerful complementary examples in this field. They have also both contributed considerably to the National Mental Health Strategy (see Table 14.1), as have other states and territories more recently, e.g. to indigenous and multicultural mental health services, consumer involvement in services, workforce competencies, remote interactive tele-conferencing, development of integrated services and early intervention services for children and adolescents. England and Scotland could be seen as partly analogous to NSW and Victoria in terms of Scotland's mental health services remaining institutionally based much longer. Potentially Scotland will now be able to draw on lessons from the English experience, when Scotland is ready to shift its substantially preserved mental health resources (Rosen, 1997).

The local level I agree with the principal authors (p. 4) that it is crucial that 'mental health services should be primarily organised at the local level', being both responsible and accountable for not just each clinical encounter or episode of care, but sometimes for lifetime care for individuals and families in the context of the larger scale of public health policy.

However, there is some confusion and dissension as to whether the local mental health service should be organised at the truly local community district service level or the Area/Regional level. A local 'area integrated' mental health service is defined in the Area-Integrated Mental Health Service (AIMHS) standards (Rosen *et al.*, 1995), from which the National Health Strategy (Whiteford, 1993) and the National Mental Health Standards' Definition is derived, as 'The service . . . responsible for the overall mental health needs of a **local** catchment population'. This **local** service is further defined as integrating community and hospital, acute treatment *and* rehabilitation into one **local** system of mental health care, with one unified management, with accountability for and flexibility of use of a defined budget. This is usually for a population of 50–250 000 people, but several Australian State mental health administrations are now intent on forming units of 500–750 000 which purport to have these characteristics.

This results in some of our 'local' level services serving populations larger than the State of Tasmania (600 000), which has several mental health catchment services. The term 'Area' was used generically because of variable terminologies for clinical and administrative mental health service entities in different Australian states, e.g. Regions, Areas, Networks, Sub-areas, Sectors, Districts, Catchments.

There is no known high quality research which determines optimal catchment size, but the investigators and directors of internationally renowned evidence-based good practice models concur that the most effective and efficient catchment size for a local urban/suburban integrated mental health service is between 50 000 and 150 000, e.g. optimal catchment size for mental health services listed below (pers. comm.):

Madison, Wisconsin, USA	100–150 000	(Stein, 1996)
Birmingham, UK	50–150 000	(Hoult, 1996)
Trieste, Italy	40 000	(Dell'Aqua, 1996)
Verona, Italy	75 000	(Tansella, 1996)
Netherlands	30–80 000	(Witters, 1996)
Oslo, Norway	30 000	
Germany	150 000	
Sydney, Australia	110 000 (Ryde) to 230 000 (Blacktown)	

Andrews (1991) has proposed ideal workforce resources, numbers, mix and organisation on the basis of a mythical urban catchment of 250 000, as a manageable unit of care. However, inner city services generally do better with a smaller catchment population.

Senior health managers may advocate or form much larger population catchment units, based on the much more mythical principle of 'economy of scale'. This is to confuse regional administrative convenience with clinical and managerial practicality at the local level. Smaller human management, work, and business units represent a more contemporary approach to achieving organisational effectiveness. In any case, smaller catchment services are usually part of some larger mental health or general health organisation, which should ideally assist in defraying per capita overheads, unless top-heavy bureaucracies are allowed to develop unfettered.

I would concur with the principal authors' implication that there is no sense in trying to form a local administrative unit larger than a maximum of 250 000 because there are no mental health laws at these local levels, but only at State levels. Further, service management and providers cannot get to know their clientele well if they are covering larger populations, so cannot ensure a humane, measured and safe response from the benefit of prior experience of individual service users and their families.

Conclusions on the Concept of 'Local' Mental Health Service

1. An 'Area' of 750 000 population cannot be accurately portrayed as a *local* secondary mental health service entity. It may be a reasonable urban geographic unit, however, in which to form collaborative networks of *tertiary* services, and from which to provide resource accountability.

2. A local catchment Mental Health Service with the responsibility for all local clinical services and a defined coherent and stable budget does not preclude having single-point accountability and transparency of mental health service resources and planning at a larger Regional or State Health Service level.

3. A clinically functional service will only work with *both* responsibility and authority for clinical services and the service's budget. The management for this local service must also be assured of the coherence, recurrent stability and discretion over the flexible use of this budget. Otherwise the service management will be left with full clinical responsibility without authority, which is untenable. Without reasonable budget predictability, strategic planning becomes impossible, and senior supervising staff who have been committed to the long-term needs of service-users, evidence-based service innovation, and service-system consolidation become disillusioned and will move on.

14.4 The input, process and outcome phases

Providing this horizontal dimension to the matrix results in a map with which it is easier to follow the systemic forces and complex interactions associated with service outcomes at different levels. Superficially it has the look and feel of a board game, although there is no one unidirectional causal arrow, and it becomes increasingly clear that it requires multilevel lateral creative systemic thinking, as well as rational linear processes and a bit of luck to arrive at a desired outcome.

On the other hand, at the population-needs and service-users level it would cause understandable dismay to perceive that decisions with such crucial impact on their lives could be played over their heads like a game. As a map, the matrix requires a third dimension, 'change through time', which would turn it into a cubic matrix. The heuristic value of this matrix organisation lies also in its allowance for qualitative as well as quantitative inputs, processes and outcomes. Consistent with contemporary Quality Improvement Methodologies, it emphasises:

(a) The importance of variables at the structural and process levels, while monitoring outcome variables. That is, that outcome focus, while important, cannot be a sole or pure preoccupation with 'the bottom line', without concern for how the end does not always justify the means.

(b) The need to focus on system errors rather than blame of individual clinicians, and to use the former as opportunities for constructive change.

There is also recognition of the need for service providers to lift our heads out of our preoccupation with the pressure of current clinical casework, and switch our mindsets to a population-needs focus. Rather than just trying to cope with the next crisis or psychiatric emergency, we should be reorganising our services to go looking for people in dire need who have never yet appeared on our doorsteps, in keeping with the emerging evidence of better outcome with earlier detection and intervention of depression and psychosis. We should be taking responsibility not only for the next clinical encounter, but for the continuity of the whole episode of care, or even whole of life care if necessary, and for the encounter with the local community.

An application of the matrix may help us understand the systemic relations and impact of quality improvement processes, and the increasing involvement of consumer and family groups in the management of our services (see Table 14.2).

The Australian National Mental Health Standards (Gianfrancesco *et al.*, 1997) were conceived from the beginning as an essential plank of the National Mental Health Strategy platform. This is because it was perceived that the historical (institutionally based) approach to mental health care had not always been conducive to achieving the high standards that

Table 14.2. *Relations and input of quality improvement services*

	Input	Process	Outcome
National/ State	National Accreditation mechanisms for all Hospitals and Community Health Organisations State Laws providing qualified privilege for Quality Assurance mechanisms involving Clinicians Statutory Watchdogs: e.g. Health Complaints Commission, official visitors	National Mental Health Standards generated following nation-wide consultations with all stakeholders	All states encourage their Mental Health Services to complete Accreditation with National Mental Health Standards Indicators
Local service	Resources and infrastructure provided by management for professional peer review mechanisms Consumer and Family Management Advisory Boards Consumer monitoring and evaluation mechanisms	e.g. QARNS file audit and review e.g. SUNS Community team or facility Surveyors e.g. Consumer Network e.g. Consumer Consultants e.g. Official visitors	Corrective response by Service to: Collated adverse events and trended data rates Consumers and family feedback to management Community visitors' survey reports Consumer satisfaction studies
Individual service -user	Explicit and openly advertised complaints and comments mechanism strongly supported by consumer and family networks	Monitoring of: (a) Ease of access for both service-user and family (b) Quality of contact (c) Information provided	Monitor and adjust service in response to consumer's, family's or clinician's perception of: Adverse outcome Good practice outcome Satisfaction with service

Australians had come to expect of their general hospitals and other health services.

Therefore, the National Standards were developed by a consortium consisting of the Area-Integrated Mental Health Service (AIMHS) Standards Project (Rosen *et al.*, 1992, 1995), which had produced outcome-oriented standards for both community and hospital components of integrated mental health services, and the two national health accreditation bodies, the Australian Council of Healthcare Standards (ACHS), and the Community Health Accreditation Standards Program (CHASP). The new standards were generated through national consultations including all professional bodies, consumers, carers, managers and government.

This has resulted in a set of outcome-oriented standards for all mental health services, whether public or private, hospital or community, with indicators for assessing whether services are meeting these standards, and an external accreditation system at least as rigorous as that for general health care. In endorsing the National Mental Health Standards, all Health Ministers and Departments are committed to encouraging strongly all mental health services and facilities to complete accreditation, with at least one state (Victoria) providing a financial incentive to services to do so. They surpass other healthcare standards in the degree of integration required of community with hospital, and acute with rehabilitation services at a local level, and the enshrining of the human rights of consumers throughout the standards. They also ensure that all services are involved in meaningful, quality improvement activities on a regular basis. Local examples of such activity in our services include:

    (a) *Quality Assurance Royal North Shore (QARNS)*, which provides a permanent team of nurse surveyors who conduct total in-patient file audits, and flag all perceived adverse occurrences on the basis of previously agreed criteria for each health field (e.g. in psychiatry include all absences without leave, suicide attempts, stays or readmissions within 30 days, etc.). All flagged files are then subjected to individual senior clinician scrutiny raising pertinent questions, and then to fully documented peer review to answer them, and to agree and implement improvements to the service system as necessary. This process allows full and frank dissection of service system errors at the local level only because at the state level legislation ensuring 'qualified privilege' protects individual clinicians engaged in a defined range of quality assurance activities from having these proceedings being used in any possible litigation. Once continuing problems, recommendations and collective trended data are extracted, peer review proceedings about individual cases are shredded. The limitation of this system is that as yet it is limited to in-patient episodes and the best result can be only the elimination of adverse events, as it does not detect or trend instances of high-quality outcomes.

(b) *Service Users North Shore (SUNS)*, which illustrates interaction between the local service and service user levels. SUNS is a standing service-user advisory committee which is an integral part of our mental health service management structure. It comprises representatives of all local consumer and family mental health advocacy organisations, including the *Consumer Network*, which has an office and a defined budget within our service, any expenditure from which the Network determines internally. SUNS meets monthly with the directors of the service, dealing with negative and positive feedback about service delivery and consumer needs. All complaints are documented and Service Directors formally report back about action they have taken. Teams or individual service providers are formally commended on instances of outstanding service. This explicit complaints and comments mechanism is advertised boldly in every public waiting area in all our facilities. SUNS nominates *consumer* representatives to other management committees, who receive training and pay for their time. SUNS consumer and family representatives also conduct quality reviews of all components of the service whether in the hospital or the community, using surveys or checklists of performance indicators derived from the AIMHS Standards.

Complaints can otherwise or also be taken formally to semi-independent bodies such as the 'Official Visitors' at the psychiatric in-patient unit or the Patient Representative at the general hospital locally, or at a State level to the Health Complaints Commission, Professional Registration Boards, or directly to the Health Minister. However, if such mechanisms were to operate to promote the full possible range of quality improvement processes, the former would be reconstituted as the 'Health Complaints and Kudos Commission'. Variations on those systems of quality improvement and consumer and carer participation in them have been developing in other Australian Mental Health Services and States.

14.5 **Relevance of service components**

The main variations in Australia on the service components described by the principal authors are the following:

1. Our service components are similar but conceived and organised somewhat differently. There is an increasingly high level of horizontal

integration between community and hospital services. Acute services integrate 24 hour community-based crisis and care management teams, hospital-based acute psychiatric in-patient unit, psychiatric triage service to the general hospital emergency department, and a consultation-liaison psychiatry service to other wards. Rehabilitation services integrate an Intensive Mobile Case Management Team, day and evening group programmes, vocational co-operative and placement services, and short- to long-term community residential and resettlement facilities, which range from weekly visit only to 24 hour supervision. Increasingly in Australia in-patient rehabilitation services are undergoing horizontal integration with community rehabilitation services, while in some states and areas the former remain separate as tertiary referral units in psychiatric hospitals.

Bridging both acute and rehabilitation strands are a unified service management, consumer and family advocacy bodies, and interface programmes with other service providers such as General Practitioner Shared Mental Health Care, Early Prevention and Intervention of Severe Psychiatric Disorder programmes (in co-operation with Adolescent Health and primary care services) and Dual Disorders programmes (e.g. with Drug and Alcohol or Intellectual Disability Services). Tertiary referral regional services include Mood and Eating Disorder Units, Adolescent Units and secure long-stay provision.

2. A high level of co-operation is expected and prevails between components, e.g. our acute extended hours community service will also provide 24 hour crisis cover to all facilities in the service, e.g. residential, or intensive mobile team clientele; when the team is off duty after 9 pm; e.g. the in-patient unit assists with initial phone triage when the Extended Hours team switches from on-duty to on-call after 10.30 pm.

3. In our service and increasingly in others, 24 hour mental health crisis response teams and community centre based case management services have been merged into one Extended Hours Team. In this way, the bond forged in crisis between service providers, users and their families can be translated relatively smoothly into a more trusting continuity of care relationship. The same professional case managers will also assist and follow individual service-users into hospital should in-patient care become necessary, continuing to play an essential role in their in-patient care team, to ensure consistency of care.

However, it is recognised in Australia that there is no one perfect way to slice the cake and organise such services, and so the distinction between a dedicated Crisis and Assessment Team in one Area or Combined Extended Hours Service Team in another can be confusing. Further confusion can arise between the roles of such teams and an

Table 14.3. *Contrasting community mental health teams responding to psychiatric crises (Hambridge & Rosen, 1994)*

	Psychiatric crisis team	Psychiatric extended hours team	Mobile community intensive-case management team
Service user type	No exclusion criteria for local residents with any psychiatric disturbance	No exclusion criteria for local residents with any psychiatric disturbance	Only service-users with severe and long term mental illness, with many previous hospitalisations
	Service-users have a wide ability range	Service-users have a wide ability range	Service-users functioning in lower range, often poor co-operation with services
Location of services	Often home centred at height of crisis	Centred at home and Community Mental Health Centre (CMHC)	All/mostly home centre plus work or leisure sites
	Separate crisis team	Crisis Service combined with CMHC	Separate intensive case management team
Case management approaches	Open-ended caseload High intensity input for a short period only	Open-ended caseload Intensity of input limited by caseload	Finite caseload (1:10) High intensity on ongoing basis (if required)
Type of services	Crisis responsive (to pressing concerns and symptoms) Short term crisis care and treatment	Crisis responsive and proactive to prevent crises Crisis care, and treatment and ongoing case management	Crisis responsive, and proactive to prevent crises Crisis care, treatment ongoing case management and intensive rehabilitation

assertive/intensive mobile long-term case management team. This is clarified in Table 14.3.

4. Our Intensive/Assertive Mobile Case Management Teams (variably available in NSW and other states, much more consistently applied in Victoria) provide home-based individual treatment and rehabilitation for individuals who have much more long-term intensive needs for daily care than can be coped with by most crisis and community case

management teams. This includes individuals who are homeless or on the brink of it, have the challenging combination of long-term psychosis and severe substance abuse, are in a dilapidated physical state, or will not take daily medication without support.

These teams usually work 7 days and evenings per week with an average staff: service user ratio of 1:10. Unlike model and research teams of this type internationally who indefinitely retain service-users who meet their criteria for needing heavy use of services, services such as ours in the real world are always under pressure to create new places in the team with finite resources. However we also find that most of these individuals no longer require such a high level of services within 1 to 2 years of intensive community rehabilitation, and we can slowly transfer them back in a quiescent stable state to our local community mental health teams within an average 2–3 years.

5. At the same time our mental health services are gradually beginning to shift our lower intensity clientele to General Practitioner Shared Mental Health Care projects, with Mental Health Teams providing ongoing monitoring of care, and as necessary clinical review and rehabilitation services.

14.6 **Relevance of the proposed steps towards reforming mental health services**

Australia has closely paralleled neither the Italian nor the English experience of deinstitutionalisation. Italy worked the political process effectively to subvert the institutions from the inside, then nationally to close the front doors of the institutions, continuing to run back-door operations, while they hurriedly started organising community mental health care.

England became administratively and economically adept at closing down psychiatric hospitals, but has not been very good at what to do next; whereas Australians, progressively from 1979, became very good at what to do next in the local communities, but did not give enough attention or apply similar talent and skill to shrinking and closing psychiatric hospitals while transferring resources, with few exceptions, e.g. Victoria. This allowed parallel hospital-based and community-based systems to coexist for too long, and considerable loss in some States of resources which should have followed patients into the community.

14.6.1. **Principles and values in terms of the seven proposed steps**

All Australian States and Services have now generally adopted the principles of the National Mental Health Strategy (see earlier section on

'Recent National Developments'). Commitment to its core values varies from very high level to lip-service, at Federal and State governmental levels, and in local services. On the whole, as you might expect, there has been a higher commitment to these principles and values in mental health than in general health bureaucracies, in public much more than private service-providers, or integrated or community based services more than remaining stand-alone psychiatric hospitals, and among consumers and family organisations more than professional and industrial organisations, at least until recently. Recent reports have proposed new mechanisms for public and private collaboration at a local level, and in future all private mental health facilities will be accredited on the basis of the National Standards based on the principles of the National Mental Health Strategy.

14.6.2 Setting Boundary Conditions

(a) *Geographical boundaries* for mental health services apply throughout Australia, though there is considerable ambiguity concerning the maximum catchment size over which one management can realistically expect to demonstrate responsibility (pp. 182–6).

(b) *Functional boundaries:* In the Richmond Implementation in NSW (1984–7) and subsequent mental health policies in this and other states, priority was squarely to be given in the public sector to individuals with 'serious mental illness' and their families. This is because it was perceived that people with milder disorders had more insight into their conditions, were often less socially deprived, and more resourceful and would more readily access assistance from general practitioners, private psychiatrists and counsellors. Further, many private mental health professionals seemed to prefer this type of clientele, who would be patient on a waiting-list and not generate out-of-hours crises or require home visiting. The term 'serious' is unfortunate when applied to mental illness, implying that we may not take all psychiatric conditions seriously. 'Severe mental illness' is preferable, but contrary to convenient misconception among some service providers, this term should not be restricted by diagnosis to only psychoses and major depression.

Severity is a function of several other 'd' words besides diagnosis: degree, duration, distress, disability, disorganisation, danger and de-family (i.e. social support or isolation), and these should be applied to any DSM-4 Axis I or II diagnosis. The term more recently being adopted refers to individuals and families 'seriously affected by mental illness'. With the advent of early prevention, detection and intervention programmes, with poorly defined prodromes, it is tempting for specialist services to offer a wide, unfocused array of primary and early secondary prevention services and to again 'try to be everything to everyone'. With finite resources, this is much less a practical clinical strategy than theological wishful thinking.

The dilemma here is that individuals with early stages of severe psychiatric disorders may present with relatively minor symptoms, and early intervention may well ultimately lessen impairment and disability. The challenge is twofold: (a) to educate primary-care clinicians to listen carefully, detect prodromal symptoms, filter and refer those with a high risk of severe disorder to specialist services, using standardised screening tools and (b) to harness the resources of the private sector to augment the public sector, so that it can widen its specialist services systematically to provide early intervention as well as ongoing care.

There is increasing concurrence among mental health planners with the principal authors' conclusion that specialist services are scarce and should be focused upon those individuals likely to have the most severe symptoms and greatest disability. This should include a shared care role in early detection and intervention strategies for these disorders. At the same time, more efforts are being made to support, retrain and supervise primary care clinicians to provide services for less severe disorders, and to do shared care with more severe disorders.

14.6.3 **Population needs assessment**

The National Mental Health Strategy has commissioned an Australian Community Epidemiological Study to compare existing knowledge of treated prevalence with a more accurate knowledge of total and untreated prevalence, rather than relying as previously on estimates based on the ECA study in the USA. To take the cautionary tale of the untargeted model a step further: Met unneed, or treated non-prevalence should also be considered here as a factor distorting patterns of use of mental health professional resources.

A = *Unmet need* = Untreated Patients or prevalence.

B and C = *Met need*   = Treated prevalence in primary and secondary care.

D = *Met unneed* = Psychiatric treatment or therapy for people with no recognised psychiatric disorder

Met unneed is a term first coined, as far as we know, in a workshop on Mental Health Service Needs Analysis in London in early 1992 (Rosen, 1992). Its prevalence in Australia is unknown because a psychiatric condition is sometimes declared by the provider for health insurance or public accounting purposes. Our fee-for-service private health system creates fertile conditions for its continued existence. The media promotion of psychotherapeutic fads and psychopharmacological quick-fixes may help it to flourish. Undoubtedly it is also alive and well in general practice. It is a form of iatrogenesis, as the impact of such therapies may generate psychological symptoms, or adverse effects from any medications used.

14.6.4 Current service provision assessment

The Annual Report of the National Strategy provides detailed comparisons on key characteristics between the States (including per capita funding for public mental health services, proportions expended in hospital and community services, degree of shift per year, etc.) and work is progressing towards a more accurate National Collated Database, with standardised massed data-collections now occurring from every state and region.

A few states have long-established state-wide psychiatric database systems which allow relatively accurate and meaningful comparisons between local services. Other states are variable in the reliability and comparability of their mental health databases at a local level, particularly in terms of their infrastructural or overhead costs. There is no national psychiatric case register with unique patient identifiers, and this is unlikely to occur under the prevailing community attitudes and laws regarding privacy.

14.6.5 Strategic planning, implementation, monitoring and review

These are considered sequential steps, but as we live in complex systems they may not always occur in a linear rational sequence. Opportunities for implementation sometimes crop up at the most inopportune time, even embarrassingly before we have thought to put them in the strategic plan. Organisational or service system building may be conceived of as requiring an amalgam between sound short- to medium-term management and staff support, good luck and making things happen. There are visionary, lateral, creative and entrepreneurial elements required, as well as fiscal responsibility and strong clinical competence and safety parameters (Rosen *et al.*, 1997). It is not just a policy or a strategic planning document we are implementing, but an essential service in time of need for a community, hopefully delivered on the basis of social equity of access. It is just as our politicians sometimes appear to need to remind each other, 'it's not just an economy we live in, but a society'.

The hydraulic metaphor presented by the principal authors is a powerful reminder of the inter-relatedness of compartments of service. Leakage occurs not only of patients, but of disillusioned family members and staff, and of vital fluid resources, when not being actively siphoned from the system by the wider health or governmental systems surrounding this 'hydraulic engine'. Like Freud's hydraulic model of the psyche (e.g. displacement) this model is too mechanistic to comprehend complex human systems, and so is heuristically limited. General Systems Theory, when applied to organisms, rapidly outgrew static homeostasis and closed loop systems, leading to dynamic equilibrium and open systems, engaged in reciprocal commerce with (i.e. both input from and output to) the surrounding environment. Human systems involve higher order cybernetics (allowing for the impact of external monitoring or the observer as an actor in the system). Larger systems are less predictable, and the possibility of discontinuous 'quantum leap' change must be anticipated rather than assuming that continuous change can be extrapolated in a linear fashion in response to particular strategic inputs (Rosen *et al.*, 1997).

While the national strategic plan flows from the National Mental Health Strategy, most Australian States and some regional and local services publish strategic plans. Implementation at the national level is contracted with the states in approximate terms through the Medicare Agreement (see previously) and monitored via the annual National Mental Health Report. Implementation from State to local level is best exemplified by Victoria, where Health Service Agreements on Price and Volume (Outputs) of Service have been in place since 1989, and monitoring occurs on the basis of a set of performance indicators with comparisons between local services being published quarterly. Key indicators include: caseload and cost per full-time equivalent staff member, contact hours per client per month, involvement of extended hours crisis services and involuntary care, as well as in-patient utilisation data.

14.7 Growing points and major issues for developing mental health services in the next 5 years in Australia

A transition must be made from reforming mental health services to consolidating change, without services becoming 'institutionalised' or habitual again. We must build in the conditions for both endurance or stability, and continuing creativity and evolution (Rosen *et al.*, 1997). We must shift from model services to widely implemented integrated service systems, with their centres of gravity in the community. To achieve this, several crucial issues must be addressed:

(a) Workforce training and supervision in specific evidence-based functional teams and micro-skills (e.g. cognitive and family interventions), to counter the over-reliance on non-specific counselling skills.

(b) Workforce planning encompassing collaborative and complementary arrangements between professional disciplines and the public, private and non-government sectors.

(c) Involving consumers and family carers more in service management and as direct service-providers.

(d) Meeting the challenge of mental health services being mainstreamed (co-located and managed) with general health services, and of forming locally integrated systems of care, and reconciling these with the progressive corporatising or partial privatising of such services; with national policy, and with demands for publicly transparent accounting, contractual and monitoring mechanisms to ensure that priorities are set on severe disorders, local access, integrated services and preservation of mental health resources.

(e) Developing funding mechanisms which provide incentives for whole episodes of care whether in the community or hospital, rather than providing incentives for hospital-based or acute episodes only.

(f) Providing systematised solutions for current gaps in services which people in need often fall through, e.g. Early Prevention and Intervention for Severe Psychiatric Disorders and Suicide Prevention, Dual Disorders or Comorbidity with physical illness, brain damage, drug and alcohol and intellectual disability, etc.

(g) Further developing in-service training, consultation services and shared mental health care arrangements with primary care clinicians.

(h) Developing more culturally appropriate and clinically effective mental health services for Australian indigenous peoples, plus particular non-English speaking background and refugee populations.

(i) Continuing national and local efforts aimed at confronting stigma and changing attitudes to mental illness in the wider community as well as in the helping professions and among potential employers; and also, community awareness campaigns to promote early access and referral to services.

(j) Progressively providing increasing access for people with mental illness to education, training, jobs and accommodation in the real or 'secular' world, rather than in dedicated 'cloistered' mental health facilities, while retaining some bridging operations (e.g. residential, vocational or leisure programmes) until full membership of the local community can be re-established, and as transitional objects while both capital and recurrent resources are devolved from institutions.

(k) Attain more accurate definitions and estimates of met need, unmet need and 'met unneed' for mental health services and their relative potentials for disability, to assist us in setting clinical and resource priorities.

To achieve these ends, it is very important that the Australian National Mental Health Strategy be continued and recurrently renewed, as it has focused and combined efforts of many stakeholders in Australia towards long overdue reforms, and must now help us focus on attaining enduring services while fostering further evolution.

Acknowledgements

To Roger Gurr, Sylvia Hands, Vivienne Miller, Liz Newton, Beverley Raphael, Andrew Stripp, Ainslie Vines and Harvey Whiteford for advice and help with the manuscript.

References

Andrews, G. (1991). *The Tolkien Report: A Description of a Model Mental Health Service.* Sydney: Caritas Research Unit for Anxiety Disorders. .

Baruch, G. & Treacher, A. (1978). *Psychiatry Observed.* London: Routledge.

Dax E. C. (1989). The first 200 years of Australian psychiatry. *Australian and New Zealand Journal of Psychiatry,* 23, 103–110.

Gianfrancesco P., Miller V., Rauch A., Rosen A. & Rotem W. (1997). *National Standards for Mental Health Services.* Canberra: Australian Health Ministers National Mental Health Working Group.

Hambridge, J. & Rosen, A. (1994). Assertive community treatment for the seriously mentally ill in suburban Sydney: a programme description and evaluation. *Australian and New Zealand Journal of Psychiatry,* **28**, 438–445.

Hoult, J., Rosen, A. & Reynolds, I. (1984). Community oriented treatment compared to psychiatric hospital oriented treatment. *Social Science and Medicine,* **18**, 1005–1010.

Hunter, E. (1997). Double talk: changing and conflicting constructions of indigenous mental health. *Australian and New Zealand Journal of Psychiatry,* **31**, 820–827.

National Mental Health Strategy (1995). *National Mental Health Report for 1994.* Mental Health Branch, Department of Human Services and Health, Commonwealth of Australia.

National Mental Health Strategy (1996). *National Mental Health Report for 1995.* Canberra: Mental Health Branch, Department of Health and Family Services, Commonwealth of Australia.

Psychiatric Services Division Department of Health and Community Services, Victoria (1996a). *Purchasing Better Mental Health Services in Victoria.* Melbourne: Hospital and Community Services Department.

Psychiatric Services Division Department of Health and Community Services,

Victoria (1996b). *Monthly Area Mental Health Service Key Performance Indicators*. Melbourne: Hospital and Community Services Department.

Richmond, D. (1983) *Inquiry into Health Services for the Psychiatrically Ill and Developmentally Disabled*. Sydney: NSW Department of Health.

Rosen, A. (1992). Identifying the Mental Health Needs of Local Populations. Presentation to workshop with Jenkins R and Dean C. In *Making It Happen: International Perspectives on Community Mental Health Care*. London: Institute of Health, King's College.

Rosen, A. (1994). 100% Mabo: De-Colonising People with Mental Illness and their Families. *Australian and New Zealand Journal of Family Therapy*, **15**, 128–142.

Rosen, A. (1997). *Mental Health Services in the Era of Quality, Service-User Focus and Human Rights*. Plenary address to 'Reading the Right Signals', 3rd Biennial Conference on Mental Health, Scotland's NHS Trusts, Glasgow.

Rosen, A., Parker, G., Hadzi-Pavlovic, D. & Hartley, R. (1987). *Developing Evaluation Strategies for Local Mental Health Services*. Sydney: NSW Department of Health.

Rosen, A., Miller, V. and Parker, G. (1989). Standards of Care for Area Mental Health Services, *Australian and New Zealand Journal of Psychiatry*, **23**, 379–395.

Rosen, A., Miller, V. & Parker, G. (1992 & 1995). *Area-Integrated Mental Health Service (AIMHS) Standards*. Sydney: Royal North Shore Hospital and Community Mental Health Services.

Rosen, A., Diamond, R., Miller, V. & Stein, L. (1997). Becoming Real: From Model Programs to Implemented Services, In *The Successful Diffusion of Innovative Program Approaches. New Directions for Mental Health Services* (ed. E. J. Hollingsworth). San Francisco: Jossey-Bass.

Stein, L. I. & Test, M. A. (1980). Alternative to mental hospital treatment. I. Conceptual model, treatment programme and clinical evaluation. *Archives of General Psychiatry*, **37**, 392 – 397.

Swan, P. & Raphael, B. (1995). '*Ways Forward': National Consultancy Report on Aboriginal and Torres Strait Islander Mental Health*. Canberra: Australian Government Printing Service.

Thornicroft, G., Ward, P. & James, S. (1993). Care management and mental health, countdown to community care series. *British Medical Journal*, **306**, 768–771.

Whiteford, H. (1993). *Help Where Help is Needed: Community of care for people with chronic mental illness*. National Health Strategy, Issues Paper No. 5. Canberra: Commonwealth Department of Health and Family Services.

Wilson, R. (1997). *Bringing them Home: National Inquiry into the Separation of Aboriginal and Torres Strait Islander Children from their Families*. Human Rights and Equal Opportunities Commission, Commonwealth of Australia.

15

Canada

ALAIN D. LESAGE

15.1 **Introduction**

Best Practices in Reforming Mental Health Services has just been launched
by Health & Welfare Canada, the Federal Ministry of Health (Health &
Welfare Canada, 1997). Since the beginning of the 1990s, many of the ten
provincial governments, all responsible for the planning, financing and
governance of health and social services, have produced new mental health
policies, with particular regard to severely mentally ill patients. Indeed, as
with many industrialised countries, Canadian planners consider that we
have entered an era of transformation for services in need of a reform. These
documents talk about moving and ensuring proper care in the community
and indicate the main service components at the patient, local and provincial levels.

But are we witnessing a social reform? Can it not be argued that this is
just another phase in the pursuit of further deinstitutionalisation and
development of community care? The deinstitutionalisation and community care movement started three to four decades ago. Consider how in most
industrialised countries there has been a steady decline of psychiatric hospitals' population (but no country has done without these facilities), the
development of general hospital psychiatric services, of ambulatory out-
patient and rehabilitation services. The movement has been fuelled, as indicated in Chapter 2, by social forces: humanitarian, clinical and economic
(see also Lesage & Tansella, 1993). Humanitarian concerns have fostered the
view that people with disabilities, physical or mental, shall not be segre-
gated and shall live as normal a life as possible in their community. The con-
troversies early in the British deinstitutionalisation movement about the
relative importance of neuroleptics and rehabilitation just underline that
these two clinical dimensions, which have enriched themselves of new
elements in the past decades, still form the basis of the treatment for
severely mentally ill patients. Finally, if current economic constraints seem

everywhere now, the 'age of innocence' (Knapp, 1997) about economic constraints in the more affluent welfare state of the 1960s seem to have blurred the recognition of this factor, but not its presence.

The outstripping of psychiatric services' resources started just there. Another social dimension rests on the implicit social contract that ties psychiatric services to both the social control and the care of mentally ill individuals, especially severely mentally ill patients. Even though the recognition and the current social prominence of each of these social forces and elements of the social contract have varied over time, they have not been challenged and are still intact. The reform is marching on, even though it has always been short on reaching its objectives of creating 'an accessible and accountable service delivery system that is designed to consolidate and flexibly deploy resources so as to provide comprehensive, continuous, cost-efficient, and effective mental health services to targeted individuals in their home communities' (Hoge *et al.*, 1994, cited by Health & Welfare Canada, 1997). So what is fuelling this current plethora of mental health reform papers by planners that seem to rediscover deinstitutionalisation and community care?

Mental health care is not alone in this respect and other health fields are also reducing the utilisation of costly bed facilities and turning to care in the community with special emphasis on the role of GPs. Much faith is put by planners and researchers, including in the present book, into an evidence-based approach to ensure better protection and pursuit of community care. It can be said that at best it remains an hypothesis to be put to the test.

In this chapter, the issues facing Canadian mental health system stakeholders and the paths used in reforming mental health services will be described. Examples will come particularly from the Province of Québec (country/region level of the matrix) and one local area (east-end Montreal) will be used as the acid-test for the matrix model and evidence-based approach. The situation in Canada, and the reference to Quebec, answers both basic criteria set in the first chapters about the matrix model: first, to be applicable to 'mental health systems of care which are provided within a public health framework', second as an 'explanatory tool, first for understanding and acting to improve services' in one Canadian province now bracing for a new phase of community care. Finally, the Canadian governments at the federal and provincial levels have all accepted the public health perspective that priority shall be given by the mental health services system to severely mentally ill patients.

The next section will provide more details on the national, provincial/regional and local context in Canada. Then, the main issues confronting the mental health services system will be presented as a proposition to see if the matrix can be of help. Next will follow comments on the three points of each of the two dimensions of the matrix. The main service components recommended by the Best Practices in Reforming Mental Health Services in Canada (Health & Welfare Canada, 1997) will be commented on in relation to what has been described in the previous chapters and what further steps may be required. The values, the importance of staff and their integration in the planning process described in Chapters 10 to 13 will be embedded in these sections. Finally, the relevance of the steps proposed to reforming mental health services will be challenged since we have already argued that the societal forces, economic, clinical and humanitarian inputs that have fuelled the deinstitutionalisation and community care reform over the past decades are still intact, undisputed and active now.

What appears to be a new reform is but at best a new phase, certainly with new actors. The issue is whether with the current emphasis on developing evidence-based approaches and fostering a matrix such as proposed here, we will harness the forces better and create knowledge-transfer, to allow better empowerment and sharing mechanisms among mental health system stakeholders to ensure better outcomes for people suffering from severe mental disorders.

15.2 **Canadian context**

In Canada, provision of health and social services is the responsibility of the provinces and in the Province of Québec, of a single government department. The population of Canada is now over 30 million; Province of Ontario is over 11 million and nearby Québec over 7 million. The public funds for health and social services come from transfer payments from the federal government and from provincial taxes. The allocation of resources is determined by the provinces. In Québec, the Ministry of Health and Social Services distributes funds to Québec's 18 Regional Health and Social Services Boards who in turn are responsible for planning and allocating resources to local hospital or community-based services. The allocation to each region takes into account socio-economic variables, which include an index of needs for mental health services, but no envelope is specifically targeted or ring-fenced for mental health services. General practitioners and medical services have a separate funding system.

As in other provinces, Québec's Health Insurance Fund does not allocate funds on a regional basis but most practitioners are paid on a fee-for-service basis. Not-for-profit provider agencies in the mental health sector are mainly funded by public funds from the Ministry of Health and Social Services, or in Ontario from a separate Social and Community Services Ministry, but they also rely on voluntary work and private donations. The private sector plays only a small part in the provision of mental health services, concentrated on residential care funded by boarding allowances from the Ministry or, as in the UK, income maintenance to individuals. The not-for-profit and private sectors have a larger market share of drug and alcohol abuse services, which have developed separately from mainstream public mental health services.

In such a system, the Provincial Government and Regional Boards have complete control of the allocation of resources. The movement towards devolution of planning and budgets to regional authorities is also accompanied by the will to organise services at a local level. In Canada, the Québec's Centres for Local Health and Social Services (CLSCs) launched in the early 1970s are considered visionary. The CLSCs have fared variously though in Québec, being generally boycotted by GPs who preferred to set up their own group practice. Currently the CLSCs are attracting new funding as general hospital beds are closed and policies favouring home-care, especially for the elderly, are brought forward.

While it is recognised that money tied up in psychiatric hospitals could be used to develop community resources in the various regions, current allocations continue to favour the psychiatric hospitals. Central provinces such as Saskatchewan have been at the vanguard of socialised medicine in Canada, and less that 50% of the mental health expenditures were spent on hospital services in the early 1990s (Rochefort, 1992). But this was more the exception that the rule in other provinces, especially Ontario and Quebec. In 1994–1995, it was estimated that in Quebec 8.8% of the Ministry of Health and Social Services' budget was spent on mental health services (about 8% in Ontario), or CDN $142 per capita. Out of this budget, 39% went to psychiatric hospitals, 25% to departments of psychiatry in general hospitals, 17% for physicians' fees; 6% for psychotropic drugs reimbursed to welfare recipients and retired people, 5% to nursing homes, 2% to rehabilitation schemes for mentally retarded people; 3% to non-profit or community agencies, and 3% to CLSCs. However, psychiatric hospitals, and to some extent departments of psychiatry of general hospitals, have developed and run residential and rehabilitation services outside the hospital, so that (excluding physicians' fees), over 37% of the resources were spent outside the hospitals.

Two publications were instrumental in encouraging the development of community-based psychiatric care in Québec; *Les Fous Crient au Secours* (Madmen cry for help), written by an in-patient of the St-Jean de

Dieu psychiatric hospital in 1961 and the Bédard, Lazure and Robarts Commission Report in 1962. This was rapidly followed by the downsizing of psychiatric hospitals alongside the development of beds in the department of psychiatry in general hospitals and the development of community-based multi-disciplinary teams and clinics. St-Jean de Dieu, now Louis-H. Lafontaine Hospital, was the largest psychiatric hospital in Canada. By 1987, it had reduced in size from about 6000 in-patients (in the late 1950s) to 2200, and now there are only 900 beds, with plans to close another 500 by 2003 (Hôpital Louis-H. Lafontaine, 1997). A similar pattern occurred elsewhere in Quebec, with a steady decline in the size of psychiatric hospitals. Complete psychiatric hospitals closure has occurred only in Saskatchewan (Lafave & Grunberg, 1974). In 1994–1995, there was about one psychiatric bed per 1000 inhabitants in Québec, compared to 0.5 in Ontario, or in the provinces of British Columbia on the west coast. However, more people are now served by community-based services; only about 15% of those in contact with psychiatric services considered long-stay in-patients and another 15 to 20% have had a short-stay in-patient admission in the last year. Most people in contact with psychiatric services (about 1.5% of the population each year in east-end Montreal) receive only ambulatory care (Lesage et al., 1997).

15.3 The main issues in Canada

As in many Canadian provinces, the recent policy paper by the Quebec government (MSSS, 1997) focuses on reforming the services for the severely mentally ill. It is presented as part of other previous or forthcoming mental health policy papers on mental health, suicide prevention, child and adolescent services. Its system analysis rests on an inquiry using focus group and key stakeholders' interviews in various regions; on budget allocation and beds ratio and comparison of the latter with the Province of Ontario. The inquiry stressed (a) a distribution of resources concentrated on hospital-based services (as described above); (b) twice as many beds, both acute and long-term care beds, as in Ontario and some other provinces; (c) great variations in regional allocation of mental health resources, by a factor of 1:4 (d) lack of co-ordination between hospital-based services and the existing community agencies for rehabilitation; (e) poor support for families. Among the solutions found in the literature, the document recommends (1) to make severely mentally ill (SMI) a priority for the mental health services system; (2) to foster the development of assertive community treatment (Deci et al., 1995); (3) to sustain further deinstitutionalisation using financial incentives such as the British dowry system (Knapp & Beecham, 1990).

The reform would involve (1) establishing in each region the array of services for SMI oriented towards community care and ensuring continuity and co-ordination of services; (2) reallocation of resources in the community from the current 60%–40% split (60% for hospitals services) to 40%–60% within 5 years. The new allocation should prioritise (a) access to basic residential and subsistence; (b) crisis interventions; (c) access to treatment; (d) access to rehabilitation; (e) support to families; (3) closing in the next five years over 50% of short- and long-stay hospital beds (currently 6000 beds excluding the 1500 beds for the mentally retarded individuals to a total of about one bed per 1000 inhabitants); the resources released being transferred to community-based services; (4) confirming the responsibility of Regional Boards to organise services, reallocate resources, providing SMI individuals with a fixed point of responsibility through designated teams, utilisation of performance contracts with community agencies and training staff. Some specific mechanisms are finally presented such as Ministry support to regions in setting and monitoring the reform, including the development of a Mental Health Information System (MHIS); and (5) evaluation and support of evidence-based practices.

In other Canadian provinces, rather similar analyses and orientations have been put forward (Goering *et al.*, 1992). In the Province of Ontario, the document *Putting People First* (Ontario Ministry of Health, 1993) stressed the lack of co-ordination by describing the three domains: psychiatric hospitals, general hospital and community-based services. The priority there, as well as in the Province of New Brunswick's 1992 Network Committee report, was on SMI.

The Canadian Best Practices recommendations stress particularly at the system level (1) that each region should develop strong mechanisms (Assertive Community Treatment teams and Mental Health Authority) for service integration with clearly designated responsibility for co-ordination and bringing the domains together; (2) the creation and protection of a separate, single funding envelope that combines various funding streams for the delivery of mental health care; (3) the setting of explicit operational targets, goals and standards. In that document, the Canadian Mental Health Association's matrix of community-based resource is described with much greater emphasis on consumers and consumer-led initiatives and the value of enpowerment.

The main issues lie in implementing these recommendations. At the national and provincial level, the creation of strong mechanisms or separate envelopes for mental health services encounter strong resistance from other health and social services sectors. First, for simple resources competition reasons. Second because a public health and systemic approach is to be pursued, then a parallel system is difficult to sustain. At a local level, the setting of targets, goals and standards require leadership and strong stakeholder participation – a difficult mixture to achieve. The current book suggests that the matrix and evidence-based approaches, counterbalanced by ethical and clinical values, would be of help in the pursuit of a community-based system of mental health care. It seems that the issue is less one of a new conceptual framework, although useful and sound that may be as we will see below, but to ensure a process of reform with the largest number of stakeholders involved and committed to its pursuits, not in isolation. Two further values should therefore be added to those suggested in the application of the matrix: (a) empowerment of stakeholders as suggested by the Canadian Mental Health Association and (b) knowledge transfer.

15.4 **The geographical dimension of the matrix**

From the above description of the Canadian context, it would appear quite easy to ascribe the matrix geographical levels to each. At the country/region level comes the provincial government, duly elected and whose Ministry of Health and Social Services plans, budgets, monitors and directs the regional boards. The federal government provides general health policies, national norms (universality, accessibility, limitations on private schemes and over-billing, transferability of entitlements between provinces) that govern transfer payments to provinces, running and commissioning innovative programme development, evaluation and guidelines (such as the Best Practices Book, Health & Welfare Canada, 1997). At this level also would fit the regional boards. The decentralisation movement has rendered this level responsible for planning, budgeting, allocating funds to various components of the regional health, social services and non-profit and community agencies. The size of the 18 regional boards in a province such as Québec with over 7 million inhabitants will vary, from over a million and a half for Montreal-centre region to less than half a million in rural or remote areas. Three Canadian government levels would therefore be included at this level of the matrix, but with their functions as described, it is quite easy to categorise them and to relate their roles.

Mental health is not entitled to a specific federal or provincial budget, nor is a specific agency responsible for the functions described above. In other provinces such as Ontario or New Brunswick, directorates or commissions existed but have been disbanded recently. The regional boards in Québec often have a mental health direction that helps with the planning, recommendation for allocation and co-ordination, but has no control on the budgets, which rest with the Board itself. At the bottom of the geographical dimension, the patient/provider level is quite straightforward and poses no problem at classification and delimitation of its domains. No, the problem rests with ensuring the leadership and the boundaries at the local level.

At first sight, if one considers the east-end Montreal, the situation would be clear in this psychiatric hospital dominated local system of services for the mentally ill. The hospital has a sub-regional responsibility for the catchment area of 341000 inhabitants, but the territorial activity is organised around community psychiatric clinics close to the CLSCs territories, on average of 50000 inhabitants. However, most clinics will tend to divide again their work around one to three teams of five mental health workers according to the needs emerging from the area's clinic.

At the provincial level in Québec, the CLSCs are now claiming responsibility and funds for home care. Some areas are moving existing out-patient psychiatric services staff into the CLSCs. In one area, there were talks of disbanding an hospital-based Assertive Community Treatment team, considered a form of home care, and to relocate staff in various CLSCs, therefore losing the central ingredient to ACT and not even ensuring that teams focus on SMI. Now it could be argued that CLSCs have a natural role for co-ordinating primary health and mental health care for the common mental disorders, but how will it ensure the necessary protection of ACT workers among the other responsibilities of CLSC (prevention, promotion, entry point and primary health and social services)?

On the other hand, many university-based hospitals and psychiatric services are rapidly moving towards the American model of specialised clinics to ensure better research, training and treatment. Even if the services keep a catchment-area responsibility, these organisations tend to desert the leadership for the care of SMI and seem quite ready to leave the responsibility to the CLSCs, and to non-profit organisations, with their own role limited to admissions, assessment, medication and consultation. Finally, some areas are so deprived of resources, for example psychiatrists, that primary care providers have long assumed the responsibility for the care of SMI. Current reorganisation would create regional GPs' departments with responsibility to ensure services in a given region or sub-region, including CLSCs territories. All these forces therefore act differently according to the local area history, geography and socio-economic and cultural context. This renders difficult the standardisation of local boundaries in Québec for services and for clear responsibilities.

Some help may come from the recognition that locally there shall be a well-identified specialised team, adequately trained, ensured of existence if continuity of care is to be maintained. This would help in delimiting what is operating best at the local area level – be it based on CLSCs' territories or other administrative boundaries such as psychiatric sectors. Also, a sub-regional territory, greater than the usual 50 000 inhabitants, maybe in the 250 000 range, would often be necessary locally to have the critical mass for some rehabilitation and residential services (such as sheltered workshop, hostel wards) or forensic services.

15.5 **The temporal dimension of the matrix**

A joint France–Québec committee has received a mandate to produce a document on the tools national, regional and local planners shall have to plan according to needs. Interestingly, the committee has also suggested a conceptual matrix of needs with one axis being needs for whom (users, families, non-profit organisations, primary care providers, specialists, local, regional and provincial/national planners). The second axis represents a temporal sequence of (1) identifying problems; (2) defining the appropriate interventions; (3) determining the services to deliver these interventions. A third axis encompasses promotion, prevention, treatment, rehabilitation. One important step of the committee was to conduct focus groups with provincial, and regional and local planners, clinicians and users, on their vision of what they require to plan and act according to needs. One key finding was not so much the lack of tools and resources, which was recognised, but rather how to use the results. In one region a major pilot epidemiological study produced quite precise rates of DSM-III-R disorders and of utilisation of services for mental health reasons, but no use was made of these data in the regional planning documents, except to mention it.

As proposed, the temporal axis presents the input, process and outcome classic dimensions stemming from public health perspective. Even though they have not been formerly identified by most respondents in our focus group, they would quite easily be accepted. The tools proposed to assess these dimensions would also raise consensus. First, there would be easy recognition that patient-based outcome tools have been well developed by evaluative research. There would also be recognition that instruments and methods need to be developed to assess the various dimensions, in particular process. There would be no dispute that a variety of tools and methods would be appropriate: at the national/provincial and regional level, key stakeholders focus group (a qualitative approach to process and outcome);

literature and other jurisdictions comparisons (qualitative and at times quantitative approaches to needs, input and process); budget analyses (quantitative economic approach to inputs and processes); beds utilisation (process).

Consider also how the local area of east-end Montreal conducted outcome studies on the impact of new residential settings and rehabilitation programs for SMI at the patient outcome and process level (Lesage & Morissette, 1993); how the hospital started quality programmes in all its administrative and clinical programmes (local outcome); how local needs were modelled according to socio-economic variables (input on needs) (Lesage *et al.*, 1997); or how recently a survey was conducted to assess the needs for acute care beds and alternatives to admission (input on needs, local and patients level). There would finally be recognition that known tools are not sufficiently implemented, the best known example being a Mental Health Information System whose absence is noticeable in all Canadian Provinces with the exception of Saskatchewan and local areas such as Kingston in Ontario.

The train is running, and the concepts will become better known and tools will be further developed towards being more user-friendly as indicated in this book. However, a limitation will persist and is related to the finding described above in the focus groups: how to use the results and how to articulate them in the dynamic process of planning and evaluation. The temporal dimension of the matrix presents an analytical, rather static approach to represent the dynamic process of evaluation and planning. If researchers may feel more at ease with such an analytical perspective, planners will be ill at ease because of their need to integrate the results in the dynamics of planning and managing services within the local, regional and national historic, socio-economic and cultural context. Models of utilisation, of development and of transferring this source of knowledge need to be researched. The Canadian Best Practices (Health & Welfare Canada, 1997) underlined the following context: skilled leadership and committed, expert staff; clearly articulated philosophy, principles and vision; infrastructure support; and political will. It has not sufficiently developed how all stakeholders shall be included in the process, how information shall be shared, transferred and developed by users, non-profit organisations and clinical staff.

15.6 **Service components**

The key services components examined by the Canadian Best Practices in Reforming Mental Health Services (Health & Welfare Canada,

1997) are presented under two headings: core services and support; system reform strategies. Core services and supports include (1) assertive community treatment/case management; (2) crisis response/emergency services; (3) housing/community support; (4) in-patient/out-patient services; (5) consumer self-help and other consumer initiatives; (6) family self-help; (7) vocational and educational. The system reform strategies would touch policy, governance & fiscal dimensions, evaluation and human resources. They imply components such as common vision, broad stakeholder involvement, covering key issues, protected, and separate funding envelope, mental health authority, fiscal incentives, monitoring of activities, continuous quality improvement, staff redeployment strategies, training and reskilling, and opportunities for consumers to be providers.

There are several similarities with many of the service components described in Chapters 1–3 of this book. The necessity of two headings also refer to the concepts of segmental and systemic approaches to planning or the horizontal versus vertical application of different values (i.e. continuity, comprehensiveness, accountability) illustrated in Chapters 10 and 11. There is no choice between these approaches; a system should possess the capacity to accommodate all of them. A good system depends on its capacity to allow a flow of information about input, processes and results, into loops from top down and from bottom up (Wing *et al.*, 1992). It depends more importantly on its capacity to allow stakeholders the power to inform and be informed, to participate in the planning, and allocation of resources and evaluation, and finally the power to act. It relies more precisely on the capacity to involve staff in the reform.

A recent study of the attitudes and opinions about psychiatric rehabilitation among staff of one of the largest psychiatric hospitals in Canada illustrates these issues (Bonin *et al.*, 1998). Using focus-group approach to elicit staff views, the analysis confronted this with known rehabilitation theories. It found ward staff holding a humanistic view centred on the importance of the relationship and practising many, but not all, principles of psychiatric rehabilitation. However, the concepts of rehabilitation are hardly recognised except by rehabilitation professionals of the same hospital, often working in isolation from ward staff. These findings challenge the values often attributed to psychiatric hospital staff, as in chapter 12.

More importantly, the reforms towards community-based services has often proceeded with little regard for the patients and staff left behind in psychiatric hospitals. Yet, despite downsizing of most and closures of many psychiatric hospitals in the years ahead, only Italy is planning to close all its psychiatric hospitals. All other countries involved in the present book plan to retain psychiatric hospitals in 10 years from now. In all cases, staff from these hospitals will continue to work inside the hospital or be deployed outside. These staff has been disempowered by lack of recognition, by stigmatisation by the community-based movement, and by lack of training and information transfer. Further organisational analysis would indicate how they have been stripped of the means to act by the decisions of other stakeholders, who are themselves much less in contact. It could therefore be argued (Bachrach, 1996) that the future of the reform lies with the integration, not the exclusion of psychiatric hospitals in a systemic, not segmental, planning of services. Such planning at the provincial, regional and local level may involve the closure of psychiatric hospitals, certainly their transformation, but not without the close participation of their staff. Secondly, it calls for the empowering of ward staff to act, and for bringing professional and administrative efforts to build a team around the key relationship with ward staff. The empowerment of staff in all service components, including psychiatric hospitals, is the key to the pursuit and renewal of a successful reform.

15.7 Steps in reforming mental health services

The first step relates to a clear vision and political will. If the former is pervasive in many federal and provincial policy documents, the latter may be lacking at the moment. In the introduction, I argued that the current deinstitutionalisation and community care was launched in the 1960s in Canada and (as can be seen in this book), in many countries with various speed, but nonetheless has been relentlessly pursued. I also stated that the movement launched with strong political and public support has never been challenged. At least in Canada, it would be difficult to state that the movement is now stirring public enthusiasm. As such it has become a quiet revolution that is being pursued by the public institutions, much without fanfare. Nobody is opposing the movement.

But this absence of enthusiasm and strong political stamina keep the public institutions from encroaching on the decentralisation movement in health and social services and ensuring strong specific mental health governance, with power at provincial and regional levels on ring-fenced budgets, and clear co-ordinating powers with fiscal incentives and clear accountability. In such a system, the matrix would be a natural conceptual and measurement tool for planners, researchers, clinicians, users and relatives. But at the moment, at best, it is just utopia. Can it be of help now for planners and clinicians, community groups, users and relatives?

It is certainly an educational tool that would help bring the system forward. First, the matrix fosters a system vision. It is implicit in this book, and it has been the foundation of the Health Systems Research Unit at the Clarke Institute of Psychiatry in Toronto that has conducted the Best Practices in Reforming Mental Health Services' study, so often referred to in this chapter to support the matrix model's relevance in the Canadian context. Thinking in terms of a system means considering components interacting, considering components with a partial vision of each other, considering components that depend on each other's coherence to deliver care adequately. The matrix itself is also educational for the various actors of the mental health system. It provides a map to identify where efforts should be directed.

But the matrix has limitations that stem from its analytical standpoint and not integrating well the dynamic perspective. Its historical perspective has failed to recognise the past accomplishments and how at any point in the past decades, tremendous advances have been achieved. A body of knowledge, theoretical and practical, has been built up about treating, rehabilitating and maintaining the majority of people with SMI in the community and relying ever less on institutional care. One could even name these advances in mental health care 'health technologies'. Yes, so much remains to be done, but so much has been accomplished over the past decades and so much is done every day. We are part of a movement started long ago and with a long way to go. Let's be modest in judging past systems and humble in what can be accomplished in our own time.

The community care and deinstitutionalisation movement has not been linear, and has moved in cycles, or maybe in quantum leaps. Evaluation and planning also work in cycles (Wing, 1986) and these dynamics are currently pushing the current evidence-based approach to the forefront because they are best suited at this point in time. Knowledge-transfer is also the new paradigm supported by the recently created Canadian Health Services Research Fund and by the Quebec Health and Social Research Funds at a time where other health research funds have been frozen or reduced. Capturing these dynamics, but also the necessary interactions between the components of the matrix, would be essential if it is to be of help. Models of this type of utilisation could come from model areas that let researchers engage in action-research, by observing and detailing the process of developing, generating and transferring knowledge. Another break-through will come from the few individuals that can assume multiple roles – researchers, planners, clinicians and clinical decision-makers (Wasylenki & Goering, 1995). These authors recommend that researchers be prepared to assume multiple roles in the service delivery field, so as to reduce the gap between science and practice. Finally, national planners and organisations shall themselves open up to scrutiny and part of action research their current mental health reforms, how to put in place an improved system of mental health care.

References

Bachrach, L. (1996). The state of the state mental hospital in 1996. *Psychiatric Services*, 47, 1071–1978.

Bonin, J. P., Lesage, A. D., Ricard, N., Demers, M., & Morissette, R. & Benoit, D. (1998). Empowering the staff in long-stay wards. *Canadian Journal of Psychiatry*, 43, 1055.

Deci, P. A., Santos, A. B., Hiott, W. B., Schoenwald, S. & Dias, J. K. (1995). Dissemination of assertive community treatment programs. *Psychiatric Services*, 46, 676–678.

Goering, P., Wasylenki, D. & MacNaughton, E. (1992). Planning mental health services: II. Current Canadian initiatives. *Canadian Journal of Psychiatry*, 37, 259–263.

Health & Welfare Canada (1997). *Best Practices in Mental Health Reform*. Prepared by the Health Systems Research Unit & Clarke Institute of Psychiatry Consulting Group. Ottawa: Health & Welfare Canada.

Hôpital Louis-H. Lafontaine (1997) *Plan de Transformation. Les Orientations et le Modèle d'Organisation des Services en Psychiatrie*. Montréal: Hôpital Louis-H. Lafontaine.

Knapp, M. (1997) Economics and mental health: a concise European history of demand and supply. In *Making Rational Mental Health Services, Epidemiologia e psichiatria sociale Monograph Supplement 1* (ed. M. Tansella), pp. 157–166.

Knapp, M. & Beecham, J. (1990) *Dowries, Report to the Cross Financing Review Group*, Discussion Paper 711, Personal Social Services Research Unit, University of Kent at Canterbury.

Lafave, H. G. & Grunberg, F. (1974). La fin de l'asile. *Information Psychiatrique*, 50(5), 525–535.

Lesage, A. D. & Morissette, R. (1993) Residential and palliative needs of persons with severe mental illness who are subject to long-term hospitalization. *Mental Health in Canada*, Spring, 13–18.

Lesage, A. D. & Tansella, M. (1993) Comprehensive community care without long-stay beds in mental hospitals: trends emerging from an Italian good practice area. *Canadian Journal of Psychiatry*, 38, 187–194.

Lesage, A. D., Clerc, D., Tourjman, V., Cournoyer, J., Fabian, J., Van Haaster, I. & Chang, C.-H. (1997) Estimating local-area needs for psychiatric care: a case study. *British Journal of Psychiatry*, 169, 49–57.

Ministère de la santé et des services sociaux du Québec (MSSS) (1997). *Orientations Pour La Transformation des Services De Santé Mentale*. Québec: Direction De La Planification et de L'évaluation, MSSS.

Ontario Ministry of Health (1993) *Putting People First. The Reform Of Mental Health Services In Ontario*. Toronto: Ontario Ministry of Health.

Rochefort, D. A. (1992). More lessons, of a different kind: Canadian mental health policy in comparative perspective. *Hospital and Community Psychiatry*, **43**, 1083–1090.

Wasylenki, D. A., Goering, P. N. (1995). The role of research in systems reform. *Canadian Journal of Psychiatry*, **40**, 247–251.

Wing, J. K. (1986) The cycle of planning and evaluation. In *The Provision Of Mental Health Services In Britain. The Way Ahead* (ed. G. Wilkinson & H. Freeman), pp 35–48. London: Gaskell.

Wing, J. K., Brewin, C. R. & Thornicroft, G. (1992). Defining mental health needs. In *Measuring Mental Health Needs* (ed. G. Thornicroft, C. Brewin, & J. Wing). London: Gaskell.

16

Central and Eastern European countries
TOMA TOMOV

16.1 Overview of the historical development of mental health services in the Region

The countries in the Region differ in the degree to which they have been involved as territories and cultural settings in the emergence of Western Civilization. Whereas the countries of Central Europe such as Poland, the Czech Republic and Hungary have been fully integrated in the processes of carving human individuality out of a diffuse primitive group identity reaching back several centuries and variously referred to as capitalist development, scientific revolution or Renaissance, the countries further East or Southeast, such as Russia, Ukraine and the Balkan states have stayed peripheral to these concerns largely because of their own major preoccupation – the Eastern Orthodox Religion and the Ottoman Empire. The resemblance between these two groups of countries, revealed to the observer when the Berlin Wall fell, turned out to be more apparent than real and quickly wore out as soon as the regimes of total control were toppled and the peoples were free once again to get in touch with their own histories and cultural processes.

For reasons of simplicity the countries of the former Eastern block will be referred to throughout the chapter as 'the Region'. The list of these countries will include the Newly Independent States (e.g. Russia, Ukraine, Belarus, Moldova), the countries of the Caucasus region (e.g. Georgia, Armenia, Azerbaijan), the countries of Central Asia (e.g. the Kirghiz Republic), the Baltic countries, the Balkan countries (e.g. Bulgaria, Yugoslavia, Romania, Albania, Croatia, Macedonia, Bosnia and Herzegovina) and the countries of Central Europe.

In spite of profound historical and cultural differences all the countries in question pledge, though in varying degree, their belonging to the cultural tradition of Europe. They regard their current mental health services as originating from the collective practice to apply to certain aberrations in human behaviour the explanatory mechanism of illness, rather than that of demonic possession, a shift usually dated in late fifteen and early sixteen century. Similarly to the rest of Europe the institutional response to this shift in beliefs in the Region was the asylum, a move motivated by concerns for the safety of the 'regular' citizens, rather than by compassion for the sick. It was initially the Church and later (second half of sevententh century) the municipalities, which were entrusted with the provision of the asylums as places primarily not intended to provide treatment, but ending up about a century later with adoption of non-restraint policies and thus becoming psychiatric hospitals (Kanabih, 1928).

The common history, which these countries shared over the past 50 years as members of the socialist family, has brought about similarities between them in the beliefs held about mental health and in the practices guided by these beliefs, which set them apart from the rest of Europe. Some of these countries, notably those of Central Europe, avoided fully complying with the organisational model imposed by the socialist health care doctrine on psychiatry. No country avoided, however, the dehumanising effects on professional attitudes of the disrespect for individual dignity propagated by socialist ideology. It should not come as a surprise, therefore, that the current psychiatric scene in the Region is dominated by concerns about psychiatric reforms, the preoccupation being with *professional ethics* and *needs assessment*.

The centrality of ethics is an expression of the will of the professional communities to take human dignity seriously, by going beyond the assertion of humanistic values to enforce the observance of patients' rights through legislative measures and legal and administrative procedures. This is very much in line with the cultural tradition of Western Civilization, and in stark contrast to the practice of totalitarianism to disempower individuals and groups by depriving them of the right to opinion, and by severely punishing impulses to self-authorisation such as taking initiative or risks.

The salience of ethical concerns among the profession in the Region at this point reflects decades of negligence of this aspect of care provision and a growing awareness of the serious biases in the service design which have resulted from this. The period between the end of World War Two and the fall of the Berlin Wall witnessed throughout the Region the unfolding of a public health doctrine known as socialist health care. It was notorious for the disregard of individual needs and the neglect of the role of human context (e.g. family life, doctor–patient relationship, etc.). Under it the mental health sector was set apart from the rest of health care: from the primary care level to the specialist care level mental health was equipped with its own structures, cadre and lines of operation which did not liaise to general health and social services. Reductionist biological theories about mental health and ill-health were imposed in the Region as part of an ideology-driven effort. Primitive and mystic attitudes to mental illness acquired in childhood were left unchallenged at all stages of the professional training of doctors. The psychiatric dispensary was brought into existence. It was designed to extend the control over the patient beyond the walls of the hospital into the community. Said to provide comprehensiveness and continuity of care, the psychiatric dispensary in fact acted as a vehicle to export custodial culture into millions of families and small communities. As a result social stigma and prejudice against the mentally ill infiltrated public attitudes even more.

The *assessment of needs* as a point of departure in setting out strategic goals for mental health is not a tradition of central planning in the Region. Rather than develop health strategies, timetables and outlines of service inputs and service processes to meet needs, health planners have been working by annual adjustments to the funds allotted to mental health. In this they were guided by forecasts of economic growth and by political concerns. Admittedly, both of these could only very crudely reflect mental health needs. The present concern with needs assessment in the Region is in response to the challenge of transition from a service-led planning to a needs-led planning. The former is dear to staff as a paragon of security. The latter requires the skill of construing the psychiatric scene realistically and on the basis of evidence, as well as the development of methods and instruments for obtaining such evidence, which work under the circumstances in the Region. In addition, awareness is growing that the perception of needs by the mental health professionals may be different from that of the care consumers, their families, the professionals from other sectors such as education and police and the public at large. Who should become involved at what level and to what degree with needs assessment is another issue which very few are as yet prepared to face constructively.

Eight years into the transition to market economy there is still very little *deliberation* among the mental health profession in the region as to how to approach health services in terms of considerations of ethics and cost-effective management. In most former Soviet countries this can be explained with the fact that health economics has not been put on the political agenda yet. The politicians in Central Europe, the Balkans and the Baltic states, however, have arrived at the conclusion that public accountability in the health field is now imperative and that the practice of decision-making should adjust to its demands. The technological solutions for this are however still not found. One would expect that their search would engage academics and researchers from the Region in a passionate professional discourse. This is hardly the case.

A search of the field reveals changes in the health *legislation* in the Region, which are driven by efforts to bring the countries' legal systems in line with EU requirements and dwell on extrapolations from studies and experiences accumulated in the West. Poland, for example, developed a programme which specified in detail the community and hospital services as well as the manpower needs, which derive from a formulated national mental health strategy turned into a law in August 1994. Russia, by comparison, changed in a far less radical way: it passed a mental health law in July 1992, which went a long way to protect the human rights of the mentally sick, but did not question the established conceptual and organisational basis of care provision in the country (Law of the Russian Federation on Psychiatric Care, 1992). Other former Soviet states followed the example of Moscow, notably Ukraine, Georgia and Lithuania. Many of the other countries in the Region introduced changes into the existing legislation. The impression which this development leaves is that reforms in the Region, to the extent to which they exist, leave out the professional and academic communities and their practices.

A review of the standard reading lists provided to students in the mental health field in the Region reveals virtually no difference between the pre-1989 period and now: there is a dominating presence of texts written in the Soviet style, i.e. authoritative statements wanting both in evidence (from research or experience) and in argumentation. Even the best specimens among them (e.g. Kabanov, 1985; Litvienko, 1989; Aleksandrowicz, 1994; Achkova, 1996; Solojenkin, 1997) betray a lack of awareness about the paradigmatic nature of scientific knowledge in general and of the explanatory schemes informing mental health action, in particular. These texts often convey a disregard for the need of authors to be aware of the position from within which they make pronouncements. An example of this would be indictments of backwardness which fail to take into account the impeding effects of the institutional arrangements within the context of which care is provided.

A regional conference on mental *health economics* held in Budapest in the summer of 1996 attracted reports from many countries in the Region. The presenters were young, had arrived to health economics as a result of non-traditional career opportunities opened by sponsors (e.g. the Open Society Institute, financed by the American billionaire George Soros), and sought to engage in a dialogue with each other in spite of lack of a common language.

Their contributions suggested the importance of a conceptual frame and tradition and revealed a lot of anxiety and uncertainty as to the future of the field.

In the course of the last 10 years a reformist movement building around the Netherlands-based Geneva Initiative on Psychiatry Foundation (Tomov, 1997) has put sharply into focus the close interrelation between *professional attitudes*, including ethical principles, and mental health practices, indicating that the divorce between obsolete values and advanced technologies witnessed throughout the Region brings about the peculiar intellectual impotence in the field of training, research and management of mental health reforms (Tomov & Butorin, 1996).

Against the background of this brief historical account it appears that the matrix model promises to be exactly the tool which is deemed necessary to the local professional communities in the Region in their attempts to address their major concerns with mental health reforms. A more detailed investigation of the application of the matrix model to the psychiatric scene in the Region will be done in the sections that follow.

16.2 **The geographical levels of the matrix model: are they applicable?**

The administrative division of the territory in the countries of the Region is of long-standing tradition and the distinction between local and central administration is clearly made and earnestly maintained. Centre-versus-periphery is a dimension of very vibrant meaning in all countries and all sectors. The denial of the right of the local representatives to be outspoken about the interests of their constituencies was brought to an end by the developments of 1989.

In almost all the countries of the Region the overwhelming emphasis on central planning has left behind a pattern of solutions found and a tradition of decision-making which have many deficiencies. These deficiencies come immediately into focus when seen against the background of the matrix model. An example here would be the uneven spread of psychiatric beds across this country's territory: three- to four-fold difference in rates will not be unusual, as is for instance the case with Bulgaria (Achkova *et al.*, 1997). The inconvenience that this creates to patients and their families, the limitations it imposes on the application of intervention methods, particularly those targeted at re-integration and various other less obvious implications, have certainly been seen before but have been dismissed as minor side-effects of an overall correct and advanced health policy. Such an interpretation of these observations is no longer possible within the matrix model framework. Within it, these facts reveal that the decision-making had been left with the wrong geographical level of the health system.

The legacy in this respect left behind in most countries from the Region is grave and may cool the enthusiasm of even the strongest supporters of reforms. To give an example, closing beds in one part of the country and opening beds at the same time in another is fully unacceptable to unenlightened central bureaucracies, and is seen as indulgence in recently acquired freedoms by the local administrations. Central bureaucracies still have a very strong grip over the countries in the Region, and impose on governments their choice of course to be followed independently of the political orientation of the cabinets.

If used to guide the allocation of decision-making to geographical levels, the matrix model could prevent further misconceptions. An immediate effect could be gained in the Region from basing the annual statistics about the utilisation of services on the territorial division of the country rather than obtaining data from each health facility separately and processing it at the national level as is often the case now. The adoption of the matrix model will ensure better use of the available information and will enhance the relevance of the decisions to the local situation. An additional effect will be the participation of middle level health managers in responsible decision-making, a practice which the total control systems deny to all, with the exception of the ones at the very top.

Regarding individual work with patients as a geographical level of activity fully comparable in terms of managerial decision-making with the local service level, and the central administration level, is certainly unusual to the culture of clinical psychiatry in the countries from the Region. The model in which psychiatrists and other staff construe their professional identities is still very much the fantasy figure of the omnipotent doctor who triumphs over death and sickness and leaves cost-effectiveness to managers and economists. Partnership (and the humility it implies) in developing the doctor–patient relationship is experienced as puzzling at best, and threatening and risky at worst. Patient behaviour, complementary as it is to that of the doctors, unsurprisingly is predominantly passive and helpless. Doctors and patients alike regard what they do in therapy only as a process of applying what others had invented, decided or ordered. This generates an unpleasant feeling of impersonal and uninvolved relating. The advent of markets in the field of health, which come unheralded and unregulated, forces changes on doctors and other staff. Entrepreneurship of all shades abounds as does the belief in the unlimited regulatory potential of the health insurance principle.

All the above observations are illustrated by material brought into the training sessions over a period of two years by a group of 15 Ukrainian psychiatric nurses, who were introduced through case-work, role-play, tutoring and supervision to case-management and team-work. Individual sessions with patients were vehemently avoided by the nurses in training until it transpired that any exchange in private between nurse and patients rendered the nurse liable to prosecution, as privacy implied objectionable conduct (Tomov *et al.*, 1995).

To conclude, the benefits of self-management by psychiatric staff are beginning to be learned in the Region; conceptualising clinical work in such terms (and the change of attitudes this implies) is spreading fast, thus rendering the matrix model's geographical dimension fully relevant to the realities in the Region.

16.3 The temporal dimension of the matrix model: is it relevant to the Region?

The temporal dimension even more than the geographical dimension implies role blurring: clinician, manager, researcher, public health man – which hat does the doctor wear and when? It is this demand for a flexible professional self-concept which the matrix model puts forth, that reveals the most unfortunate deficit of the human resources in the Region – the *rigidity of minds*.

The temporal dimension of the matrix model assumes that innovation is a permanent component of all levels and that what is at stake is how to proceed with it in a systematic way. Thus one's preoccupation with the positive change in one's performance and the better outcome of one's work is taken for granted. This assumption dwells on the world view espoused by professionals in market economies. In economies of central planning this world view is virtually extinct. An example could clarify this comment. In many of the countries of the Region psychiatry comes in two varieties: hospitals and dispensaries. No matter how insistently you ask a doctor employed by one such institution about the service profile of his hospital or dispensary, you will not get a description, because all dispensaries are believed to be virtually identical and so are all hospitals. They have been made to be identical. If one of them changes, it will not be because the doctors employed there chose to introduce one programme, rather than another, for a certain reason. The only conceivable way to change is as a result of following directives to that effect from the Centre.

A special issue here is that what was called 'rigidity of minds' above and what was traced to a social (and professional) arrangement known as 'central planning', has an attitudinal as well as a cognitive component. Whereas at the cognitive level awareness of the limiting effects of one's rigidity of mind on one's social (and professional) participation can be gained and its maladaptive effects in a market economy setting can be comprehended, this does not imply that at the attitudinal level similar progress can be made as easily. Attitudes change only gradually: the more fully one is involved in a new practice the faster the process of change will be. It is this reasoning which renders the matrix model and its temporal dimension in particular a very appropriate tool to the tasks now at hand on the mental health scene in the Region: it puts change permanently on the agenda and supplies the method for managing it.

The activities in the Input Phase of the temporal dimension are about to become possible in many countries of the Region as a result of their transformation into democracies. Public debates on health budgets, legislation and needs assessment are being held now in practically all of the countries and create a growing demand for evidence-based argumentation.

The Process and Outcome Phases suggest analyses and use of indicators. This was a widely misused practice under the total control regimes. The managerial culture created by the planned economy encouraged a process whereby positive indicators took on normative functions (Murray, 1996) virtually overnight. This need not be blamed on the individuals involved since they were compelled to present reports pleasing to the ear. The attitude of mind of all engaged in the collecting, handling and analyses of the data was nevertheless heavily influenced by this injunction. It is therefore imperative that a very different professional culture be brought into existence in the countries of the Region for collection of evidence, and for evidence-based decision-making to become established.

To summarise, the applicability of the temporal dimension of the matrix model to the countries in the Region is conditional on several preliminary steps and to precipitate them is a real challenge. These steps have to do with the removal of obstacles left as a legacy of the regimes of total control. They concern the managerial culture in health care in general. One such obstacle is the tradition to base decisions on beliefs rather than evidence. Another obstacle is the disavowal of the differences in the clinical profiles of institutions: making the existing clinical profiles explicit will legitimise variability and will facilitate doctors in taking authority for the work they do and for changing it. Yet another obstacle arises from the need for the accumulation of a critical mass of like-minded individuals for a paradigmatic shift in the managerial culture of health care to occur in the Region. The reform-minded psychiatrists are in the minority in each country and meet with very strong opposition from the conservative academic establishment. The chances for reformers lie in investing heavily in networking with the reformist groups in the Region and with the rest of European psychiatry.

16.4 **The relevance of the service components to the countries from the Region**

In most of the clinical settings in the Region the notion of service does not imply humility on the part of the providers, contiguous upon the centrality of the sick individual to the whole practice of mental health care and its superstructures. The prevalent attitude is rather one of impassive paternalistic condescension. The projection of this attitude in the practice of health management is often demonstrated in the expectation on patients to adjust their problems to the existing programmes and to self-censure themselves with respect to needs which are not legitimised by the existence of provisions to meet them.

Even a scant inspection of the affairs in the Region in the field of service provision reveals the lack of discourse based on correct reasoning and probability as a prelude to accountable decision-making in this most difficult area. Interestingly, ideas of community mental health and the range of new skills, practices and infrastructures that can make it happen are discussed and the general familiarity with the key notions of reformed psychiatry is quite high. This knowledge does not translate, however, into practical action but remains limited to academic debates. A crucial societal mechanism whereby authority is lent to individuals to undertake change with due awareness of the risks involved, somehow fails bitterly and results in severe diffidence which blocks action.

In the field of service provision more than in any other the Matrix Model reveals the amount of work that needs to be done in every country of the Region for accountable mental health care to become possible. At present, there is a general recognition of the fact of confusion though no clear idea of the degree of mismanagement exists yet. An assessment of mental health needs as a basis for planning can provide a big impetus to the service development in the Region. The methodology should, however, take into account the general paucity of societal and institutional structures, the low level of managerial sophistication of the average professional and the necessity to introduce by way of training the paradigm within which such an exercise makes sense.

The service provision and service utilisation data, as already mentioned, available though they are in the Region, are of unknown validity and come in sets and combinations which render them of little use for improving the capacity and variety of the service components. There is an obvious need throughout the Region to adopt classifications of service components, which derive from notions of reformed practice.

To summarise, the Matrix Model suggests the methodology needed for the countries in the Region to streamline their efforts when and if they decide to establish a sound base for mental health services.

16.5 Steps to reforming mental health in the region: is the matrix model relevant?

The political will to re-form mental health care does not derive necessarily from logical reasoning on the basis of facts about abominable conditions in institutions and abuse of individual freedoms and rights. The political will to re-form in the Region is generated by pressure from professional groups, concerned with restoring the independent status of their profession, by activities of consumer groups driven by unmet needs, by economic interests of all sorts and by many other factors.

The question faced by the countries in the Region is how to translate all this will into the coordinated effort that the seven-step procedure of the matrix model implies. Traditionally, the most common approach has been to enforce top-down. This creates a serious risk that the mental health reform may be approached in a similar doctrinaire fashion.

Caution against such developments suggests that step one put forward by the matrix model – establishing the service principles – is of more than trivial importance in the Region. To those who have first-hand experience with psychiatric practice there it should be clear that this step has been taking place in an unpremeditated way for several years already in most of the countries and is far from finished. It can be argued that forcing too ambitious a programme or too fast a pace at too early a stage can easily compromise the whole exercise. The political development in Russia, for instance, as a result of which a new mental health act was passed, is an illustration of a very positive step which came too early – a mismatch which thwarted much of the positive effect the legislation might have had if similar developments at the service level had taken place simultaneously.

An analysis of developments in the Region points to the importance of confronting those who are motivated in one way or another to challenge the institution of psychiatry with the attitude they hold. This attitude shows not so much in the contents of their arguments, as in the methods by which they argue. Disclosures occur in the course of group and inter-group inter-actions which constitute the human process of the incipient reform in the Region. A not uncommon result from the awareness gained from facing one's own attitudes is a shift in emphasis towards changing the internal structure of one's own mind, rather than the institution of psychiatry.

To summarise, the matrix model of the reform process beautifully captures the complexity of this process, and reveals the need of a sufficient level of structural complexity within professional and other communities as well as within the human mind to guide the reform process properly.

16.6 **The main issues to be addressed in the Region over the next five years**

Gaining awareness of attitudes and their role as well as recognition of needs as perceived by health consumers and others outside the psychiatric profession are two overlapping domains, which need to be opened in the public discourse on reforms in the Region. The effect of such a development will be mostly in establishing, in much more detail than is possible now, the differences that have been accumulated over the years in the Region as a result of the disavowal of the ethical foundations of psychiatric practice. It is against this background that plans for reform can be safeguarded against the distorting effects of the legacy of central planning.

International collaboration at all levels – individual, local and central – with countries which have advanced considerably with reforming their mental health systems can be of particular value.

References

Achkova, M. (ed.) (1996). *A Textbook of Psychiatry* (in Bulgarian). Sofia: Znanie Publishers.

Achkova, A., Tomov, T., Yadkova, L., Velinov, V., Gerdjikov, I., Jivkov, L., Boyadjiev, B., Radev, K., Sedefov, R. and Arsenov G. *Report to the Minister of Health*. Bulletin of the Bulgarian Psychiatric Association (in Bulgarian), 1,27.

Aleksandrowicz, J. (1994). *Psychotherapia Medyczna* (in Polish), Wydawnictwo Lekarskie. Warszawa: PZWL.

Kabanov, M. (1985). *Rehabilitation of Psychiatric Patients* (in Russian) Leningrad: State Medical Publishing House.

Kanabih, U. (1928). *History of Psychiatry.* Leningrad: State Medical Publishing House (in Russian).

Law of the Russian Federation on Psychiatric Care and the Guarantees of Citizens' Rights in Providing It (1992). Ussuriysk: ALGO (in Russian).

Litvienko, V. (1989). *Formation of Therapeutic Environments in Psychiatric Wards: A*

Methodological Guide. Poltava (Ukraine): Poltava Publishers.

Murray, C. (1996). Rethinking DALY's. In *The Global Burden of Disease*, Vol. 1 (ed. C. Murray and A. Lopez), p. 2. Geneva: WHO.

Solojenkin, V. (1997). *Psychological Foundations of Therapeutic Activity*. Kirghiz Republic (printed in Moscow): Soros Fund (in Russian).

Tomov, T. (1997). *Mental Health Care in Bulgaria*. Mental Health Reforms, 3, vol. 2. Hilversum: Geneva Initiative Publishers.

Tomov, T. & Butorin, N. (1996). *Views Held by Psychiatrists of Their Profession: Are there Differences between East and West?* Paper presented at the Fourth Meeting of Reformers in Psychiatry, Madrid, August 29–31.

Tomov, T., Fercheva, A. & Mihova, Z. (1995). *Professional Training for Psychiatric Nurses in Ukraine*. CEBEMO sponsored project. (Text available upon request).

Nordic European countries

POVL MUNK-JØRGENSEN

17.1 Brief historical overview of Danish psychiatry

In Denmark organised psychiatric treatment dates back to the beginning of the nineteenth century, with the establishment of the first asylum, now Sct. Hans Hospital, which opened in a former manor house in Roskilde southwest of Copenhagen, serving the capital, Copenhagen. In 1852 the asylum idea had gained much ground, and a new asylum was established north of Aarhus, the second largest town in Denmark. The asylum was built for the purpose and was designed by one of the leading Danish architects. It is my opinion that the ideas behind the asylums were far more epoch-making and visionary compared with the organisation, practice, knowledge and attitudes dominating in the mid-1800s than anything else which has been seen in psychiatric organisation since then. The asylum model dominated in Denmark until the Second World War.

Denmark had a psychiatric law (1938) and a social reform (1933), however, without a radical change in the concept of treatment. In Denmark this period was marked by the same progress within treatment as the rest of Europe, progress that I will not mention here, but a specifically new way of thinking which resulted in an important treatment facility, namely home care. Long-term patients from the psychiatric hospitals lived with private families, often farmers, under the inspection of the hospitals. This model faded out in the 1960s and the 1970s.

The asylum model was still in use in the post-war period when we in Denmark, in parallel with the beginning of the psychopharmacological era at the end of the 1950s, started establishing psychiatric departments at the general hospitals. The idea behind this development was a governmental order which emphasised the importance of an equality between psychiatry and the general medical specialities. From the 1960s and up to the 1980s this development was marked by the establishment of such departments at general hospitals alongside a gradual reduction of the capacity of the asylums.

The next phase, in the post-war period in the 1960s and 70s, was in its first part marked by an increasing extension of the psychopharmacological concept and towards the end a vehement conflict between established psychiatry and the anti-psychiatric movement. In this period psychiatric treatment in Denmark was mainly based on psycho-pharmacology. Psychotherapeutic treatment took place on an elitist basis in a few places in Denmark, mostly in Copenhagen and Aarhus, without noticeable spread. A governmental order from the 1950s, and another from 1977, in relation to the transfer of psychiatry from the State to the counties, recommended the decentralisation of psychiatry. The first stage of reform in the 1950s recommended the co-ordination of psychiatry with the other medical specialities, as mentioned above, and resulted in the establishment of many psychiatric departments at general hospitals, while the second, which more or less recommended a community psychiatric model, was without impact. Community psychiatry in Denmark was only instituted in a few research projects, of which the internationally best known was the Samso-project, which was abolished in 1993.

The last years of the 1970s and 1980s can be characterised as the psychotherapeutic era, although this approach varied a great deal throughout the Nordic countries. Norwegian psychiatry had, over several years and much more intensively than Danish psychiatry, practised a psychodynamic psychotherapy, with the main stress on individual and group therapy, a model that Denmark to a lesser extent followed, while Finland has attached more importance to a family therapeutic model. The psychotherapeutic era in Denmark has almost had the character of a monopolised psychodynamic model, and only in the last few years, the mid-1990s, did the cognitive model, with an emphasis on the psycho-educative method, gain importance. The development of these cognitive methods now almost has the character of a flood.

The era of decentralisation/social psychiatry can be dated to the last years of the 1980s and until the present (1998). A Government Order in 1977 recommended that the counties, which had just taken over the responsibility for psychiatry in 1976, move towards decentralisation (in the terminology of that time: community psychiatry). It is hardly wrong to conclude that nothing really happened until the Minister of Health in 1988 demanded that all the Danish counties (14 in total, plus two municipalities, Frederiksborg and Copenhagen, which have the status of counties) create plans for the development of psychiatry in their areas. These plans, which were published in 1989, were marked by the inexperience of psychiatry in the counties. Several years went on before decentralisation changed from being plans and became reality, and only in the recent past (1995–98) have decentralised treatment and service facilities reached such a quality and quantity as to have assumed any importance in treatment.

The reduction of beds, mainly in the former asylums, which from having regional functions until 1976, afterwards served the counties in which they were located, began in the early 1970s and continued until the mid-1990s. From 1987 The Danish Medical Organisation and The Danish Psychiatric Society warned against continuous reduction in beds without the establishment of decentralised functions. The debate in Denmark took place between, on the one hand, the political organisations and administrative functions, and on the other hand the psychiatrists who were vehement, especially in the light of the appearance of a range of negative indicators such as an increasing number of suicides among psychotics compared with the general population, more homeless mentally disordered persons, increasing use of coercion in the psychiatric wards, and increasing criminality among psychiatric patients.

A new period seems to have begun in these years (1995–98), namely a neo-Kraepelinean, new-biological era, seen in a specialisation of functions with a consequent centralisation. This theme will be discussed in the last section of this chapter.

17.2 The three geographical levels

The three geographical levels model fits like a glove to the conditions existing in Denmark. Since the end of the 1980s the care concept in Danish psychiatry has been geography. Critics of the system ironically mention that mentally ill patients are treated according to their postal code instead of to their diagnosis. I will try to introduce a little more nuance into the discussion.

The authors of this book mention the country/regional level, the local level, and the patient level. In Denmark we employ more levels: the country level, the regional level, the county level (which is the local level), a sector level, further broken down in local area levels, and only hereafter the patient level. From a Danish perspective the country level is of minor importance. It has been like that since 1976, when the responsibility for psychiatry was transferred from the State to the counties. The counties were established in 1970, and immediately after they became responsible for the general hospital service and for psychiatry six years later. There are 14 counties in Denmark, of a size varying from about 200 000 to more than 600 000 inhabitants with the little county covering the island of Bornholm with only 45000 inhabitants constituting an exception. Two municipalities, namely Copenhagen with about 0.5 million inhabitants, and the small Frederiksberg which is surrounded by Copenhagen, have the same status as counties.

The State's influence on psychiatry is very limited. The Ministry of Health has limited direct influence. In the Danish counties the Ministry of Health is somewhat cheerfully referred to as the 'Ministry of Attitudes'. The Minister has, through the National Board of Health, a supervising function, however, with limited possibilities of intervention and sanction. Not even by economic means has it been possible for the State to control psychiatry. For instance, the State can not even assure that increasing subsidies to counties, granted with the direct purpose of consolidating psychiatry, will actually be used according to their intentions.

The 14 counties, and the two Copenhagen municipalities with county status, are fully responsible both for psychiatry and for other hospital services, and the counties have a right to the independent imposition of taxes. In some ways the transfer of psychiatry to the counties has been a great advantage. The close local organisation has been of benefit to psychiatry, mainly in terms of social services. The young counties' lack of experience in running hospitals seems to have resulted in a distinct lack of an empirical and scientific foundation in tracing, treatment and aftercare initiatives. Therefore, a marked heterogeneity is seen in the various counties' ways of performing these tasks, a heterogeneity that forms a contrast to the small geographical distances in Denmark, with a maximum of 350 kilometres from the east to the west, and from the north to the south, and to the small population of 5.2 million inhabitants. A tender beginning of co-operation between some neighbouring counties on the solutions to these issues on a regional level can be seen faintly, e.g. organisation of forensic psychiatry.

The autonomy of the counties can be exemplified by the organisation of the psychiatric services. Twelve counties, including the two Copenhagen municipalities, have organised their psychiatric services together with the rest of the secondary health care system, while four counties have disconnected psychiatry from the other health services; in two counties psychiatry has been transferred to social services, in another county a joint organisation has been established, including both a large part of the former social service and of psychiatry, and yet another county has established an equal model, but has now taken psychiatry back to the health service. A joint organisation together with the social service has been shown to be an advantage for increased resources, but not in terms of its cultural removal from the other medical specialities. This is an adverse development in a period where more and more evidence of a biological genesis of mental disorders accumulates.

The counties are further divided into sectors. For instance, the County of Aarhus is divided into five sectors, each with 110–130 000 inhabitants. These sectors are responsible for both hospital based and decentralised services for the mentally ill. The goal of sectorisation was to limit the catchment areas in geographical extent and number of inhabitants, so that the professionals who treat the patients could get the greatest possible local knowledge of the neighbourhood and of the patients and their network.

The disadvantages of the establishment of sectors have proved to be limited capacity in the hospital departments of the sectors. As a sector can only maintain a few wards, it has been necessary to treat acute and severe cases of different illness categories in the same physical settings, such as young severely maladjusted hebephrenic schizophrenics together with middle-aged, severely inhibited and anxious depressive patients. From this situation has arisen the ironical characteristic, as formerly mentioned, that patients are not treated according to diagnosis but to postal code. Recently, the problem is being addressed by the establishment of specialised functions and specialised wards, but as the resources for these establishments are mainly being taken from the already existing wards this causes further deterioration in the situation.

This becomes even more problematic when the sectors are subdivided. It has become the practice in Denmark to subdivide sectors into local areas with about 30–40 000 inhabitants. As for the sectors, the ideology is to promote the work of integration in the patient's environment. Although staff benefit from the advantages that such local knowledge brings about, it is a problem in that in the long run they may lose expertise. For example, in Denmark with about 5 million inhabitants there are 500 new cases of schizophrenia per year, i.e. one per 10 000 inhabitants. So in a local area of 30–40 000 inhabitants there will be 3–4 new cases of schizophrenia per year, and as the distribution is considerably skewed, with approximately half of the new cases in Copenhagen, it means that some rural areas may expect one or a maximum of two new cases of schizophrenia per year, not at all enough to maintain an expertise. Even more seldom will new cases of for example, eating disorders occur.

In terms of the patient level it might be appropriate to mention some figures. In 1996 the Danish psychiatric hospital service, including out-patient services and community services, was in contact with almost 70 000 persons, corresponding to between 13 and 14 per 1000 total inhabitants (1.3%–1.4%). If the approximately 30–40 000 persons who are treated in private practice are included, the figure will be about 100 000 corresponding to 19–20 per 1000 total population (1.9%–2.0%). In the Danish population approximately 18 000 persons diagnosed schizophrenic have at any time of their life been in contact with the public treatment system – corresponding to a prevalence of 0.3–0.4%. The public psychiatric system was in 1996 in contact with less than the half of these persons either at admission, out-patient treatment or community based service.

Although approximately 28% of the total of 1.5 million bed-days used in Denmark were used in treatment of schizophrenics, there is still a sharp contrast between the relatively few schizophrenic patients in treatment and the one-sided focus on treatment of schizophrenics in Denmark at present. In sum, it can be postulated that Danish psychiatry is organised with special reference to treatment of schizophrenia, which constitutes less than 10% of the diagnoses.

The possibility of longitudinal treatment, especially of schizophrenia and other long-lasting psychotic conditions, has been considerably improved during the last ten years, although some negative factors are observed. These patients are increasingly looked on as partners in a collabo-ration, rather than as objects of treatment, and this tendency is supported by the law of psychiatry (1989), which at present is being revised (1998) and social legislation (1976), revised 1998, which secure the patients' rights and existential basis.

In Danish psychiatry it is still discussed that the hospital model has neg-ative effects. Also in the present book it has been opportune to list these neg-ative consequences. In my opinion, the negative factors associated with the large mental hospitals in most of the Western world is now history, or soon will be.

That the negative factors still have such a large space in textbooks, such as the current book, is in my opinion caused by the fact that the authors who write the textbooks mentally are caught in a time and a treatment model which they themselves devotedly revolted against and tried to change. This is quite parallel to the fact that, for instance, tertiary syphilis is described in detail, in many textbooks although no psychiatrists below the age of 50 have met such a patient.

In Denmark we aim at longitudinal treatment, modified according to each patient's immediate need, such as admission to closed wards, open wards, stay in social psychiatric institutions, shared households or sheltered accommodation, work initiatives, leisure activities and other conditions aiming to achieve social integration. The basic principles in Denmark are that each level has its own staff, who communicate with the staffs of other levels, as opposed to the model with staff who are responsible at all levels. There are two reasons for this: to avoid the complicated organisation of the staff's daily timetable, and to cultivate professionalism within specific areas, instead of diluting their know-how by demanding effort on many different levels of function.

As regards relatives, very active organisations have been established alongside the numerous discharges during the 1980s and the beginning of the 1990s. For instance, approximately 450 000 schizophrenia bed-days (approximately 50% of the initial level) were 'exported' from hospitals to the immediate environment, which in practice means to relatives. But after a turbulent beginning, co-operation between relatives' organisations and the psychiatric health services is now fruitful and mutual rewarding.

To sum up, on the patient level there are professional and theoretical possibilities for a balanced emphasis between biological, psychotherapeutic, and social psychiatric treatment, delivered by professionals in a longitudinal model. On the other hand, the available resources are insufficient. Consequently, general practitioners have a central position as gatekeepers, and must rather drastically filter patients to be referred for psychiatric treatment.

Due to our large illness and population registers in Denmark we at the Psychiatric Central Register (Munk-Jørgensen *et al.*, 1993) have long been able to take a comprehensive view of the occurrence of mental disorders (Munk-Jørgensen *et al.*, 1996) on an in-patient and day-patient level, and since 1995 on an out-patient level as well. However, exact knowledge about mental illness in the community – on a population level – is scarce.

17.3 Productivity of the system

If a model has a common validity, it must be applicable to other systems than the one in which it is developed, systems functioning according to the same principles as the original. Applied to such parallel systems, the model, with acceptable sensitivity and specificity, must be able to deliver statements on, for example, the outcome of the system or to pick up new knowledge and new hypotheses.

The model described by the authors is very broad and non-specific. Therefore, it can by and large be applied to a wide variety of human service systems. The sensitivity of the model is at a maximum and it can be used in any psychiatric region from Camberwell through Regio Veneto to Kazakhstan. Its specificity is close to zero. It is difficult quite to understand the practical relevance of the model. As indicated, it describes without difficulties any existing system. As used by the authors it describes a system which is already in existence the world over. The authors mention that 'In psychiatry as compared with other medical specialities, a relatively small contribution towards visible inputs in expenditure on medication, supplies, equipment and investigations'. This attitude to psychiatry describes the ideology of the 1960s and the practice of the 1980s/1990s.

Looking at the recent years' progress in research the authors' view could be quite provocatively formulated as tomorrow's '*Welt von Gestern*'. Future psychiatry must be presumed to be highly specialised and technologised, with specific treatment and hopefully/possibly/probably with specific prevention of the psychiatric diseases of the brain. The best of what is developed today for the treatment of social complications to the psychiatric brain diseases might be useful in the social care system, when the present era's model has assumed the character of anachronistic nonsense. But for some years the present priority to legions of caregivers may still be a reality, meaning that more resources are spent on staffing.

A model which does not automatically catch new possibilities, as is the case at the present, is too vague to be applicable in a science-based speciality. At the most it will be useful in giving an ideological/political-based system a touch of scientific legitimisation. In its seductive details it will be suitable as a heuristic method for spreading the present ideology, just as both Adam Smith's and Karl Marx's 'theories' in periods have been capable of founding schools without any of them, by scientific methods, being able to document their validity.

In other words: the model fits, mainly due to its vagueness, the Danish system in every detail. It will be suitable for teaching psychiatrists, other staff, patients, clients, users or whatever the politically proper designation at any time might be. This was the case when moral psychiatry was predominant, when the asylum model was right, when psycho-pharmacological treatment was the only proper method, as is the case today when the official ideology is decentralisation and social psychiatry, and obviously 'tomorrow' when gene technology and neuro-physiology will be the prevailing ground for psychiatry.

However, if taken as an instrument to catch new hypotheses, to test these against existing methods and quickly implement them in a balanced relation to already existing methods, including the political–administrative level and in society in general, the matrix model is, in my opinion, less usable. This is documented by the authors' view of the model as a careful description of a system that today already in principle is on its way to be 'yesterday'.

17.4 **Service components**

The most important component of all within psychiatric treatment is a qualified staff of both academic and non-academic members. A trend in psychiatry has been to emphasise the psychiatrists' and other staff groups' humanistic, empathic, and holistic attitudes. Of course, these are necessary qualities, but not without a profound professional expertise. The tendency for staff to work in a cross-disciplinary model in which each person should be able to function within more areas, is dying out, for instance that the psychiatrists should master both psychotherapy and psycho-pharmacology, have a knowledge of the social legislation, and be a skilled chauffeur when driving around to the patients' homes. This role-blurring is a disrespectful attitude towards the mentally ill, a tendency that now luckily is fading away. Cross-disciplinary co-operation must take place in such a way that top professionals, psychiatrists and staff from other professions, each make their contribution to an overall solution. In a total treatment service the specific high technology acute hospital ward is as necessary as the long-term socially oriented rehabilitation effort, and vice versa.

In a listing of service components it might seem absurd when a list of basic components includes, for instance, 'police' and 'prison', necessary authorities in special and rare cases, but not necessarily the first choice when good clinical practice in treatment of mental disorders is the goal. As previously mentioned, in creating models one must ensure that high sensitivity, i.e. to identify as many of the necessary services as possible, does not cause low specificity, so that the model fits any organisation. As the authors mention the basic service components in Table 10.3 one could argue that, if it was turned upside down, it would describe the fight against criminality in a certain country, with police and prisons as important components and self-help and user-groups' unsupervised housing with administrative protection, and crisis houses as necessary supplements. The list in Table 10.3 is very comprehensive, and I will not spontaneously be able to mention missing components. Nevertheless, in the near future, or in relation to a non-Western European culture, the model will probably be insufficient. What is needed in establishing a treatment service is a list of all the possibilities the authors present but also an indication of the minimum that must be available. Personally, I would not be afraid to take the responsibility for establishment of a psychiatric service in a certain Danish county without presence of, for example, 'voluntary groups', 'prisons', 'domiciliary care (e.g. cleaning)', as opposed to establishment of a service without the presence of, for example, 'sheltered workshops', 'specialised units for specific disorders', 'group homes', and 'collaboration with primary care (GPs)'.

An important feature in establishing a psychiatric service is availability. I use the word 'availability' as a term instead of the word 'continuity' that often has been misinterpreted as a continuous co-operation between patient and a staff member. The term continuity is far more broad. It is of the utmost importance to emphasise that psychiatric patients are also biological beings. Recent studies have shown that almost 50% of the psychiatric patients have physical disorders, from mild to severe, and many of these are unrecognised and untreated. Many physical disorders show psychiatric symptoms and vice versa. Consequently, in a listing of service components the need for close co-operation with other medical specialities must be strongly emphasised.

In recent years, advances within neuro-physiological and neuro-biological diagnoses and psychopharmacological treatment of the psychiatric disorders of the brain, e.g. schizophrenia, bipolar disorders and others, has demanded access to specialised technology and qualified expertise within, for instance, pharmacology, biochemistry, and laboratory facilities. A social rehabilitation which is not based upon a maximum utilization of the biological advances within diagnosis and treatment is of no value and vice versa. Therefore, I must react against a statement as it is mentioned in Table 12.8, that in the community-based model the therapeutic orientation among the staff is one which 'may neglect physical diagnoses and treatment'. Any treatment without a background in a science-based diagnosis, biological, psychological or social, is a problem and must be considered unqualified and unethical.

17.5 **The process of re-forming**

The authors elevate seven steps to reform community services: Establishing the service principles, setting the boundary conditions, assessing population needs, assessing current provision, formulating a strategic plan for a local system of mental health services, implementing the service component at the local level, and monitoring and review cycles. These seven steps are hardly distinguishable from the classical spiral of evaluation, only more complicated. In the classical spiral the problems are formulated and based on these and intervention with special reference to changes is made.

Before, during and after the intervention relevant parameters are monitored, and based on these parameters the result of the change is evaluated. Subsequently, the problems are reformulated and a possible new intervention can be planned with matching monitoring before, during and after.

The authors' 'seven steps' are very detailed, however, without consideration for practical conditions. By 'establishing the service principles' and 'setting boundary conditions' the political factor has not been heard. The authors mention 'colleagues sharing common ground', 'planning groups', 'planners', 'planning process', and in the point concerning boundary conditions they point to two types of boundary of primary concern, the 'geographical' and the 'functional'. These theoretical based principles are in the best of all worlds fully sufficient and relevant to formulating problems. However, in the organisation of psychiatry the word 'reason' has a weak ambience. Psychiatry has been the playground for politics and ideology, as no other medical sciences and organisations, and professionals occupied with the reform of psychiatric service must all the time be aware of this political factor.

I started this section with a remark that the model seems to be a complication of the classical spiral of evaluation. I should like to illustrate this complication by, for instance, point 4 'assessing current provision' for which, after several readings, I still do not understand the meaning. A more sophisticated theorising of a practical way of presenting the problems is a necessity from an academic angle. Only by sophisticated analyses is it possible to expose complicated problems, but we risk that practical clinicians, planners, and politicians who are responsible for reforms do not have time, insight, and/or patience to acquaint themselves with the available background knowledge in the present book before they act, and instead they resort to easy, seductive slogan-based management models. The authors, with their model, face such a danger.

In their steps for reforming the services the authors point at a very essential question, namely where to put the threshold for access to treatment. We know that between 25 and 30% of the adult population have mental health problems in any year, and that a maximum of 2–3% of the population during a year reach specialised treatment. These 2–3% represent too few, as 5–8% of a population at any time suffer from anxiety and/or depression to a degree that demands treatment. As opposed to this there is no doubt that a referral of the 25–30% with mental health problems would be mostly inexpedient, both because normal psychological reactions would be perceived as morbid and because from an economic angle it would be disastrous.

To the question of who should be involved in writing the strategic plan, the authors list 13 authorities or groups starting with health service managers and ending with external advisors. If the authors really mean, rather than just speaking in politically correct terms, that all these authorities are to be involved, they have most probably secured themselves against the likelihood that anything sensible will happen. The creation of a strategy with so many partners would be such a morass of different interest groups, treatment ideologies, and impotent results of consensus seeking, that a plan would be unspecified and action-preventing.

If, however, the authors want to obtain guidance from these many authorities, then this puts a different complexion on it. A small, strong decision-making group would get access to the necessary information, and in a phase of planning use this in the best possible way in which to plan services for the mentally ill. Finally, the authors remind us of the necessity of monitoring and assessment, a step that is often forgotten.

In the discussion of the reform process we should remind ourselves of the many possibilities in such a process. Previously, I hinted that it is my impression that the authors are inflexible in an either–or attitude to hospitals/asylums. This attitude is illustrated by their comment on two ways to change an asylum, either the Italian model of 'closing the front door' or the English one of 'closing the hospital'. In Denmark all the large asylums have been 'recycled'. In, for example, the Psychiatric University Hospital in Aarhus, which originally was a large hospital with approximately 800 beds, we have after a reduction of the catchment area, gradually changed the hospital to an intensive diagnosis and treatment centre with a few hundred beds. The hospital now serves three catchment areas with a total population of 160 000, 125 000, and 125 000, respectively. The beds, declined in number from 670 in total in 1977 to a total of 330 in 1997, representing 6.0, 7.6, and 6.3 per 10 000 inhabitants in the three catchment areas, respectively. They function as acute closed wards, a few rehabilitation wards, and as 'district' wards working in close collaboration with the community mental health centres (CMHCs) and the community team. A psychogeriatric unit with 30 beds (0.5 per 10 000 total population) serves the entire county.

The free capacity is now used for therapy of many types, patient information centres, practice rooms, exercise rooms, research units, studios and rooms for art exhibitions, different patient workshops, and restaurants, all in a fruitful growing co-operation with the surrounding environments and their inhabitants.

In the Nordic countries (Munk-Jørgensen *et al.*, 1995), among which the situation in Denmark has already been described, the most radical decreasing number of beds was seen in Finland, mainly because Finland started with many more beds than the other countries. Therefore, Finland has been in the turmoil of drastic organisational changes. Until a few years ago, the model was dominated by the psychoanalytic approach, but now a social-psychiatric model is dominant, focusing on family-centred psychiatry.

Iceland has the highest number of psychiatrists per 1000 inhabitants in the Nordic countries. The predominant treatment model has been a biological and social-psychiatric approach in the public system, whereas the approach in private psychiatric practice mainly is psychodynamic.

In Norway the treatment models and the organisation of psychiatry are very similar to what is seen in Denmark. The major difference is in the approach. In Norway psychodynamic thinking has been in the forefront, but a more regular social-psychiatric way of organising psychiatry is gaining ground. Because of the dominating psychoanalytic basis for Norwegian psychiatry, the biologically based treatment has a relatively weak position ideologically as well as in research, but this situation is now changing rapidly.

Sweden, the largest of the Nordic countries, has for many years based its psychiatry on the biological model. Therefore, Sweden is also very strong in biological psychiatric research, but during the past 15–20 years psychodynamic and social-psychiatric treatment models have forged ahead. More national programmes have aimed at heightening the integration of bio-psycho-social treatment models. Swedish psychiatry has focused intensively on ethics and human rights in building up modern psychiatry.

In all five Nordic countries the authorities have tested a series of organisational models, trying to integrate primary and secondary health services and health services with social care. In the same way as the matrix model fits the present Danish psychiatry it is also applicable to the psychiatric services in the other Nordic countries.

17.6 **The near future of Danish psychiatry**

As previously mentioned, Denmark has in the last 10 years passed through a period during which social psychiatry and decentralisation have been given a high priority on the grounds that have been emotional, ideological, political, and economical, and to a very limited extent professional and scientific. Psychiatry has been the playground for organisational experiments and psychiatrists and psychiatric staff have hardly been heard in these developments. No doubt, these developments have been an advantage for many, but there has been a shortage of a qualified scientifically based evaluation of social psychiatric efforts in Denmark. Only in a few centres has such research been done. A thorough non-biased scientific evaluation is missing from the social services angle, not only from the medical scientific side.

On the other hand, a series of negative indicators exists, as mentioned before, more homeless mentally ill (Brandt, 1992), increasing suicide rates among mentally ill compared with the general population (Sundhedsministeriet, 1994), increased criminality among mentally ill (Kramp & Gabrielsen, 1996), more coercion in the psychiatric departments, (Sundhedsstyrelsen, 1996) and perhaps most seriously a vehemently increasing drug and alcohol abuse among psychiatric patients, especially psychotic patients (Hansen, 1997). It is impossible with absolute certainty to determine whether decentralisation is the reason, as we cannot make causal conclusions based on aggregated data. However, it is necessary to investigate and prove which groups of patients who benefit from a social psychiatric, decentralised effort, and which types of social psychiatric efforts are effective, which types of treatment are possible to decentralise, and which are not. Based on such studies, what can be used must be strengthened and the ineffective must be consistently eliminated. The romantic, ideological part of social psychiatry must as fast as possible be abolished and the resources spent on other purposes.

As regards the present social psychiatric era it is possible to draw a parallel to the psychopharmacological era in the 60s and the 70s, and to the psychotherapeutic era in the 70s and 80s. Firstly, there has been the appearance of these methods, followed by an uncritical widespread and excessive use of the method, and subsequently a reduction in its use, to include only that shown to be effective. Consequently, the psycho-pharmacology has become a unique tool in long-term treatment of psychotics and psychotherapy is no longer used as one-sided dynamic methods in Denmark. Instead, cognitive methods have been shown to be applicable in more short-term courses of treatment, and the psychodynamic methods are used as a basis for contact and alliance with the patients, as well as in more environmental therapeutically oriented settings.

It seems to be a paradox that all medical specialities except psychiatry increasingly centralise their functions, while psychiatry has become deprofessionalised and decentralised. However, a gradually increasing specialisation of functions is also occurring within psychiatry. It is still not quite acceptable to discuss this process on the organisational or political level, but the development is impossible to stop and it is a question of time before the political level, patients and their relatives, will favour the development. A specialisation and centralisation of the forensic psychiatry is already being seen, lithium clinics for prophylactic treatment of bipolar affective disorders are established, as are centres for treatment of eating disorders. Child psychiatric treatment is specialised and centralised in a few centres in Denmark, as is forensic psychiatry, and in autumn 1997 the establishment of special clinics for psychotics with associated drug abuse was discussed.

Thus, a development seems to have been started that is a natural reply to patients' and their relatives' needs and to the science-based development of the medical profession of psychiatry. Furthermore, in future a development must be anticipated in which neuro-physiological, neuro-anatomic, and genetic research increasingly will bring the neuro-specialities, especially neurology, and psychiatry closer together, and subsequently even an amalgamation of psychiatry and neurology in a neuro-psychiatric speciality, as was the case at the beginning of this century. At the same time hopefully we can expect that social services will be qualified to handle the social care and rehabilitation for the mentally disordered, realising that these have needs different from the average population.

All these possibilities, some of which have already started, may demand flexibility, visionary reasoning and scientificity both among the professional groups within psychiatry, the social service, organisers, and politicians.

References

Brandt, P. (1992) *Yngre hjemløse i København. Disputats. (Young homeless in Copenhagen. Thesis)*. København, Aahus, Odense: FADL's Forlag.

Hansen, S. S. (1997). Drug abusers in Danish mental hospitals. *Addiction* **92**, 429–435.

Kramp, P. & Gabrielsen, G. (1996). Antallet af psykisk syge kriminelle er fordoblet på ti år. (The number of mentally ill criminals has doubled within ten years). *Nyt fra Kriminalforsorgen,* **5**, 4–5.

Munk-Jøgensen, P., Kastrup, M. & Mortensen, P. B. (1993). The Danish psychiatric register as a tool in epidemiology. *Acta Psychiatrica Scandinavica*, Suppl. 370, 27–32.

Munk-Jøgensen, P., Lehtinen, V., Helgason, T. Dalgard, O. S. & Westrin, C. G. (1995) Psychiatry in the five Nordic Countries. (1995) *European Psychiatry*, **10**, 197–206.

Munk-Jøgensen, P., Kastrup, M. & Mortensen, P. B. (1996). The epidemiology of mental disorders in Denmark. *Nordic Journal of Psychiatry*, **50**, Suppl 36, 15–24.

Sundhedsministeriet. (1994) *Udvikling i selvmordsd ø delighed i Danmark 1955–1991. (The Ministry of Health. Development in suicide mortality in Denmark 1955–1991)*. København: Sundhedsministeriet.

Sundhedsstyrelsen. (1996) *Registrering af indberetring af brug af tvang i psykiatrien. (The National Board of Health. Registration of coercion in psychiatry)*. Copenhagen: Sundhedsstyrelsen.

18
United States
RICHARD WARNER

18.1 **Historical Overview**

The end of the institutional era in psychiatry (the transition from Period 1 to Period 2 proposed by the authors of this book) arrived later in the USA than in northern Europe. While Britain, Norway and the Netherlands were experimenting successfully with the therapeutic community, open-door hospitals, early discharge, and other forms of institutional reform in the early 1950s, in the USA people with psychosis generally were still locked away in archaic asylums. Only after the antipsychotic drugs and Medicaid health insurance for the indigent were introduced in the middle of the 1950s did deinstitutionalisation take off in America, and, even then, it was primarily effected by transferring people with psychotic illness from hospital to such 'community' facilities as nursing homes and massive boarding homes where treatment was often inadequate or non-existent (Warner, 1994).

Medicaid is a health insurance programme funded jointly by the federal and state governments which covers treatment of recipients with mental illness in the community but not in free-standing psychiatric hospitals. State hospitals, are entirely supported by the state budget. This arrangement created an unusual fiscal incentive for state governments to transfer patients out of state hospitals to access federal funding, and promoted radical deinstitutionalisation policies. The elimination of public psychiatric beds, after the advent of Medicaid, progressed further and faster in the USA than anywhere else in the world at that time.

Large federal grants in the 1960s established a network of community mental health centres across the nation, but these, through an excess of zeal for the emerging concepts of primary prevention in psychiatry, focused on providing treatment to citizens with less severe levels of psychiatric disturbance and largely failed to meet the needs of newly discharged mentally ill people. Many ex-hospital patients, in consequence, found themselves numbered among the homeless and jail inmates. Their experience of psychiatric treatment was often as 'revolving-door patients'.

The National Alliance for the Mentally Ill – a network of local organisations of relatives and friends of people with mental illness – was spawned in the late 1970s in reaction to these problems, and their advocacy had much to do with subsequent reforms in community care for the mentally ill. The Community Support Project was a federal effort in the late 1970s to establish model community treatment programmes for people with serious mental illness. Changes in federal reimbursement in the 1980s outlawed the use of nursing homes for most people with functional psychoses and directed federal dollars to the care of the most seriously disturbed patients in the community as a matter of priority.

One might date the authors' Period 3 as beginning in the 1970s when increasingly complex and effective community support systems developed under the heightened awareness generated by advocacy groups. This transition was a little earlier than in Britain, in part because the plight of the seriously mentally ill was more dire in the US and reform was urgently needed. It is also true that progress in rehabilitation psychiatry in Britain was dealt a blow by the introduction of the Seebohm Report in the early 1970s. The report created legislation which transferred much responsibility for the community support of people with mental illness from health service to social service agencies, which were ill-equipped to meet the needs of the new clientele. British community psychiatry, hitherto among the most vigorous in the world, stalled at this point and has struggled to recover.

Although one may find examples of good service systems for seriously ill patients across America, treatment resources are very limited in large cities where numbers of mentally ill people live in desperately inadequate surroundings – incarcerated in jails, and living under bridges, in homeless shelters and in single-room-occupancy hotels (Warner, 1994; Torrey *et al.*, 1990).

The structure of US medicine has led to a characteristic distribution of responsibility for services. Since most people with psychotic disorders are indigent, they receive care from the public agencies – community mental health centres. When acutely disturbed, some may be treated, under Medicaid or Medicare health insurance, in general hospital wards, but for longer-term care they are usually transferred to the state public hospital. University hospitals are rarely involved in the treatment of the mentally ill except in the acute phase, and university departments of psychiatry have few links to public treatment facilities such as state hospitals and community mental health centres. As a result, there is little academic involvement in the USA in rehabilitation psychiatry, in social factors affecting the course of illness, or in the study of epidemiological issues which inform the provision of psychiatric services to a community population. This bias is reflected in the publications on mental illness in US journals (Morlino *et al.*, 1997).

Through the early decades of the community mental health era community agencies were quite de-medicalised; they were seen as primarily *social* agencies. Psychiatrists were marginalised and 'medical model' was a term of disparagement. In the authors' period 3, with the increased focus on long-term care of the seriously mentally ill, psychiatrists have been integrated more fully as members of the treatment team. To this day, however, users of community mental health services are referred to as 'clients' rather than 'patients'. The role of the various mental health disciplines has also been minimised, and an unusual degree of role-blurring and simplification of professional roles continues to be the rule. Staff are often hired into generic 'mental health worker' jobs, regardless of discipline. A nurse may supervise a psychologist or vice versa. Some professions, such as occupational therapists and activity therapists, are almost non-existent. Psychologists are few and they often function much like social workers. Nurses generally have a distinct role, but sometimes do the same work as other therapists. Staff with no specific mental health training are not uncommon.

18.2 Geographical levels

18.2.1 National level: socio-political context

The USA is a federation of states each with considerable autonomy. Consequently, there are marked geographical differences in the provision of care. The mental illness statute varies considerably from state to state. In some, the process for obtaining and sustaining an order for involuntary treatment is so rigorous and complex that many patients go untreated.

The written constitution of the USA sets an overall libertarian tone. In the late 1970s, case law based on constitutionally guaranteed rights, established the principle that, while the presence of mental illness and an imminent risk of dangerousness were grounds for involuntary confinement, they were not, of themselves, grounds for the involuntary administration of medication. A further showing, at a special hearing, was ruled necessary to establish that the mentally ill person lacked competence to take decisions about his or her psychiatric treatment. This change in the law, originally heralded by prominent psychiatrists as 'the profession's dark hour' (Ford, 1980), leading inevitably, it was thought, to patients 'rotting with their rights on' (Gutheil, 1980), has not had the dire results predicted. Some cases come to court, but many are settled by a more thorough progress of negotiation between patient and doctor than existed before the change in the law. The extra legal hurdle means, however, that some patients who might benefit go untreated.

State autonomy leads to substantial differences in mental health policy and service structure. In some states, mental health centres are private non-profit entities, in others, they are city or county agencies, and in yet others they are state-run. There is an eight-fold difference between the most generous and most miserly states in per capita spending on mental health services (Torrey *et al.*, 1990).

Geography and demographics play a role in service delivery. Rural and thinly populated states like Idaho, Mississippi, and Arizona have few psychologists or psychiatrists per capita; mentally ill residents may travel for hours and, even then, receive services from non-specialists. Small, compact states like Vermont, New Hampshire, and Rhode Island, have highly rated mental health systems, while large, thinly populated states like Texas, Wyoming and Montana have poorly developed systems of care (Torrey *et al.*, 1990)

Economic factors

While the introduction of governmental health insurance shaped service development by promoting a radical, uncoordinated shift to 'community care' in the 1950s and '60s, the competitive market in health care has also had a major impact on service development. The unrestricted growth of the health care market to 14% of the nation's gross domestic product forced a reaction. In the 1980s, manufacturing industries became concerned that the high cost of health insurance premiums, provided as a fringe benefit to workers, was pricing American goods out of the global market. Similarly, government has become concerned at the uncontrolled growth in the cost of the federal Medicaid and Medicare programmes resulting from skyrocketing payments to private providers.

The free market in health care, lack of cost controls under private and public insurance, and imprecision in the diagnosis of psychiatric conditions allowed an explosion in the provision of in-patient psychiatric care in private for-profit psychiatric hospitals in the 1980s. The treatment of multiple personality disorder, for example, almost entirely an American epidemic, was big business for chains of for-profit hospitals across the country. Another common diagnosis at such for-profit hospitals was post-traumatic stress disorder, sometimes for supposed abuse by such bizarre practices as satanic ritual abuse. Child and adolescent hospital care also ballooned at this time. Medicaid pays for inpatient treatment of children and adolescents (but not adults) at free-standing psychiatric hospitals. Seizing this market opportunity, private hospitals advertised in local newspapers for concerned parents to bring their offspring in for psychiatric evaluation; many were hospitalised, some diagnosed with bipolar disorder for symptoms which, a few years earlier, would have been considered to represent disorders of attention or conduct.

Pressures such as these led to the development of managed-care mechanisms to define appropriate treatment and to control costs. These mechanisms have promoted the development of health maintenance organisations (HMOs) and other managed-care entities, and have also led to the development of capitated funding mechanisms for government insurance programmes, like Medicaid.

Managed care has drastically changed the face of USA psychiatry. Many for-profit hospitals have gone out of business. Many private office-based practitioners have been forced to change their styles of practice and contract with managed-care companies to provide short-term focused therapy. Young professionals often choose salaried work with public agencies or HMOs over the uncertainties of private practice. As a result, staffing and quality of care at public agencies have improved. Community mental health centres, traditionally required to exercise cost control due to the limitations of public funding, have found themselves on the cutting edge of managed care. Many public agencies have been able to market their services to managed-care companies, based on superior cost-efficiency, and contract to provide in-patient, out-patient or emergency services for local subscribers. Others have amalgamated to form their own managed-care entities.

Staffing and training

Despite the present-day prominence of community-based public agencies, academic training programmes for work in these settings continue to be inadequate. The gulf between academic and community settings is diminishing, but slowly. The best community agencies provide their own training for new staff and students. In the recent past, training for psychiatrists in the USA was directed towards office-based psychotherapy. In the 1970s, for example, 80 percent of psychiatric residents in the USA underwent personal psychoanalysis as part of their training. Contact with seriously mentally ill people was primarily in the acute in-patient setting, and, as a discipline, psychiatrists had a poor understanding of rehabilitation or social interventions. Community-based training for psychiatrists has increased in recent years and contemporary graduates can work effectively in public settings.

Doctoral level psychologists are still not extensively employed in community psychiatry, and their training is not much spent in community settings or with long-term mentally ill clients. As a result, psychological testing and treatments which are usually the domain of psychologists, such as cognitive and interpersonal therapy, are under-used in the USA, especially in the management of the adult mentally ill.

18.2.2 Local level

The private marketplace in health care has created a certain amount of fragmentation of services at the local level. In some states, subcontracting of programme elements to small providers by state or local funding agencies is quite common. One agency may provide residential services for the seriously mentally ill; another will offer emergency evaluation; another, in-patient care; another, intensive case management; and yet another, a psycho-social clubhouse with a continuous supported employment programme. Consequently, continuity of care can be a problem. Ensuring that subcontractors meet their obligations to the service system and maintain smooth working relationships with other providers requires a good deal of administrative commitment and expense.

On the other hand, where the care provider is relatively independent of government, considerable efficiencies can result. Independent non-profit treatment agencies can respond rapidly to changing circumstances and use available funding sources to create programmes which meet community and individual needs. Independent agencies do not have to adhere to government job categories and pay scales, and they are rarely unionised. Each agency will determine its own pay rates, raises and benefits based on local market conditions.

Colorado is an example of a state which avoids the pitfalls of excessive subcontracting and maximises the entrepreneurial advantages of independence. The state is divided into catchment areas by county or region, and the community mental health centre for each area is a private non-profit agency which provides all or most of the publicly funded care without subcontracting to other entities except for in-patient care. When the federal government recently issued waivers allowing states to create capitated funding schemes under Medicaid, these Colorado agencies were able to respond rapidly, submitting proposals to transform the treatment system in the space of a few months; some agencies subsequently generated increases in efficiency which allowed savings to be rechanelled for the care of medically indigent clients.

On the negative side, these community agencies have largely based their programme decisions on funding opportunities rather than socio-demographic indicators. When psychiatric services to the elderly increase, for example, it is more likely to be due to success in billing Medicare (the government health insurance plan for elderly Americans) than to using demographic and public health data to identify clinical needs in that population. An interest in social indicators is developing, however. As agencies come to recognise that their continued operation may require them to compete with large for-profit entities for their operational contracts, they have become increasingly interested in service assessment, not only in such domains as service accessibility, consumer satisfaction, clinical change and quality of life, but also in social indicators like out-of-home placement of children and adolescents.

In many parts of Colorado, the community mental health agencies have good links to other agencies or services, but in other areas such collaboration may be tentative or non-existent. All have a continuity-of-care liaison to the state psychiatric hospital, most have good working relationships with consumer advocates (such as the local Alliance for the Mentally Ill), many have well-organised services to the county jail or to homeless shelters, and some have programmes in the district schools. The trend is towards even more 'horizontal integration' and one may find multi-agency programmes which effectively combine mental health, public health and social service resources to combat child abuse and neglect in high-risk families (Huxley & Warner, 1993), to reduce out-of-home placement of adolescents and children in foster homes or correctional facilities, or to provide coordinated services to substance abusers.

One of the areas of weakest collaboration is between the general health sector and public mental health. Primary health care is under-developed in the U.S., and most referrals to public psychiatric agencies come, not from family doctors or other physicians, but through self-referral, the police, private therapists or emergency-room staff. A community physician may suggest that his or her patient 'go to the mental health centre,' but communication between physicians and public psychiatrists is rare. This relationship reflects the perceived status of mental health centres as social agencies rather than health agencies.

18.2.3 Individual level

Only about 10 to 20 per cent of people with serious mental illness in the US are employed (Anthony *et al.*, 1988). By way of contrast, 60 per cent of a sample of people with schizophrenia in Bologna were found to be employed (Warner *et al.*, 1998). One reason for the low US employment rate of the mentally ill is the work disincentive created by public entitlement programmes. Patients who work part-time gain only a slight increase in their real income, because the increase in their earned income is accompanied by a loss of disability pensions, rent subsidies and other supports. To overcome this disincentive, most patients require a higher wage than they can actually command in the marketplace (Polak & Warner, 1996). These disincentives to work are less severe in Italy but worse in countries such as Britain and New Zealand.

18.3 The temporal dimension

18.3.1 Input

The visible inputs in mental health services across the USA are widely variable. We have referred above to the eight-fold difference in per capita funding between states which invest well or poorly in mental health services. In practice, this leads to huge differences in staffing for essentially similar types of service. In Boulder, Colorado, for example, the caseload for a case manager on an intensive treatment team (treating outpatients with unstable psychosis) is around 12 to 15 patients; on a standard outpatient team therapists are responsible for about 35 to 40 clients. In Dallas, Texas, by way of contrast, a therapist on an out-patient team can have a caseload of 300 clients. Under such circumstances the treatment provided is very limited.

The largest category of staff in community mental health is master's degree social workers, though many staff have a bachelor's degree or a lower level of academic training. Due to role-blurring, most patients will never know the discipline or training of their therapist, and there may be a moderate degree of institutional resistance to revealing this information. It will, however, be clear who is their treating psychiatrist, if they see one. Psychiatrists are relatively few – about one for every 250 clients in a well-staffed agency – and they are used selectively for second-level evaluation of clients, formulating treatment plans, prescribing medication, and training staff.

The invisible inputs in US mental health can be powerful. For example, the libertarian culture and liberal mental illness statutes make it more difficult to treat seriously mentally ill people who are resistant to treatment. Within the month prior to writing this chapter there were two national news stories which illustrate this point. In one, an elderly woman with paranoid delusions who held the police at bay with a shotgun when they arrived to take her in for hospital treatment received considerable community support for her resistance to 'government intrusion' during a stand-off which lasted several days. In another story, a young woman who was brought to a hospital emergency room, naked and illogical, was released 'against medical advice' because her friends in the Church of Scientology objected on principle to psychiatric treatment. She died within a few days from complications of dehydration. Although the state mental illness statute would have allowed involuntary treatment in such a case, the cultural bias led to her release.

Another invisible factor influencing mental health services is the individualism of US culture. American consumers expect complete information about their medical and psychiatric treatment and do not lightly accept the authority of physicians or other treatment staff. European practice, by comparison, is more paternalistic. Paternalism may have advantages, especially when someone with an acute psychotic illness could benefit from treatment but refuses it, but it carries certain negative consequences. It may limit the patient's sense of competence, reinforcing a stereotype of disability and leading to reduced functioning. On the other hand, US mental health procedures for involuntary treatment are more legalistic and litigious and disrupt long-term therapeutic relationships.

The violence and the availability of firearms in American society is another input shaping mental health services. Visitors from abroad comment on the lack of mobility of American emergency psychiatric services. Most acutely disturbed patients are brought in for evaluation by the police or family members. Evaluations outside the agency are likely to be done at another institution – for example, a jail or emergency room. Emergency staff rarely venture into people's homes to do an evaluation, and if they do, it is likely to be with a police escort. Attempts to change this pattern of practice are met with stiff resistance from staff who fear being confronted by armed and aggressive people.

Direct family support is a crucial input which is absent for many American patients. In Boulder, Colorado, only 13% of people with schizophrenia live with a family; in Bologna, Emilia Romagna, 70% of a similar patient population are living with family (Warner *et al.*, 1998). This difference reflects a larger cultural variation. In Bologna, adult offspring are much more likely to live with their family of origin than in Boulder. Nearly 60% of single Bolognese men in their early thirties still live at home (Barbagli & Pisati 1995); in Boulder, the equivalent figure is around 3 per cent (Miller & Caldwell 1995). The value placed on staying close to family runs deep in Italy. As one Italian sociologist remarked, 'If in the States a young person doesn't want to leave home, everyone wonders what is wrong with the person. Here (in Italy), if a young person wants to leave home, everyone wonders what is wrong with the family' (Bohlen, 1996).

18.3.2 Process

Compared to a country such as Italy there is little emphasis in the USA on patient rehabilitation in the treatment process. Most efforts are expended in establishing financial support, housing, practical daily support and adequately monitored psychiatric treatment. The absence of direct family support may force this role upon the treatment system. For those living at home, families meet many needs like accommodation, food, house-cleaning, and budgeting. Consequently, service systems in Italy do not have to invest as many resources in meeting basic needs as in the USA, making it easier for Italian services to develop home-based counselling and comprehensive employment opportunities (Warner *et al.*, 1998).

An important recent change in the process of delivery of public psychiatric services in the USA has been the development of pilot projects for capitated funding under Medicaid health insurance – a large component of the funding for the treatment of serious mental illness. According to a recent Bazelon Center (1996) report, 43 states had, at report time, obtained waivers of federal Medicaid rules to allow capitated funding on a pilot basis. Under this mechanism, instead of billing for every service provided, agencies receive a predetermined amount for each Medicaid recipient in the catchment area.

Capitated funding creates incentives for agencies to develop cost-efficient treatment approaches for Medicaid recipients (Yank *et al.*, 1992) and allows savings to be used for other purposes, clients and programmes. Proponents argue that it makes possible treatment methods which were not funded under the previous fee-for-service mechanism (Warner, 1989), and that it promotes more client-centred, flexible, timely and community-based treatment (Godshalx, 1996). Critics are concerned that the new financial incentives could lead to reduced service quality and worse outcome for seriously disturbed clients (Lehman, 1987; McFarland, 1994).

There is little research available on the outcome of the pilot efforts. A small study in Washington, DC (Harris & Bergman, 1988) indicated reduced hospitalisation but no decrease in service utilisation. Studies in New York and California demonstrated reduced hospital use and lower treatment costs but no difference in functioning or symptomatology (Cole *et al.*, 1994; Reed *et al.*, 1994; Chandler *et al.*, 1996). More recently, a study in Boulder, Colorado, reported lower psychopathology and hospitalisation and improved quality of life (in the domains of work, finances and social relations) for people with schizophrenia, with no increase in the amount of outpatient treatment, suggesting improved cost-efficacy (Warner & Huxley, 1998).

18.3.3 Outcome

There is no agreement at a national level on indicators of outcome for mental health services. The one effort at a nationwide assessment of mental health services, Fuller Torrey *et al.*'s (1990) rating of state programmes, used only input and process measures. Some states are making efforts to develop co-ordinated state-wide measures. A recent shortlist of proposed assessment measures for the Colorado mental health system comprises one input measure (consumer participation in governance), eight process measures and nine outcome variables. The outcome measures include patient housing and employment status, hospital readmission rates, patient functioning level and mental health problem scores. There are many problems with the reliability of therapist-rated measures of patient functioning and pathology which need to be addressed before the assessment package can be used for programme comparisons.

Service satisfaction and quality of life instruments such as those developed by Lehman (1983) and Oliver *et al.* (1996) are gaining prominence. In using these measures, however, a question hangs over the value of subjective reporting. Quality of life studies often find that subjective satisfaction bears little relation to objective life circumstances (Skantze *et al.*, 1992). Satisfaction tends to be high regardless of the population (Barry & Crosby, 1996) and is disappointing in detecting differences between patients in different or changing circumstances (Warner *et al.*, 1998). The same event may result in opposite evaluations from the same person, depending on the person's emotional state (Schwarz *et al.*, 1994), and interventions that produce objective improvements may lead to a *decrease* in life satisfaction as patients become aware of how their lives might be better (Lehman, 1996). In Colorado, this concern has led to an emphasis on more objective measures; of the shortlist of 19 proposed state-wide measures only three are subjective satisfaction ratings.

18.4 Service components

The most significant differences in service components in the USA in comparison to other developed countries are:

- crisis intervention teams are less mobile;
- public hospital beds are very few; in Colorado there are six adult public psychiatric beds per 100 000 population;

- assertive outreach case-management teams are the primary model for achieving low hospital utilisation;
- the psychosocial clubhouse model has been widely adopted and provides much of the vocational rehabilitation;
- day treatment centres are rare and are considered somewhat institutional and not sufficiently goal-specific;
- carer support is better developed than in years past, but family psycho-educational intervention has not caught on;
- cognitive therapy is not widely utilised;
- liaison to primary medical practitioners is virtually unknown;
- physical and dental care for the seriously mentally ill is sorely deficient;
- user advocacy groups are prominent and generally respected; primary and secondary consumers are often involved in service governance (as board members) and sometimes in service provision (as staff);
- comprehensive services for children and adolescents are widely available.

18.5 **Reforming services**

How can the authors' matrix model be applied to the analysis of service reform? A specific example, the use of crisis homes, helps illustrate the applicability of the model.

Under the crisis home model, acutely disturbed adults are placed in short-term foster-family homes and treated by a mobile psychiatric team. The first programme of this type was developed by Paul Polak and his colleagues (1995) at Southwest Denver Mental Health Center in Colorado, during the 1970s, where it decreased the annual use of hospital beds to 1 per 100000 population. Similar systems are now in operation at Dane County Mental Health Center in Madison, Wisconsin and, on a smaller scale, in Boulder, Colorado. These programmes provide care to a variety of people in crisis, most of whom would otherwise have spent time in hospital. Many of these clients suffer from acute psychotic illness and some are actively suicidal. Violence and safety are almost never a problem, in part because of careful selection of appropriate clients and in part because clients feel pleased to be invited into another person's home and try to behave with the courtesy of house guests. For this reason, people with difficult personality disorders behave better in a crisis home than they would in a hospital ward.

Using the matrix model to analyse the viability and success of such a model in a new locale, we would consider the following factors:

A: Input level

1: Country/regional level

- The programme can be cost-effective if hospital expenses are diverted into it as hospital use decreases (as under Medicaid capitation or other systems where 'the dollar follows the patient').
- The programme will be heavily utilised and affordable if few hospital beds are available in the region.
- It is easier to launch an innovative programme of this type if the sponsoring agency is sufficiently independent to avoid external administrative interference.

2: Local level

- The programme requires that there be enough households available with an empty spare bedroom (a factor which prevented success of the programme in Blacktown, New South Wales).
- The programme is particularly valuable in rural areas where the hospital is far removed, and the crisis home is closer to the patient's own community.
- The community should be liberal and accepting, so that neighbours' concerns do not prevent host family enrolment.
- Staff should be flexible and training programmes adequate.

3: Patient level

- The programme presupposes that the patient's own family is not readily available (making the programme acceptable in Boulder, Colorado, but out of place in Bologna, Italy).
- Patients and their relatives must be able to tolerate the idea of family care instead of hospital care (making the programme less suitable for first episodes of illness).

B: Process level

1: Country/regional level

- The programme should be acceptable to the regional health authority and consumer groups.

2: Local level

- The programme requires a co-ordinator to ensure smooth working relationships between the crisis/admission team and the mobile team which will treat the patient.
- The programme co-ordinator must be available to provide immediate support and consultation to host families.
- One process measure is the numbers of users placed in crisis homes.

3: Patient level

- Process measures include patient, family and staff acceptance of the programme and length of patient stay in the crisis home.

C: *Outcome Level*

1: Country/regional level

· The programme should be actively promoted as a model by the regional health authority and consumer groups.

2: Local level

· Measures of success include frequent utilisation, a high retention rate of host families in the programme, good cost-efficiency compared to other forms of in-patient care, and reduced levels of hospital use.

3: Patient level

· Outcome measures include clinical change and patient and family satisfaction (in comparison to prior hospital admissions), readmission rates, and incidents of violence, suicide attempts or other problems.

The matrix model provides a framework for programme developers to set out the preconditions and assessment measures for a novel project in a comprehensive way so that its viability in a new setting can be more fully determined. The model allows us to see, for example, that the crisis-home model is unlikely to be viable in:

· highly bureaucratised and centralised service systems;
· systems which are rich in in-patient beds or where treatment funds do not 'follow the patient.'
· working class areas where there are few households with spare bedrooms;
· cultures where most mentally ill people live with their own families.

18.6 **Future concerns**

A looming issue for the USA health system is attaining cost-efficiency. Various forms of managed care have clearly come to stay. A concern in public mental health is the extent to which for-profit managed-care entities are moving into the potentially profitable area of Medicaid capitation and converting clinical resources into shareholder profit in return for setting up cost-control mechanisms. If public mental health agencies are to avoid corporate take-overs they need to develop (1) their own cost- and utilisation-control mechanisms, and (2) outcome measurement systems for demonstrating cost-efficiency when they compete for contracts to serve their communities. In the new competitive environment consumers and fundholders will be studying whether managed care leads to reduced choice and outcomes or improved programming as the system abandons the restrictions of fee-for-service regulations.

If patient outcomes are to improve, the USA should continue to develop successful rehabilitation models. Vocational rehabilitation efforts are hampered by work disincentives inherent in the USA disability pension schemes (Supplemental Security Income and Social Security Disability Income). The income restrictions of these programmes need to be changed if employment rates of people with disability are to improve, and with US unemployment rates at their lowest since the 1970s, this is a good time to address the issue. As university departments of psychiatry increasingly recognise that the main focus of activity of psychiatric care is in the community they should attempt to revive academic interest in rehabilitation technology.

Certain intervention models have not gained prominence in the USA; these include family intervention and cognitive therapy. The failure to disseminate family intervention is understandable, since, in most areas, few Americans with mental illness continue to live with their families. In those subcultures where families are more involved in ongoing care of their mentally ill relatives, there would be a benefit to intensified training on this approach. Cognitive therapy could be more broadly used throughout the system, but the health system itself must promote the treatment model. Unlike drug treatment, which is intensively marketed both by the industry and by the research in professional publications, social models of intervention have few advocates.

To improve the care of the mentally ill in the USA, it will be important to rectify the acute shortage of resources in the large cities. Rootless people with mental illness tend to drift into city centres where resources are inadequate to meet their needs and psychiatric caseloads are often very high. It is here that the deficiencies in care are most apparent – large numbers of homeless people with mental illness roam the streets behaving strangely and dying of exposure in back alleys. There are few studies of morbidity and mortality among the mentally ill in the USA, in part because there is not a strong constituency representing the interests of the homeless mentally ill. Treatment agencies do not wish to attract attention to their service inadequacies, nor are they keen to develop outreach programmes that will further increase caseloads. Consumer advocacy groups such as the Alliance for the Mentally Ill have promoted improvements in service and research, correctional agencies complain about the increase in the numbers of mentally ill people in jail and prison, city mayors struggle with the problem of mentally ill people in shelters for the homeless, but no group has succeeded in placing the plight of the untreated, homeless and incarcerated mentally ill high on the nation's political agenda.

References

Anthony, W. A., Cohen, M. R. & Danley, K. S. (1988) The Psychiatric Rehabilitation Model as applied to vocational rehabilitation. In *Vocational Rehabilitation of Persons with Prolonged Psychiatric Disorders* (ed. J. A. Cardiello & M. D. Bell), pp. 59–80. Baltimore: Johns Hopkins University Press.

Barbagli, M., Pisati, M. (1995). *Rapporto sulla Situazione Sociale a Bologna*. Bologna, Italy: Il Mulino.

Barry, M. M. & Crosby, C. (1996). Quality of life as an evaluative measure in assessing the impact of community care on people with long-term psychiatric disorders. *British Journal of Psychiatry*, **168**, 210–216.

Bazelon Center for Mental Health Care (1996). *Managed Mental Health Care: Survey of the States*. Washington, DC: Bazelon Center for Mental Health Care.

Bohlen, C. (1996). For young Italians, there's no place like home. *International Herald Tribune*, March 14, p. 1.

Chandler, D., Meisel, M. B. A., McGowen, M. *et al*. (1996) Client outcomes in two model capitated integrated service agencies. *Psychiatric Services*, **47**, 175–180.

Cole, R. E., Reed, S. K., Babigian, H. M. *et al*. (1994). A mental health capitation program: I. Patient outcomes. *Hospital and Community Psychiatry*, **45**, 1090–1096.

Ford, M. D. (1980). The psychiatrist's double bind: The right to refuse medication. *American Journal of Psychiatry*, **137**, 332–339.

Godshalx, S. (1996). Advantages of working in a capitated mental health system. *Psychiatric Services*, **47**, 477–478.

Gutheil, T. G. (1980). In search of true freedom: drug refusal, involuntary medication, and 'rotting with your rights on.' *American Journal of Psychiatry*, **137**, 327–328.

Harris, M. & Bergman, H. (1988). Capitation financing for the chronic mentally ill: a case management approach. *Hospital and Community Psychiatry*, **39**, 68–72.

Huxley, P. & Warner, R. (1993). The primary prevention of parenting dysfunction in high-risk cases. *American Journal of Orthopsychiatry*, **63**, 582–588.

Lehman, A. F. (1983). The well-being of chronic mental patients: assessing their quality of life. *Archives of General Psychiatry*, **40**, 369–373.

Lehman, A. F. (1987). Capitation payment and mental health care: a review of the opportunities and risks. *Hospital and Community Psychiatry*, **38**, 31–38.

Lehman, A. (1996). Measures of quality of life among persons with severe and persistent mental disorders. In *Mental Health Outcome Measures* (ed. G. Thornicroft & M. Tansella), pp. 75–92. Berlin: Springer.

McFarland, B. (1994). Health maintenance organizations and persons with severe mental illness. *Community Mental Health Journal*, **30**, 221–242.

Miller, M. Caldwell, E. (1995). *Boulder Citizen Survey: 1995*. Boulder, Colorado: City of Boulder.

Morlino, M., Lisanti, F., Goggliettino, A. & De Girolamo, G. (1997). Publication trends of papers on schizophrenia: a 15–year analysis of three general psychiatric journals. *British Journal of Psychiatry*, **171**, 452–456.

Oliver, J., Huxley, P., Bridges, K. & Mohamad, H. (1996). *Quality of Life and Mental Health Services*. London: Routledge.

Polak, P., Kirby, M. W. & Deitchman, M. S. W. (1995). Treating acutely psychotic patients in private homes. In *Alternatives to the Hospital for Acute Psychiatric*

Treatment (ed. R. Warner), pp. 213–223. Washington D.C.: American Psychiatric Press.

Polak, P. & Warner, R. (1996). The economic life of the mentally ill in the community. *Psychiatric Services*, **47**, 270–274.

Reed, S. K., Hennessy, K., Mitchell, O. S. *et al.* (1994). A mental health capitation program: II. Cost-benefit analysis. *Hospital and Community Psychiatry*, **45**, 1097–1103.

Schwarz, N., Wänke, M. & Bless, H. (1994). Subjective assessments and evaluations of change: some lessons from social cognition research. In *European Review of Social Psychology* (ed. W. Stroebe & M. Hewstone), pp.181–210. New York: John Wiley.

Skantze, K., Malm, U., Dencker, S. J. *et al.* (1992). Comparison of quality of life with standard of living in schizophrenic outpatients, *British Journal of Psychiatry*, **161**, 797–801.

Torrey, E. F., Erdman, K., Wolfe, S. M. & Flynn, L. M. (1990). *Care of the Seriously Mentally Ill: A Rating of State Programs*. Washington, DC: Public Citizen Health Research Group and National Alliance of the Mentally Ill.

Warner, R. (1989). Deinstitutionalization: How did we get where we are? *Journal of Social Issues*, **45**, 17–30.

Warner, R. (1994). *Recovery from Schizophrenia: Psychiatry and Political Economy*, 2nd edn. London: Routledge.

Warner, R. & Huxley, P. (1998) Outcome for people with schizophrenia before and after Medicaid capitation. *Psychiatric Services,* **49**, 802–807.

Warner, R., de Girolamo, G., Belelli, G. *et al.* (1998) The quality of life of people with schizophrenia in Boulder, Colorado, and Bologna, Italy. *Schizophrenia Bulletin,* in press.

Yank, G. R., Hargrove, D. S. & Davis, K. E. (1992). Toward the financial integration of public mental health services. *Community Mental Health Journal*, **28**, 97–109.

PART VI **A working synthesis**

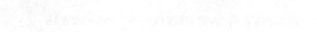

19

The matrix model as a pragmatic guide to improve services

19.1 **The purpose of the matrix model**

In describing the matrix model in this book we have four aims: (i) to provide a framework which simplifies the *description* of mental health services, (ii) to offer a way to *order* complex events, which can happen at different times, as well as concurrently, (iii) to assist *understanding* of these events, and (iv) to help to identify service deficits and to *prioritise actions* for service improvement.

First, we have attempted to simplify a *description* of the structure and functions of mental health services, because their complexity often prevents comparative assessments, and may mean that those involved in providing or receiving services do not have a shared terminology with which to communicate. We are aware that simplicity, while it encourages the initial appeal of the model, is bought at the expense of specificity. On the other hand, this question of balance is one that needs to be answered in any theoretical model that seeks to represent complex reality.

Second, with the matrix model we have sought to bring *order* by choosing time and space as the classical Cartesian axes for our two-dimensional model. We have selected these dimensions because, in our view, they are largely independent and because their interactions offer the richest array of domains useful to reflect the astonishing degree of variability in actual mental health services.

This model is therefore intended as an integrative tool. This is especially fit for its purpose within mental health services as they are characterised by several processes that tend to produce disintegration. The variety of agencies and organisations involved will often produce fission not fusion. The relative historical financial neglect of mental health services in many areas, compared with physical health services, has encouraged their decay. The competing ideological accounts of mental illness can lead to disunity in service provision. The sometimes conflicting imperatives of psychiatrists, and their colleagues, both to treat individual patients *and* to reassure the public as a whole, can fragment their identity and lead to contradictory actions. In addition, the nature of the work, involving direct contact with the apparent chaos of madness, and the deep demoralisation of depression, can be forces to oppose coherence among working clinicians. In this context, we see the matrix model as one method to increase coherence.

Third, we describe the matrix model in this book as an aid to *understanding* how mental health services operate. It seeks to explain events of clinical relevance in terms of their location in time and space, that is the 'where' and 'when', which may help our understanding of the 'how' and 'why'!

Fourth, we have entitled this book 'a pragmatic guide' since we want to stress the need to proceed from diagnosis, to *prioritising actions*, to intervention. Our aim is that this model will assist clinicians and non-clinicians (including planners, administrators and the recipients of services) to use a fuller understanding of their local services as a basis for action. The actions necessary in each local area will be quite specific to local circumstances, and will depend upon an evaluation of the current status of services. One of the issues likely to require action in many areas is to ensure that quality standards, equivalent to those used for physical health services, are applied to mental health services. Surprisingly the need to insist upon higher standards is required even in countries which spend relatively heavily upon health services as a whole, where the quality of mental health care, both in hospital and in community facilities, is sometimes unacceptable and often lower than in any other field of health care.

19.2 **The applicability of the matrix model**

An evaluation of the applicability of this model can be undertaken in several stages. As a first step we have subjected it to initial 'field-testing' at the country / regional (or multi-regional) level, using a largely theoretical approach, by asking five colleagues in different parts of the world to comment upon how far the model applies to their situation. In doing this we have asked them to adopt a critical stance. We value their expert assessments, although we do not necessarily agree with all the points they have made. In particular we disagree with many of the opinions expressed in the chapter on Nordic European countries, especially (i) with the view that the negative factors associated with large mental hospitals in most of the Western world are, or soon will be, history. In our opinion many such asylums continue to induce institutionalisation. (ii) With the low weight attached to the scientific evidence *for* some types of decentralised services, and (iii) with the expectation that technological advances will make community-orientated services decreasingly relevant in the foreseeable future. Nevertheless, the points of view expressed in these five chapters represent the range of current opinion, and indicate that among psychiatrists different visions of the future exist.

The next stages of this evaluation process will consist of the application of the matrix model to a variety of sites at the local and the patient levels. Judgement on its relevance will then be made both in terms of its usefulness for understanding unsatisfactory services, and for improving them.

At the initial assessment stage, several common themes have emerged in these five preceding chapters. In economically developed countries all around the world: (i) There is an increasing focus upon the need to apply the principles and methods of evidence-based medicine to mental health. Relating research to practice is an issue of considerable challenge. To reach this goal some degree of mutual understanding between four different cultures is necessary: the scientific research world; those who abstract and review the primary research literature; staff who produce local treatment guidelines and protocols; and clinical practitioners themselves. Each culture has its own different priorities and taken for granted assumptions. As yet we know far more about the effectiveness of patient treatment interventions than about effectiveness in the dissemination of these research findings (Dawson, 1997). (ii) The question of how far reductions in psychiatric bed numbers should proceed is becoming more and more pertinent, and suggests that many developed countries have already reduced to, or even beyond, a reasonable level of in-patient provision. (iii) The pressures for cost-containment are ubiquitous and will continue to bear down on average length of stay for admissions, and upon interventions which have not been justified by scientific evidence. (iv) Services for younger, long-term and severely disabled patients are in many sites seen to be inadequate, especially for psychotic patients with concurrent substance abuse. (v) The boundary and inter-relationships between health and social services is a recurrent line of friction, and is rarely resolved satisfactorily. (vi) An ever-present paradox for specialist mental health services in many areas is that they have the capacity to assist about 2% of the population, while ten times that number suffer from mental health problems each year, so which ten per cent of those suffering should be treated by the specialists? Who should assess and sometimes treat the remaining 90%? Any answer to this central question requires close collaboration with other services, and in particular an effective interface with primary care (Goldberg & Gournay, 1997). If the matrix model is to prove useful, it will do so by providing a common conceptual framework and terminology for tackling such widespread and important challenges to mental health services.

19.3 **Mental health services in future**

Predictions age quickly. Even so, we expect that many economically developed countries will face a similar set of questions in the near future. The role of mental health services needs to be seen here in the wider context of all health services, for in some ways the former have prefigured developments in the latter, and will probably continue to do so. The importance of *patient and carer involvement* is already better developed in many mental health services than elsewhere. The recognition of the wider range of *social needs* of those with severe illnesses has long been recognised by mental health professionals, and may be applied more closely in future to other chronic disease management programmes. Similarly, *the trend to move services away from expensive hospital sites*, except for acute treatment episodes, is already well developed in mental health and learning disabilities, and it is now developing in other disciplines managing long-term disorders.

But there is also a countervailing tendency, towards the location of highly specialised diagnostic and treatment techniques in centralised referral centres. This is likely to lead to an increasing polarisation between the proliferation of community services, and a fewer number of more expensive acute beds in large supra-regional specialist treatment centres. The functions carried out there will *only* be those which need treatment in hospital, and all other health services will be delivered by primary care or decentralised secondary care staff, as is the case at present in many types of mental health service.

In terms of research, the most pertinent questions in relation to mental health services will be of two types: which are the main *active ingredients* of effective treatments, and, in terms of *substitution,* how far can such effective treatments be used either in-hospital to make episodes of in-patient care shorter, or in community settings? This implies that the stage of 'naive community mental health', in which it was possible to argue that community services would replace all hospital services, is now past, and that in the newly emerging paradigm we shall recognise the value of facilities both at hospital and at community sites, as part of a well-integrated mental health system of care. The longer-term future is almost impossible to predict, so we shall not!

References

Acheson, E. D. (1985). That over-used word community. *Health Trends,* 17, 3.

Adams, C. Freemantle, N. & Lewis, G. (1996). Meta-analysis. In *Mental Health Service Evaluation* (ed. H.-C. Knudsen & G. Thornicroft). Cambridge: Cambridge University Pres.

Allebeck, P. (1989). Schizophrenia: a life-shortening disease. *Schizophrenia Bulletin,* 15, 81–89.

Amaddeo, F., Gater, R., Goldberg, D. & Tansella, M. (1995). Affective and neurotic disorders in community-based services: a comparative study in South-Verona and South-Manchester. *Acta Psychiatrica Scandinavica,* 91, 386–395.

Amaddeo, F., Bonizzato, P. & Tansella, M. (1997). A psychiatric case register for monitoring service evaluation and evaluating its costs. In *Making Rational Mental Health Services* (ed. M. Tansella), pp. 177–198. Epidemiologia e Psichiatria Sociale Monograph Supplement 1. Roma: Il Pensiero Scientifico Editore.

Angermeyer, M. C. & Matschinger, H. (1996). Public attitudes towards psychiatric treatment. *Acta Psychiatria Scandinavica,* 94, 326–336.

Audit Commission. (1986). *Making a Reality of Community Care.* London: HMSO.

Audit Commission (1994). *Finding a Place. A Review of Mental Health Services for Adults.* London: HMSO.

Bachrach, L. (1976). *Deinstitutionalisation: an Analytical Review and Sociological Perspective.* Rockville, Maryland: U.S. Department of Health, Education and Welfare, NIMH.

Bachrach, L. (1984). *The Homeless Mentally Ill and Mental Health Services: An Analytical Review of the Literature.* Washington: U.S Dept. of Health and Human Services.

Balestrieri, M., Bon, M. G., Rodriguez-Sacristan, A. & Tansella, M. (1994). Pathways to psychiatric care in South-Verona, Italy. *Psychological Medicine* 24, 641–649.

Banton, R., Clifford, P., Frosch, S., Lousada, J. & Rosenthall, J. (1985). *The Politics of Mental Health.* London: Macmillan.

Barham, P. (1992). *Closing the Asylum.* Harmondsworth: Penguin.

Barton, R. (1959). *Institutional Neurosis.* John Wright: Bristol.

Basaglia, F. (1968). *L'Istituzione Negata.* Torino: Giulio Einaudi Editore.

Basaglia, F. & Basaglia Ongaro, F. (1969). (eds) *Morire di Classe.* Turin: Einaudi.

Beaglehole, R. & Bonita, R. (1997). *Public Health at the Crossroads.* Cambridge: Cambridge University Press.

Bennett, D. (1978). Community psychiatry. *British Journal of Psychiatry,* 132, 209–220.

Bennett, D. & Freeman, H (1991). *Community Psychiatry. The Principles.* Edinburgh: Churchill Livingstone.

Ben-Tovim, D. (1987). *Development Psychiatry.* London: Tavistock.

Bierer, J. (1951). *The Day Hospital.* Lewis: London.

Biggeri, A., Rucci, P., Ruggeri, M. & Tansella, M. (1996). Multi-dimensional assessment of outcome: the analysis of conditional independence as an integrated statistical tool to model the relationships between variables. In *Mental Health Outcome Measures* (ed. G. Thornicroft G. & Tansella), pp. 207–216. Heidelberg: Springer.

Bindman, J. Johnson, S. Wright, S., Szmukler, G., Bebbington, P. Kuipers, E. & Thornicroft, G. (1997). Integration between primary and secondary services in the care of the severely mentally ill: patients' and general practitioners' views. *British Journal of Psychiatry*, **171**, 169–174.

Breakey, W. (1996). *Integrated Mental Health Services*. Oxford: Oxford University Press.

Brown, B. (1975). *Deinstitutionalisation and Community Support Systems*. Statement by Director, National Institute of Mental Health, 4 November. Bethesda, Maryland: NIMH.

Brown, P. (1985). *The Transfer of Care: Psychiatric Deinstitutionalisation and its Aftermath*. London: Routledge & Kegan Paul.

Bulmer, M. (1987). *The Social Basis of Community Care*. London: Allen & Unwin.

Busfield, J. (1986). *Managing Madness: Changing Ideas and Practice*, p. 246. London: Hutchinson.

Canosa R. (1979). *Storia del Manicomio in Italia dall'Unità ad Oggi*. Milano: Feltrinelli.

Chalmers, I., Enkin, M., Keirse, M. J. (1993). Preparing and updating systematic reviews of randomized controlled trials of health care. *Millbank Quarterly*, **71**, 411–437.

Clare, A. (1976). *Psychiatry in Dissent*, 1st edn. London: Routledge.

Clark, D. (1974). *Social Therapy in Psychiatry*. Harmondsworth: Pelican.

Cochrane, A. (1971). *Effectiveness and Efficiency: Random Reflections on Health Services*. Leeds: The Nuffield Provincial Hospitals Trust.

Cochrane Database of Systematic Reviews (1996). (ed. C. Adams, J. Anderson & J. Mari), available in *The Cochrane Library* (database on disk and CD ROM). The Cochrane Collaboration; Issue 3. Oxford: Update Software; 1996. Updated quarterly. Available from BMJ Publishing Group: London.

Cohen, J. (1960). A coefficient of agreement for nominal scales. *Educational and Psychological Measurement*, **20**, 37–46.

Concise Oxford Dictionary (1993). Oxford: Oxford University Press.

Cook, T. & Campbell, D. (1976). The design and conduct of quasi experiments and time experiments in field settings, pp. 266–279. In *Handbook of Industrial and Organisational*. (ed. M. Dunnette). Rand McNally: Chicago, Ill.

Cooper, B. (1979). Demographic and epidemiological methods in psychiatric research. In *Psychiatrie der Gegernwart*, 2nd edn. (ed K. P. Kisker, J.-E. Meyer, C. Mueller & E. Strómgren), pp. 685–710. Heidelberg: Springer.

Cooper, B. (1993). Single spies and battalions: the clinical epidemiology of mental disorders. *Psychological Medicine*, **23**, 891–907.

Cooper, B. (1995). Do we still need social psychiatry? *Psychiatria Fennica*, **26**, 9–20.

Cooper, D. (1974). *The Grammar of Living*. London: Allen Lane.

Creer, C. & Wing, J. (1974). *Schizophrenia at Home*. Surbiton, Surrey: National Schizophrenia Fellowship.

Davidge, M., Elias, S., Jayes, B. & Yates, J. (1993). *Survey of English Mental Illness Hospitals March 1993. Inter-Authority Consultancy and Comparisons*. Birmingham: University of Birmingham.

Davies, L. M. & Drummond, M. F. (1994). Economics and schizophrenia: the real cost. *British Journal of Psychiatry*, Suppl. **25**, 18–21.

Dawson, S. (1997). Inhabiting different worlds: how can research relate to practice? *Quality in Health Care*, **6**, 177–178.

de Girolamo, G. (1997). Evidence-based psychiatry: verso un nuovo paradigma della pratica clinica. *Rivista Sperimentale di Freniatria*, **121**, 147–178.

Dear, M. & Wolch, L. (1987). *Landscapes of Despair*. Cambridge: Polity.

Department of Health (1989). *Working for Patients*. Working Paper 6, Medical Audit. London: HMSO.

Department of Health (1990). *The Care Programme Approach for People with a Mental Illness*. Referred to as the specialist psychiatric services 1990. London: Department of Health

Department of Health (1993). *The Health of the Nation*. Key Area Handbook, Mental Illness. London: Department of Health.

Department of Health (1994). *The Health of the Nation*, 2nd edn. London: HMSO.

Department of Health (1996). *Spectrum of Care. Local Services for People with Mental Health Problems*. London: NHS Executive.

Department of Health and Social Security (1975). *Better services for the Mentally Ill*. London: HMSO.

Desjarlais, R., Eisenberg, L., Good, B. & Kleinman, A. (1995). *World Mental Health. Problems and Priorities in Low-Income Countries*. Oxford: Oxford University Press.

Dixon, L & Lehman, A. (1995). Family interventions for schizophrenia. *Schizophrenia Bulletin,* **21**, 631– 643.

Donabedian, A. (1992). The role of outcomes in quality assessment and assurance. *Quality Review Bulletin*, **181**, 356–360.

Early, D. (1978). Twenty years of industrial therapy in Britain. *International Journal of Mental Health*, **6**, 80–87.

Eisenberg, L. (1984). Rudolf Ludwig Karl Virchow, where are you now that we need you? *American Journal of Medicine*, **77**, 524–532.

Eisenberg, L. (1997). Past, present and future of psychiatry: personal reflections. *Canadian Journal of Psychiatry,* **42**, 705–713.

Endicott, I., Spitzer R., Fleiss J. L. & Cohen J. (1976). The Global Assessment Scale. *Archives of General Psychiatry*, **33**, 766–771.

Faulkner, A., Field V. & Muijen M. (1994). *A Survey of Adult Mental Health Services*. London: Sainsbury Centre for Mental Health.

Finer, S. (1952). *Life and Times of Edwin Chadwick*. London: Methuen.

Frank, J., Frank, J. & Cousins, N. (1993). *Persuasion and Healing*, 3rd edn. Johns Hopkins University Press.

Freeman, C. & Tyrer, P. (1989). *Research Methods in Psychiatry*. London: Royal College of Psychiatrists, Gaskell.

Freudenberg, R. (1967). Psychiatric care. *British Journal of Hospital Medicine*, **19**, 585–592.

Furedi, F. (1997). *Culture of Fear: Risk-Taking and the Morality of Low Expectation*. London: Cassell Academic.

Gater, R., De Almeida, E., Sousa, B., Burrientos, G., Caraven, J., Chandrashekar, C. R., Dhadphale, M., Goldberg, D., Al Kathiri, A. H., Mubasshar, M., Silhan, K., Thong, D., Torres-Gonzales, F. & Sartorius, N. (1991). The pathways to psychiatric care: a cross-cultural study. *Psychological Medicine*, **21**, 761–774.

Gater, R., Amaddeo F., Tansella, M., Jackson, G. & Goldberg, D. (1995). A comparison of community based care for schizophrenia in South Verona and South Manchester. *British Journal of Psychiatry*, **166**, 344–352.

Geddes, L. & Harrison, P. (1997). Closing the gap between research and practice. *British Journal of Psychiatry*, **171**, 220–225.

George, L. (1989). Definition, classification and measurement of mental health services. In *The Future of Mental Health Service Research* (ed. C. Taube, D. Mechanic and A. A. Adiman), pp. 303–319. DHSS Publication number (ADM) 89–1600. Washington DC: NIMH.

Gibbons, J. L., Jennings, C. & Wing J. K. (1984). *Psychiatric Care in Eight Register Areas*. Southampton: University Department of Psychiatry.

Gilman, S. (1996). *Seeing the Insane*. New York: Carlson.

Glover, G. (1996). Health service indicators for mental health. In *Commissioning Mental Health Services* (ed. G. Thornicroft & G. Strathdee), pp. 311–318. London: HMSO.

Glover, G. & Kamis-Gould, E. (1996). Performance indicators in mental health services. In *Commissioning Mental Health Services* (ed. G. Thornicroft & G. Strathdee), pp. 265–272. London: HMSO.

Goffman, E. (1961). *Asylums*. Harmondsworth: Pelican.

Goldberg, D. & Gournay, K. (1997). *The General Practitioner, the Psychiatrist and the Burden of Mental Health Care*. London: Institute of Psychiatry.

Goldberg, D. & Huxley, P. (1992). *Common Mental Disorders. A Bio-Social Model*. London: Routledge.

Goldberg, D. & Huxley, P. (1980). *Mental Illness in the Community*. Tavistock: London.

Goldberg, D. & Tantam, D. (1991). The public health impact of mental disorders. In *Oxford Textbook of Public Health*, 2nd edn. (ed W. Holland), pp 268–280. Oxford: Oxford University Press.

Goldman, H. (1981). Defining and counting the chronically mentally ill. *Hospital and Community Psychiatry*, **32**, 21–27.

Granville, J. (1877). *The Care and Cure of the Insane*. London.

Grob, G. (1991). *From Asylum to Community. Mental Health Policy in Modern America*. Princeton, New Jersey: Princeton University Press.

Gunn, J., Maden, A. & Swinton, M. (1991). Treatment needs of prisoners with psychiatric disorders. *British Medical Journal*, **303**, 338–340.

Haefner, H. & an der Heiden, W. (1986). The contribution of European case registers to research on schizophrenia. *Schizophrenia Bulletin*, **12**, 26–51.

Hall, J. (1979). Assessment procedures used in studies on long-stay patients. *British Journal of Psychiatry*, **135**, 330–335.

Hall, J. N. (1980). Ward rating scales for long-stay patients: a review. *Psychological Medicine*, **10**, 277–288.

Handy, C. (1976). *Understanding Organisations*. London: Penguin.

Hanlin, G. & Picket, J. (1984). *Public Health Administration and Practice*. St. Louis: Mosby.

Hansson, L. (1989). Utilisation of psychiatric in-patient care. *Acta Psychiatrica Scandinavica*, **79**, 571–578.

Haynes, R., McKibbon, K. & Kanani, R. (1996). *Systematic Review of RCTs of the Effects of Patient Adherence and Outcomes of Interventions to Assist Patients to Follow Prescriptions for Medications*. The Cochrane Library: BMJ updated 30 August 1996.

Henderson, A. S. (1988). *An Introduction to Social Psychiatry*. Oxford: Oxford University Press.

Henderson, A. S. (1996). The present state of psychiatric epidemiology. *Australian and New Zealand Journal of Psychiatry*, **30**, 9–19.

Hill, A. B. (1965). The environment and disease: association or causation? *Proceedings of the Royal Society of Medicine*, 295–300.

Hirsch, S. (1988). *Psychiatric Beds and Resources: Factors Influencing Bed Use and Service Planning*. London: Gaskell, The Royal College of Psychiatrists.

Holland, W. & Fitzsimons, B. (1990). Public health concerns: how can social psychiatry help? In *The Public Health Impact of Mental Disorder* (ed. D. Goldberg & D. Tantum), pp. 14–19. Toronto: Hogrefe & Huber.

Horn, G. ten., Giel, R., Gulbinat, W. & Henderson, A. S. (eds) (1986). *Psychiatric Case Registers in Public Health. A Worldwide Inventory, 1960–1985*. Elsevier: Amsterdam.

House of Commons (1985). *Second Report from the Social Services Committee, Session 1984–85, Community Care*. London: HMSO.

House of Commons Health Select Committee (1994). *Better Off in the Community? The Care of People Who Are Seriously Mentally Ill*. London: HMSO.

Houston, F. (1955). A project for a mental-health village settlement. *Lancet*, November 26, 1133–1134.

Hunter, R. & McAlpine, I. (1974). *Psychiatry for the Poor*. London: Dawsons.

Ingelby, D. ed. (1981). *Critical Psychiatry. The Politics of Mental Health*. Harmondsworth: Penguin.

Institute of Medicine (1994). *Reducing Risks for Mental Disorders: Frontiers for Preventive Intervention Research*. Washington DC: National Academy Press.

Israel, L., Kozarevic, V. & Sartorius, N. (1990). *Source Book of Geriatric Assessment*. Geneva: World Health Organization.

Jarman, B. (1983). Identification of underprivileged areas. *British Medical Journal*, **286**, 1705–1709.

Jarman, B. & Hirsch, S. (1992). Statistical models to predict district psychiatric morbidity. In *Measuring Mental Health Needs* (ed. G. Thornicroft, C. Brewin & J. K. Wing), pp. 62–80. London: Royal College of Psychiatrists, Gaskell Press.

Jarvis, E. (1850). The influence of distance from and proximity to an insane hospital on its use by any people. *Boston Medical Surgical Journal*, **32**, 409–422.

Jenkins, R. (1990). Towards a system of outcome indicators for mental health care. *British Journal of Psychiatry*, **157**, 500–514

Jenkins, R., Brooksbank, D. & Miller, E. (1994). Ageing in learning difficulties: the development of health care outcome indicators. *Journal of Intellectual Disability Research*, **38**, 257–264.

Johnson, S., Kuhlmann, R. & the EPCAT group. (1997a). *The European Service Mapping Schedule*. Version 3, February 1997. Available from the Section of Community Psychiatry, Institute of Psychiatry, London.

Johnson, S. Prossor, D. Bindman, J. & Szmukler, G. (1997b). Continuity of care for the severely mentally ill: concepts and measures. *Social Psychiatry and Psychiatric Epidemiology*, **32**, 137–142.

Jones, K. (1972). *A History of the Mental Health Services*. London: Routledge and Kegan Paul.

Jones, S. H., Thornicroft, G., Coffey, M. & Dunn, G. (1995). A brief mental health outcome scale–reliability and validity of the Global Assessment of Functioning (GAF). *British Journal of Psychiatry*, **166**, 654–659.

Kavanagh, S. (1994). Costs of schizophrenia. In *Unit Costs of Community Care* (ed. A. Netten), Canterbury: PSSRU, University of Kent.

Kessler, L. G., Steinwachs, D. & Hankin, J. (1980). Episodes of psychiatric utilisation. *Medical Care*, **18**, 1219–1227.

Knapp, M. (1995). Community mental health services: towards an understanding of cost-effectiveness. In *Community Psychiatry in Action: Analysis and Prospects* (ed. P. Tyrer & F. Creed), pp. 121–130. Cambridge: Cambridge University Press.

Knapp, M. (1996). What is community care? *Journal of Health Services Research and Policy*, 1, 254.

Knudsen, H. C. & Thornicroft, G. (1996). *Mental Health Service Evaluation*. Cambridge: Cambridge University Press.

Kovel, J. (1976). *A Complete Guide to Therapy. From Psychoanalysis to Behavior Modification*. New York: Pantheon Books.

Kramer, M., Brown, M., Skinner, A., Anthony, J., German, P. (1987). Changing living arrangements and their potential effect on the prevalence of mental disorder: findings of the Eastern Baltimore mental health survey. In *Psychiatric Epidemiology* (ed. B. Cooper), pp. 3–26. Beckenham: Croom Helm.

Kuhn, T. S. (1962). *The Structure of Scientific Revolutions*. Chicago: University of Chicago Press.

Kuipers, L. & Bebbington, P. (1991). *Working in Partnership: Clinicians and Carers in the Management of Long-Term Mental Illness*. London: Heinemann.

L'Abbe, K. A., Detsky, & A. S. O'Rourke, K. (1987). Meta-analysis in clinical research. *Annals of Internal Medicine*, 107, 224–233.

Laing, R. (1966). *The Divided Self*. Harmondworth: Penguin.

Lamb, H. (1994). A century and a half of psychiatric rehabilitation in the United States. *Hospital & Community Psychiatry*, 45, 1015–1020.

Last, S. L. (1972). *Lancet*, i, 630 (letter).

Lehman, A. F. (1996). Measures of quality among person with severe and persistent mental disorders. In *Mental Health Outcome Measures* (ed. G. Thornicroft & M. Tansella), pp. 75–92. Heidelberg: Springer.

Lelliot, P., Audini, P., Johnson, S. & Guite, H. (1997). London in the context of mental health policy. In *London's Mental Health* (ed. S. Johnson, L. Brooks, G. Thornicroft et al.). London: King's Fund.

Levine, M. (1981). *The History and Politics of Community Mental Health*. London: Oxford University Press.

Lewis, A. (1959). The impact of psychotropic drugs on the structure, function and future of psychiatric services in hospitals. In *Neuropsychopharmacology* (ed. P. Bradley, P. Deniker & C. Radonco-Thomas), p. 207. Amsterdam: Elsevier.

Light, D. W. (1991). Effectiveness and efficiency under competition: the Cochrane test. *British Medical Journal*, 303, 1253–1254.

Lindholm, H. (1983). Sectorised psychiatry. *Acta Psychiatrica Scandinavica*, 67, Supplement 304.

Locke, J. (1690). Second Treatise of Civil Government. Cited in *Oxford Dictionary of Quotations*.

Lynch, J. W. (1996). Social position and health. *Annals of Epidemiology*, 6, 21–23.

Lynch, J. W. Kaplan, G. A. & Shema, S. L. (1997). Cumulative impact of sustained economic hardship on physical, cognitive, psychological and social functioning. *New England Journal of Medicine*, 337, 1889 – 1895.

McLean, E. & Liebowitz, J. (1989). Towards a working definition of the long-term mentally ill. *Psychiatric Bulletin*, 13, 251–252.

Maden, A., Taylor C. Brooke, D. & Gunn, J. (1995). *Mental Disorder in Remand Prisoners: A report commissioned by the Directorate of Prison Health Care*. Home Office unpublished. Cited in Special Hospitals Service Authority, Service Strategies for Secure Care 1995.

Mann, N. C. (1993). *Improving Adherence Behaviour with Treatment Regimes*. Geneva: World Health Organization.

Mari, J. J. & Streiner, D. (1996). Family intervention for those with schizophrenia. In *Schizophrenia Module of The Cochrane Database of Systematic Reviews* (updated 10 September 1996) (ed. C. Adams, J. Annderson & J. J. Mari). Available in *The Cochrane Library* (database on disk and CD ROM), The Cochrane Collaboration, Issue 3. Oxford: Update Software, 1996. Updated quarterly. Available from BMJ Publishing Group: London.

Martin, L. (1984). *Hospitals in Trouble*. Blackwell: Oxford.

Maslach, C. & Jackson, S. (1979). Burned-out cops and their families. *Psychology Today*, **12**, 59–62.

Masur, F. T. (1981). Adherence to health care regimes. In *Medical Psychology. Contributions to Behavioural Medicine* (ed. C. K. Prokop & L. A. Bradley), pp. 441–469. New York: Academic Press.

Mechanic, D. (1986). The challenge of chronic mental illness: a retrospective and prospective view. *Hospital and Community Psychiatry*, **37**, 891–896.

Meltzer, H. Gill, B., Pettigrew, M. & Hinds, K. (1995). *The Prevalence of Psychiatric Morbidity among Adults Living in Private Households*. London: HMSO.

Mental Health Foundation (1993). *Mental Health: the Fundamental Facts*. London: MHF.

MIND (1983). *Common Values*. London: MIND.

MIND (1995). *Proposed Community Care (Rights to Mental Health Services) Bill*. London: MIND.

Mosher, L. & Burti, L. (1989). *Community Mental Health. Principles and Practice*, 2nd edn. revised. New York: Norton.

Mosher, L. & Burti, L. (1994). *Community Mental Health. Principles and Practice*, 2nd edn. Revised. New York: Norton.

Mueller, C. (1973). L'avenir de l'institution psychiatrique, utopie ou realite? *Social Psychiatry*, **8**, 185–191.

Murray, C. J. L. & Lopez, A. D. (eds.) (1996a). *The Global Burden of Disease, Volume 1. A Comprehensive Assessment of Mortality and Disability from Diseases, Injuries and Risk Factors in 1990, and Projected to 2020*. Cambridge Mass.: Harvard University Press.

Murray, C. J. L. & Lopez, A. D. (1996b). Evidence-based health policy – lessons from the global burden of disease study. *Science*, **274**, 740–743.

Murray, C. J. L. & Lopez, A. D. (1997a). Global mortality, disability, and the contribution of risk factors: Global Burden of Disease Study. *Lancet*, **349**, 1436–1442

Murray, C. J. L. & Lopez, A. D. (1997b). Alternative projections of mortality and disability by cause 1990–2020: Global Burden of Disease Study. *Lancet*, **349**, 1498–1504.

Murray, R., Hill, P. & McGuffin, P. (eds.) (1997). *Postgraduate Psychiatry*. Cambridge: Cambridge University Press.

National Institute of Mental Health (1985). *Measuring Social Functioning in Mental Health Studies: Concepts and Instruments*. Rockville: NIMH.

National Institute of Mental Health (1987). *Toward a Model Plan for a Comprehensive Community-Based Mental Health System*. Washington DC: NIMH.

Newton, J. (1992). *Preventing Mental Illness in Practice*. London: Routlege.

O'Driscoll, C. (1993). The TAPS Project 7. Mental hospital closure – a literature review of outcome studies and evaluative techniques. *British Journal of Psychiatry*, **162**, (supplement 19), 7–17.

Ødegaard, O. (1962). Psychiatric epidemiology. *Proceedings of the Royal Society of Medicine*, **55**, 831.

Organisation for Economic Co-operation and Development (1997). *Health Data '97*. Paris: OECD.

Parry, G. & Watts, F. (1989). *Behavioural And Mental Health Research: A Handbook Of Skills and Methods*. London: Lawrence Erlbaum Associates Ltd.

Patmore, C. & Weaver, T. (1990). Rafts on an open sea. *Health Service Journal*, 11th October, 1510–1512.

Phelan, M., Slade, M., Thornicroft, G., Dunn, D., Holloway, F., Wykes, T., Strathdee, G., Loftus, L., McCrone, P. & Hayward, P. (1995). The Camberwell Assessment of Need (CAN): the validity and reliability of an instrument to assess the needs of people with severe mental illness. *British Journal of Psychiatry*, **167**, 589–595.

Phelan, M., Wykes, T. & Goldman, H. (1996). Global function scales. In *Mental Health Outcome Measures* (ed. G. Thornicroft & M. Tansella), pp. 15–25. Heidelberg: Springer.

Poor Law Commission (1842). Quoted in *Report of Metropolitan Commissioners in Lunacy, 1844*, pp 95–96.

Powell, R. & Slade, M. (1996). Defining severe mental illness. In *Commissioning Mental Health Services* (ed. G. Thornicroft & G. Strathdee), pp. 13–27. London: HMSO.

Prosser, D., Johnson, S. Kuipers, E., Szmukler, G., Bebbington, P. & Thornicroft, G. (1996). Mental health, 'burnout', and job satisfaction among hospital and community-based mental health staff. *British Journal of Psychiatry*, **169**, 334–337.

Ramsay, R., Thornicroft, G., Johnson, S., Brooks, L. & Glover, G. (1997). Levels of in-patient and residential provision throughout London. In *London's Mental Health* (ed. S. Johnson *et al.*), pp. 193–219. London: King's Fund.

Rehin, G. & Martin, F. (1963). Some problems for research in community care. In *Trends in the Mental Health Service* (ed H. L. Freeman & J Farndale), pp. 34–43. Oxford: Pergamon Press.

Report on the Royal Commission on Mental Illness and Mental Deficiency (1957). Cmnd 169. London: HMSO.

Reynolds, A. & Thornicroft, G. (1999). *Managing Mental Health Services*. Open University Press (in press).

Robins, L. N. & Regier, D. A. (1991). *Psychiatric Disorders in America*. New York: Free Press.

Robinson, M. (1991). Medical audit: basic principles and current methods. *Psychiatric Bulletin*, **15**, 21–23.

Rose, G. (1992). *The Strategy of Preventive Medicine*. Oxford: Oxford University Press.

Rose, G. (1993). Mental disorder and the strategies of prevention. *Psychological Medicine*, **23**, 553–555.

Roth, A. & Fonagy, P. (1996). *What Works, For Whom? A Critical Review of Psychotherapy Research*. New York: Guildford Press.

Ruggeri, M. (1996). Satisfaction with psychiatric services. In *Mental Health Outcome Measures* (ed. G. Thornicroft & M. Tansella), pp. 27–51. Heidelberg: Springer.

Ruggeri, M. & Dall'Agnola, R. (1993). The development and use of Verona

Expectations for Care Scale (VECS) and the Verona Service Satisfaction Scale (VSSS). *Psychological Medicine*, **23**, 511–524.

Sabshin, M (1966). Theoretical models in community and social psychiatry. In *Community Psychiatry* (ed. L. M. Roberts, S. L. Halleck & M. B. Loeb). Madison: University of Wisconsin Press.

Sackett, D., Rosenberg, W., Muir Gray, J., Haynes, R. & Richardson, W. (1996). Evidence based medicine: what it is and what it isn't. *British Medical Journal*, **312**, 71–72.

Salvador-Carulla, L. (1996). Assessment instruments in psychiatry: description and psychometric properties. In *Mental Health Outcome Measures* (ed. G. Thornicroft & M. Tansella), pp. 189–206. Heidelberg: Springer Verlag.

Sartorius, N. (1988). Future directions: a global view. In *Handbook of Social Psychiatry* (ed A. S. Henderson & G. D. Burrow), pp. 341–346. Amsterdam: Elsevier.

Sartorius, N. & Janca, A. (1996). Psychiatric assessment instruments developed by the World Health Organisation. In *Mental Health Outcome Measures* (ed. G. Thornicroft & M. Tansella), pp. 153–177. Heidelberg: Springer.

Sartorius, N., Jablenksy, A., Korten, A., Ernberg, G., Anker, G., Cooper, J. & Pay, R. (1986). Early manifestations and first-contact incidence of schizophrenia in different cultures. *Psychological Medicine*, **16**, 909–928.

Sartorius, N., de Girolamo, G., Andrews, G., Allen German, G. & Eisenberg, L. (1993). *Treatment of Mental Disorders. A Review of Effectiveness*. Washington DC: American Psychiatric Press.

Schene, A., Tessler, R. & Gamache, G. (1994). Instruments measuring family or care giver burden in severe mental illness. *Social Psychiatry and Psychiatric Epidemiology*, **29**, 228–240.

Scott, J. (1988). Chronic depression. *British Journal of Psychiatry*, **153**, 287–297.

Scull, A. (1979). *Museums of Madness*. London: Allen Lane.

Scull A. (1984). *Decarceration*, 2nd edn. Cambridge: Polity.

Sedgwick, P. (1982). *Psychopolitics*. London: Pluto Press.

Serban, G. (1977). *New Trends of Psychiatry in the Community*. Cambridge, Mass.: Ballinger.

Shapiro, S., Skinner, E. A., Kramer, M. *et al.* (1985). Measuring need for mental health services in a general population. *Medical Care*, **23**, 1033–1043.

Shepherd G. (1984). *Institutional Care and Rehabilitation*. London: Longman.

Shepherd, M. (1983). The origins and directions of social psychiatry. *Integrative Psychiatry*, September / October, 86–88.

Shepherd, M. & Sartorius, N. (eds.) (1989). *Non-specific Aspects of Treatment*. Toronto: Hans Huber.

Shepherd, M., Goodman, N. & Watt, D. (1961). The application of hospital statistics in the evaluation of pharmacotherapy in a psychiatric population. *Comprehensive Psychiatry*, **2**, 11–19.

Shinfuku, N., Sugawara, S., Yanaka, T. & Kimura, M. (1998). Mental health in the city of Kobe, Japan. In *Mental Health in Our Future Cities* (ed. D. Goldberg & G. Thornicroft), pp. 125–146. London: Psychological Press.

Slade, M. (1994). Needs assessment: who needs to assess? *British Journal of Psychiatry*, **165**, 287–292.

Social Services Committee 1984/85 session, second report. (1985). *Community Care with Special Reference to Adult Mentally Ill and Mentally Handicapped People*. London: HMSO.

Sowden, A., Tilford, S., Delaney, F., Vogels, M., Gilbody, S. & Sheldon, T. (1997). Mental health promotion in high risk groups. *Quality in Health Care*, **6**, 219–225.

Stevens, A. & Gabbay, J. (1991). Needs assessment, needs assessment. *Health Trends*, **23**, 20–23.

Strathdee, G. & Thornicroft, G. (1992). Community sectors for needs-led mental health services. In *Measuring Mental Health Needs* (ed. G. Thornicroft, C. Brewin & J. K. Wing), pp. 140–162. Royal College of Psychiatrists, Gaskell Press.

Strathdee, G. & Thornicroft, G. (1997). Community psychiatry and service evaluation. In *The Essentials of Psychiatry* (ed. R. Murray, P. Hill & P. McGuffin), pp. 513–533. Cambridge: Cambridge University Press.

Streiner, D. & Norman, G. (1989). *Health Measurement Scales*. Oxford: Oxford University Press.

Susser, M. (1973). *Causal Thinking in the Health Sciences*. London: Oxford University Press.

Sytema, S., Micciolo, R. & Tansella, M. (1997). Continuity of care for patients with schizophrenia and related disorders: a comparative South-Verona and Groningen case register study. *Psychological Medicine*, 1355–1362.

Szmukler, G. & Bloch, S. (1997). Family involvement in the care of people with psychosis. *British Journal of Psychiatry*, **171**, 401–405.

Talbott, J. A. (1996). Re-inventing community psychiatry in the United States. *Epidemiologia e Psichiatria Sociale*, **5**, 14–18.

Tansella, M. (1986). Community psychiatry without mental hospitals – The Italian experience: a review. *Journal of the Royal Society of Medicine*, **79**, 664–669.

Tansella, M. (ed.) (1991). *Community-based Psychiatry: Long-term Patterns of Care in South Verona*. Psychological Medicine, Monograph Supplement 19. Cambridge: Cambridge University Press.

Tansella, M. (ed.) (1997). *Making Rational Mental Health Services*. Roma: Il Pensiero Scientifico Editore.

Tansella, M. & Micciolo R. (1998). Unplanned first-ever contact as a predictor of future intensive use of mental health services. *Social Psychiatry and Psychiatric Epidemiology*, **33**, 174–180.

Tansella, M. & Ruggeri, M. (1996). Monitoring and evaluating a community-based mental health service: the epidemiological approach. In *Scientific Basis of Health Services* (ed. M. Peckham & R. Smith), pp. 160–169. London: BMJ Publishing Group.

Tansella, M. & Zimmermann-Tansella, C. (1988). From mental hospitals to alternative community services. In *Modern Perspectives in Clinical Psychiatry* (ed. J. G. Howells), pp. 130–148. New York: Brunner Mazel.

Tansella, M., De Salvia, D. & Williams, P. (1987). The Italian psychiatric reform: some quantitative evidence. *Social Psychiatry*, **22**, 37–48.

Tansella, M., Micciolo, R., Biggeri, A., Bisoffi, G. & Balestrieri, M. (1995). Episodes of care for first-ever psychiatric patients. A long-term case-register evaluation in a mainly urban area. *British Journal of Psychiatry*, **167**, 220–227.

Taylor, R. & Thornicroft, G. (1996). Uses and limits of randomised controlled trials in mental health services research. In *Mental Health Outcome Measures* (ed. G. Thornicroft & M. Tansella), pp. 143–152. Springer Verlag: Heidelberg.

Thompson, C. (1989). *The Instruments of Psychiatric Research*. Chichester: Wiley.

Thornicroft, G. (1991). Social deprivation and rates of treated mental disorder: developing statistical models to predict psychiatric service utilisation. *British Journal of Psychiatry*, **158**, 475–484.

Thornicroft, G. & Bebbington, P. (1989). Deinstitutionalisation – from Hospital Closure to Service Development. *British Journal of Psychiatry*, **155**, 739–753.

Thornicroft, G. & Strathdee, G. (1994). How many psychiatric beds. *British Medical Journal*, **309**, 970–971.

Thornicroft, G. & Tansella, M. (eds.) (1996). *Mental Health Outcome Measures*. Heidelberg: Springer Verlag.

Thornicroft, G., De Salvia, G. & Tansella, M. (1993). Urban–rural differences in the associations between social deprivation and psychiatric service utilisation in schizophrenia and all diagnoses: a case-register study in Northern Italy. *Psychological Medicine*, **23**, 487–496.

Thornicroft, G., Strathdee, G., Phelan, M., Holloway, F., Wykes, T., Dunn, G., McCrone, P., Leese, M, Johnson, S. & Szmukler, G. (1999). Rationale and design: the PRiSM psychosis study (1). In *The Outcomes of Community Mental Health Services for Epidemiologically Representative Cases of Psychosis in South London* (ed. G. Thornicroft) (submitted for publication).

Tooth, G. & Brooke, E. (1961). Trends in mental hospital population and their effect on future planning. *Lancet*, **i**, 710–713.

Tyrer P., Morgan, J., Van Horn, E., Jayakody, M., Evans, K., Brummell, R., White, T., Baldwin, D., Harrison-Read, P. & Johnson, T. A. (1995). Randomised controlled study of close monitoring of vulnerable psychiatric patients. *Lancet*, **345**, 756–759.

United Nations (1992). Protection of persons with mental illness and improvement in mental health care. Resolution UN/GA/46/119. New York, United Nations, 17 December 1991, and *International Digest of Health Legislation*, **43**, 2.

Warner, R. (1994). *Recovery from Schizophrenia*, 2nd edn. London: Routledge.

Warr, P. (1987). *Work, Unemployment and Mental Health*. Oxford University Press: Oxford.

Watts, F. & Bennett, D. (1983). Management of the staff team. In *Theory and Practice of Psychiatric Rehabilitation* (ed F. N. Watts & D. Bennett), pp. 313–328. Chichester: John Wiley and Sons

Wetzler, S. (1989). *Measuring Mental Illness*. Washington DC: American Psychiatry Press.

Wiersma, D. (1996). Measuring social disabilities in mental health. In *Mental Health Outcome Measures* (ed. G. Thornicroft & M. Tansella), pp. 110–122. Heidelberg: Springer.

Wing, J. (1960). Pilot experiment in the rehabilitation of long-hospitalised male schizophrenic patients. *British Journal of Preventative and Social Medicine*, **14**, 173–180.

Wing, J. (1971). How many psychiatric beds? *Psychological Medicine*, **1**, 189–190.

Wing, J (1972). The Camberwell Register and the development of evaluative research. In *Evaluating a Community Psychiatric Service* (ed. J. Wing & A. Hailey), pp. 3–10. Oxford: Oxford University Press.

Wing, J. (1986). The cycle of planning and evaluation. In *Mental Health Services in Britain: the Way Forward* (ed. G. Wilkinson & H. Freeman), pp. 35–48. London: Gaskell.

Wing, J. (ed.) (1989). *Health Services Planning and Research. Contributions from Psychiatric Case Registers*. London: Gaskell.

Wing, J. K. (1992). *Epidemiologically Based Needs Assessments. Review of Research on Psychiatric Disorders*. London: Department of Health.

Wing, J. (1996). SCAN (Schedule for Clinical Assessment in Neuropsychiatry and the PSE (Present State Examination) tradition. In *Mental Health Outcome Measures* (ed. G. Thornicroft & M. Tansella), pp. 123–130. Heidelberg: Springer Verlag.

Wing, J. & Brown, G. (1970). *Institutionalism and Schizophrenia*. Cambridge: Cambridge University Press.

Wing, J. & Lelliot, P. (1994). Number of psychiatric beds (letter). *British Medical Journal*, **309**, 1516.

Wing, J. K., Brewin, C. R. & Thornicroft, G. (1992). Defining mental health needs. In *Measuring Mental Health Needs* (ed. G. Thornicroft, C. Brewin & J. Wing). Royal College of Psychiatrists, London: Gaskell.

Wing, J. K. Beevor, A. S., Curtis, R. H., Park, S. B., Hadden, S. & Burns, A. (1998). Health of the Nation Outcome Scales, (HoNOS). Research and development. *British Journal of Psychiatry*, **172**, 11–18.

Wittchen, U. & Nelson, C. B. (1996). The Composite International Diagnostic Interview, an Instrument for Measuring Mental Health Outcome? In *Mental Health Outcome Measures* (ed. G. Thornicroft & M. Tansella), pp. 179–187. Heidelberg: Springer Verlag.

World Health Organization (1980). *International Classification of Impairments, Disabilities and Handicaps*. Geneva: WHO.

World Health Organization (1983). *Psychiatric Case Registers*. Report on a Working Group (5–6.5.1983). Copenhagen: WHO Regional Office for Europe.

World Health Organization (1990). *International Classification of Mental Health Care*, 2nd edn. WHO Regional Office for Europe and WHO Collaborating Centre for Research and Training in Mental Health, University of Groningen.

World Health Organization (1996a). *Mental Health Law: Ten Basic Principles*. Geneva: WHO.

World Health Organization (1996b). *Public Mental Health: Guidelines for the Elaboration and Management of National Mental Health Programmes*. Geneva: WHO, Division of Mental Health and Prevention of Substance Abuse.

World Psychiatric Association (1978). Declaration of Hawaii. *Journal of Medical Ethics*, **4**, 71–73.

World Psychiatric Association (1983). *Declaration of Hawaii/II*. WPA General Assembly, Vienna, 10th July 1983. WPA document.

World Psychiatric Association (1996). *Declaration of Hawaii/III*. Revised at the General Assembly of Madrid in 1996. WPA document.

Glossary

Accessibility A service characteristic, experienced by users and their carers, which enables them to receive care where and when it is needed.

Accountability The complex, dynamic relationships between mental health services and patients, their families and the wider public.

Admission rates for patients in contact with the services In-patients prevalence divided by total treated prevalence, expressed as a percentage.

Annual treated incidence Total number of patients who had a first-ever contact with a psychiatric service during the specified year.

Annual treated prevalence Total number of patients who had a contact with psychiatric services during the specified year.

Autonomy A patient characteristic consisting of the ability to make independent decisions and choices, despite the presence of symptoms or disabilities.

Basic Service Profile (BSP) The basic services necessary for any system of mental health care.

Case registers Health information systems of a geographically defined area that record contacts between patients and designated services.

Community-based mental health service A service which provides a full range of effective mental health care to a defined population, and which is dedicated to treating and helping people with mental disorders, in proportion to their suffering or distress, in collaboration with other local agencies.

Comprehensiveness A service characteristic, comprising how far a service extends across the range of mental illness severity and patient characteristics (horizontal comprehensiveness), and the availability of the basic components of care and their use by prioritised patient groups (vertical comprehensiveness).

Continuity The ability of services to offer an uninterrupted series of contacts over time (longitudinal continuity) and between service providers (cross-sectional continuity).

Co-ordination A service characteristic, manifested by coherent treatment plans for individual patients.

Country/regional level The level with a shared government, which passes mental health laws, sets overall policy and minimum clinical standards, and organises professional training.

DALY Disability-Adjusted Life Years, the sum of years of life lost because of premature mortality plus the years of life lived with disability, adjusted for the severity of disability.

Effectiveness The proven, intended benefits of treatments (at the patient level) or services (at the local level) provided in real life situations.

Efficiency A service characteristic, which minimises the inputs needed to achieve a given level of outcomes, or which maximises the outcomes for a given level of inputs.

Equity The fair distribution of resources.

First ever admissions Total number of first-ever hospital psychiatric admissions in the specified year.

Geographical dimension A dimension of the Matrix model, comprising country/regional, local and patient levels.

In-patient prevalence Total number of patients who spent at least one day in hospital in the specified year.

Input phase The resources which are put

into mental health care, comprising visible (e.g. budget, staff, facilities) and invisible (e.g. skills of staff, organisational arrangements) inputs.

Local level The catchment area for which an integrated system of care for general adult mental health can be provided.

Matrix model A conceptual model (comprising geographical and temporal dimensions) to help formulate service aims and the steps necessary for their implementation.

Outcome phase Changes in the health status of patients (either individually or aggregated), comprising measures before and after a clinical intervention.

Patient level The therapeutic domain, which includes interventions for patients (individually or in groups), families or carers.

Planning A linked series of actions designed to achieve a particular goal, and which requires the completion of increasingly specific tasks within a given timescale.

Primary prevention Measures which stop the genesis or expression of the disorder.

Primary service goals Interventions intended to give treatment, care and assistance to patients.

Process phase Those activities which take place to deliver mental health services, the vehicle for the delivery of health care.

Public health approach An approach to applying research findings to improve the health of populations and to allocate resources appropriately.

Randomised controlled trial (RCT) A study in which patients are randomly allocated to intervention or control groups, and then followed up to determine the effect of the intervention.

Readmissions Total number of hospital psychiatric readmissions in the specified year.

Reliability The extent to which an instrument is consistent and minimises random error.

Secondary prevention Early detection of cases, where early treatment can significantly improve the course and outcome of the disorder.

Secondary service goals Measures which are addressed to the needs of staff.

Segmental approach An approach to categorising service components, in which each facility or programme is viewed as a separate entity.

System approach An approach to categorising service components, in which each facility or programme is viewed as part of a wider system of care, with interrelationships explicitly considered.

Temporal dimension A dimension of the matrix model, comprising input, process and outcome levels.

Tertiary prevention Measures designed to reduce disabilities which are due to the disorder.

Total admissions Total number of hospital psychiatric admissions with a date of admission in the specified year.

Validity The extent to which an instrument measures what it is intended to measure.

Index

THE
CRYSTAL
PRISON

Book Two of
THE DEPTFORD MICE

Written and Illustrated
by Robin Jarvis

Purnell

A PURNELL BOOK

Text and illustrations copyright © Robin Jarvis 1989

First published in Great Britain in 1989
by Macdonald Children's Books
The Deptford Mice and all
character names and the distinctive likenesses
thereof are trademarks owned by Robin Jarvis

British Library Cataloguing in Publication Data

Jarvis, Robin
The Crystal Prison.
I. Title   II. Series
823'.914 [J]

ISBN 0-361-08574-5
ISBN 0-361-08575-3 Pbk.

Typeset in Palatino by 🅰 Tek Art Ltd
Printed in Great Britain by
BPCC Hazell Books Ltd
Member of BPCC Ltd
Aylesbury, Bucks, England

Macdonald Children's Books
Simon & Schuster International Group
Wolsey House, Wolsey Road
Hemel Hempstead HP2 4SS

CONTENTS

THE DEPTFORD MICE

AUDREY BROWN
Tends to dream. She likes to look her best and wears lace and ribbons. Audrey cannot hold her tongue in an argument, and often says more than she should.

ARTHUR BROWN
Fat and jolly, Arthur likes a scrap but always comes off worse.

GWEN BROWN
Caring mother of Arthur and Audrey. Her love for her family binds it together and keeps it strong.

ARABEL CHITTER
Silly old gossip who gets on the nerves of everyone in the Skirtings.

OSWALD CHITTER
Arabel's son is an albino runt. Oswald is very weak and is not allowed to join in some of the rougher games.

PICCADILLY
A cheeky young mouse from the city, Piccadilly has no parents and is very independent.

THOMAS TRITON
A retired midshipmouse. Thomas is a heroic old salt – he does not suffer fools gladly.

MADAME AKKIKUYU
A black rat from Morocco. She used to tell fortunes until her mind was broken in the chamber of Jupiter.

KEMPE
A travelling trader mouse – he journeys far and wide selling his goods and singing lewd songs.

THE STARWIFE
A venerable old squirrel who lives under the Greenwich observatory. Her motives are good but her methods are cruel.

THE
FENNYWOLDERS

WILLIAM SCUTTLE or "Twit"
A simple fieldmouse who has been visiting his mother's kin.
Twit is a cheerful fieldmouse who looks on the bright side.

ELIJAH AND GLADWIN SCUTTLE
Twit's parents, Gladwin is Mrs Chitter's sister but ran away
from Deptford when she was young when she found Elijah
injured in the garden.

ISAAC NETTLE
A staunch Green Mouser. He is a bitter, grim figure but
many of the fieldmice listen to his ravings.

JENKIN NETTLE
A jolly mouse who suffers at the paws of his father.

ALISON SEDGE
A country beauty who flirts with all the boys. She is vain and
loves to preen herself.

YOUNG WHORTLE, SAMUEL GORSE, TODKIN, HODGE
AND FIGGY BOTTOM
Five young friends who delight in climbing the corn stems
and seeking adventure.

MAHOOOT
A wicked barn owl who loves mouse for supper.

MR WOODRUFFE
A very sensible mouse who has been elected to the
honourable position of The King of the Field.

NICODEMUS
Mysterious spirit of the fields who is trying to get free from
limbo.

THE GREEN MOUSE
A magical figure in mouse mythology. He is the essence of all
growing things whose power is greatest in the summer.

THE DARK PORTAL

The Crystal Prison *is the second book in the story of the Deptford Mice, which began with* The Dark Portal. *In Book One, Audrey and Arthur Brown, two innocent town mice, are drawn into the sewers beneath the streets of Deptford in search of Audrey's mousebrass – a magical charm given to her by the Green Mouse, the mystical spirit of Spring. Deep within the underground tunnels, the two mice discover the nightmare realm of Jupiter, the unseen but terrifying lord of the rats.*

Audrey and Arthur are helped by a number of characters: Oswald, a sickly albino mouse often mistaken for a rat; Twit, Oswald's cousin and a simple country mouse; Piccadilly, a cheeky young mouse from the city; and Madame Akkikuyu, a black rat who ekes out a living peddling potions and telling phoney fortunes.

The Deptford Mice discover that Jupiter is concocting a terrible plan – to release the Black Death upon London once again. However, with the help of the Green Mouse, the mice confound Jupiter's plot and lure him out of his lair. To their horror, they discover that Jupiter is not a rat at all, but a monstrous cat, grown bloated and evil by years of hatred in the sewers.

Audrey throws her mousebrass into Jupiter's face; it explodes and sends the giant cat tumbling into the deep sewer water. As he struggles to save himself, the souls of his many victims rise out of the waves and drag him down to a watery death.

SMOKE OVER DEPTFORD

It was a hot day in Deptford. A terrible stench hung over the housing estates, and increased as the sun rose higher in the sky. It was strongest on a building site near the river. There the air was thick and poisonous. The builders themselves choked and covered their faces with their handkerchieves.

At the edge of the site, next to the river wall was an untidy pile of yellowing newspapers. They lay in a mouldering heap amongst the loose bricks and spreading nettles. It was here that the stink began.

One of the builders came trudging up, his worn, tough boots waded through the weeds and paused at the newspaper mound. A scuffed toe tentatively nudged some of them aside and a dark cloud of angry, buzzing flies flew out. Revealed beneath the papers was the rotting body of a horrific giant cat.

*　　　*　　　*

Jupiter was dead. The evil lord of the rats had met his end weeks before in the deep, dark sewer water. His immense body had sunk to the muddy bottom where underwater currents pulled and swayed his corpse this way and that. Slowly he rolled out of the altar chamber and through a submerged archway.

Into the tunnels he had drifted, turning over and over in the water. One minute his grisly unseeing eyes would be staring at the arched ceiling above and the next glaring down into the cold dark depths. As he rolled over in this way his great jaws lolled open lending him the illusion of life. Like a snarling demon he turned. But he was dead. For some days Jupiter bobbed up and down in the sewer passages until stronger forces gripped him and suddenly, with a rush of water he was flushed out into the River Thames. The gulls and other birds left him well alone, and for a while all fish abandoned that stretch of the river.

One night nature took a hand in ridding the river of the dreadful carcass. A terrible storm blew up: the wind and the rain lashed down from the sky, and the river became swollen and crashed against its walls with shuddering violence.

On one such surging wave was the corpse of Jupiter, carried along until with a thundering smash the wave smote the wall and the cat's body was hurled over onto the building site.

*   *   *

The builder who had found him hurried away quickly but soon returned dragging behind him a great shovel caked in cement. With a grunt he lifted the sagging corpse into the air. Jupiter's massive claws dangled limply over the sides of the shovel and what was left of his striped ginger fur blazed ruddily in the sunlight.

Surrounded by the thick buzzing cloud the builder stepped carefully over to the site bonfire and tossed Jupiter into its heart.

The flames licked over the cat greedily. For a while the fire glowed purple and then with one final splutter there was nothing left of the once mighty lord of the sewers.

Only a thick dark smoke which had risen from the flames remained, and this stayed hanging stubbornly in the air over Deptford for two days until a summer breeze blew it away on the third morning.

x

1

THE SUMMONS

Oswald was ill. As soon as the white mouse had returned from the sewers he had felt unwell. When the small group of mice who had confronted the terrifying Jupiter had emerged from the Grill and climbed the cellar steps Oswald's legs had given way and sturdy Thomas Triton had carried him the rest of the way. Although the albino coughed and spluttered no-one realised how serious his condition would become.

For weeks he had stayed in bed. At first the mice thought he had merely caught a cold, and his mother Mrs Chitter had fussed and scolded him over it. But the cold did not improve and his lungs had become inflamed so that when he coughed the pain made him cry. Steadily he grew weaker. Mrs Chitter tended to him day and night, and made herself ill in the process, until she too became a poor reflection of what she had once been.

Oswald's father, Jacob Chitter, had moved his favourite chair into his son's room next to his bed. He held his son's paw throughout, shaking his head sadly. Oswald was slipping away; bit by painful bit the white mouse became more frail. Then one day Mrs Chitter could take no more. As she was carrying away the soup that Oswald had been unable to swallow the bowl fell from her paws and she fell heavily to the floor – soup and tears everywhere.

From then on Gwen Brown took charge of Oswald and his mother whilst Twit the fieldmouse looked after his uncle, Mr Chitter.

All was silent in the Skirtings. The empty old house was filled with quiet prayers for the Chitter family. All the mice helped as much as they could: those on the Landings forgot their snobbery and offered food and blankets. Gwen Brown's own children Arthur and Audrey collected all the donations and messages of goodwill and it was the job of a grey mouse from the city called Piccadilly to keep everyone informed of Oswald's condition.

All the mice owed a great deal to this small group of friends. It was they who had finally rid them of the menace of Jupiter, and all their lives were now easier. No more did they have to dread the cellar and the strange Grill which was the entrance to the dark sinister rat world. All the cruel rats had been killed or scattered and a mouse could sleep soundly at night, fearing no sudden attacks or raids. Only the older mice still looked at the cellar doubtfully and would not pass beyond its great door.

So, when they had been told of Jupiter's fall – and when they finally believed it, there was tremendous excitement and they had cheered the brave deeds of these mice. But now the youngest of the heroes was dying.

*   *   *

Piccadilly swept the hair out of his eyes and got out of bed. The sunlight shone on the city mouse and warmed him all over but he hardly noticed it. For the moment, he was sharing a room with Arthur, and Audrey was sleeping in her mother's bed, as Gwen was at the Chitter's all the time now.

"Arthur," Piccadilly whispered to the snoring

2

bundle, "wake up." He shook his friend gently.

The plump mouse on the bed blinked and drew his paw over his eyes. "How is he?" he asked directly.

Piccadilly shook his head. "I've just got up – how was he last night when you left him?"

"Bad!" Arthur swung himself off the bed and stood in the sunlight as was his custom. He stared at the clear blue sky outside. "Mother doesn't think it will be long now," he sighed and looked across to Piccadilly. "Will you stay here, afterwards?"

The grey mouse sniffed a little. "No, I've made up my mind to stay just until . . ." he coughed, "then I'm off – back to the city."

"We'll miss you, you know," said Arthur. "I won't know what to do around here when you've gone. I think Twit's decided to leave as well . . . afterwards." Arthur turned back to examine the summer sky and then remarked casually. "I think Audrey will miss you most though."

Piccadilly looked up curiously. "She's never said anything."

"Well you know what she's like: too stubborn to say anything! I know my sister, and believe you me, she likes you a lot."

"Well, I wish she'd tell me."

"Oh I think she will when it suits her." Arthur stretched himself and rubbed his ears. "He doesn't even take the milk any more you know. Mother can't get him to drink it and if he does, it won't stay down. Maybe he would be better off . . ." his voice trailed away miserably.

"I'm dreading it," murmured Piccadilly. "These past few days he's sunk lower an' lower – I don't know what keeps him going."

Arthur touched him lightly on the shoulder. "Let's go and find out."

3

Audrey was already up and waiting for them. She had not bothered to tie the ribbon in her hair as she usually did and it hung in soft chestnut waves behind her ears.

Outside the Chitter's door they stopped, and Arthur glanced nervously at the others before knocking. They waited anxiously as shuffling steps approached on the other side of the curtain.

The curtain was drawn aside, and the small features of Twit greeted them solemnly. He looked back into the room, nodded, then stepped out and let the curtain fall back behind him.

"He's still with us," he whispered. "'Twere touch 'n go for a while last night: thought we'd lost 'im twice." The fieldmouse bit his lip. "Your mum's all in; she's 'ad a tirin' time of it. What with 'im and Mrs Chitter, she's fit to drop."

"I'll tell her to lie down for a bit," nodded Arthur.

"And I'll take over," added Audrey. "You look like you could do with a rest as well Twit."

"Well, Mr Chitter, he just sits an' mopes, his wife an' son bein' so bad. I can't do anything with 'im." Twit wiped his brimming eyes. "Heck we tried – me an' your mum, but all three of 'em are slidin' downhill fast. I really think this be the last day – no I knows it. None of 'em'll see the sunset." Big tears ran down the fieldmouse's little face. He was exhausted and felt that all his efforts had been a waste of time – this branch of his family was about to wither and die.

Audrey bent down and kissed Twit's forehead. "Hush," she soothed. "Piccadilly, put Twit in Arthur's bed. I'll wake you if anything happens," she reassured the fieldmouse.

"Thank 'ee." Twit stammered through a yawn and he followed Piccadilly back to the Brown's home.

4

Arthur turned to his sister. "Right," he said. "I'll tackle Mother, you see to the Chitters. I'll come and help once Mother's gone to bed." Gingerly he pulled back the curtain.

It was dark beyond: the daylight had been blocked out for Oswald's sake.

Arabel Chitter's bric-a-brac was well dusted, her pieces of china ornament, bits of sparkling brooches and neatly folded lace shawls and headscarves had all been seen to by Gwen Brown. Mrs Chitter had always been house-proud and if things were not "just so" she would fret.

Arthur and Audrey slowly made their way to Oswald's room. Arthur coughed quietly and their mother came out to them.

"Hello dears," she breathed wearily. Dark circles ringed her brown eyes and her tail dragged sadly behind her. "No ribbon today, Audrey?" she asked, stroking her daughter's hair. "And you Arthur, have you had breakfast?"

"Have you Mother?" he took her paw in his. "No, I didn't think so. Come on, you're going to get some sleep." He would hear no protests and Gwen Brown was too tired to make any.

"Audrey, promise me you'll wake me if . . ." was all she managed.

"I promise Mother."

"Yes, good girl. Now, come Arthur, show me to my bed or I'll drop down here."

Audrey watched them leave then breathed deeply and went inside.

Illness has a smell all of its own and it is unmistakable. Sweet and cloying, it lingers in a sick room, waiting for the patient to recover or fail. Audrey had grown accustomed to this smell by now though it frightened her to enter the room.

It was a small space almost filled by the bed in

which Oswald lay. Beside him on a chair was Mr Chitter, his head bent in sleep. He was a meek mouse, devoted to his wife and son, but this had broken him.

Oswald was quite still. His face was gaunt and drained, paler now than ever before. His eyelids were closed lightly over his dim pink eyes. His fair albino hair was stuck close to his head and his whiskers drooped mournfully. The blankets were pulled up under his chin but one of his frail paws was wrapped inside his father's.

Audrey felt Oswald's forehead: it was hot and damp. A fever was consuming his last energies, burning away whatever hope there had been for him. Sorrowfully she picked up a bowl from the floor. It contained clean water and a cloth, and with them she began to cool his brow.

Next to Oswald's bed, on the wall, was a garland of dried hawthorn leaves which he had saved from the spring ceremony and preserved carefully. He had adored the celebrations and was impatient for the following year when he too would come of age and be entitled to enter the mysterious chambers of summer and winter to receive his mousebrass. To Audrey it seemed long ago that she had taken hers from the very paws of the Green Mouse. She thought of him now, the mystical spirit of life and growing things. How often she had prayed to him to spare Oswald! Now it looked as if nothing could save him.

There was a small table near her and on it were some slices of raw onion. Mrs Chitter believed this would draw out the illness from her son, and out of respect for her wishes Gwen Brown made sure that the onion was fresh every day. Audrey only regarded this superstition as one more addition to the eerie smell of illness.

6

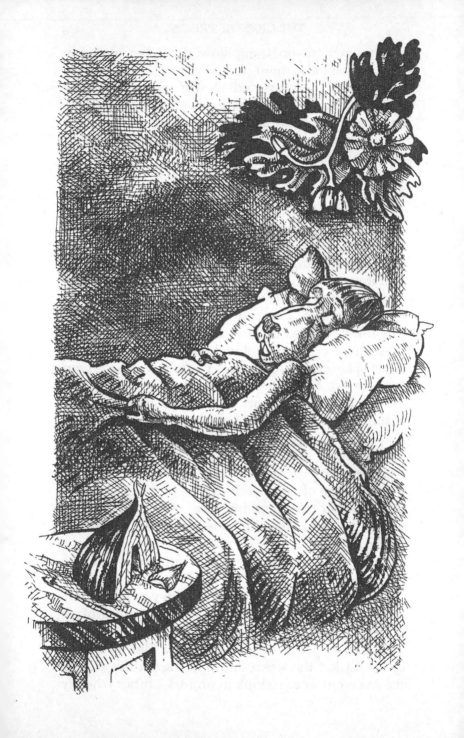

A movement on the pillow drew her attention back to the patient.

Oswald's eyes opened slowly. For a while he gazed at the ceiling, then gradually he focused on Audrey. She smiled at him warmly.

"Good morning, Oswald," she said.

The albino raised his eyebrows feebly and tried to speak. It was a low, barely audible whisper and Audrey strained to hear him.

"What sort . . . of day is it . . . outside?" His sad eyes pierced her heart and she struggled to remain reassuring when all the time she wanted to run from him sobbing. She could not get over the feeling that it was mainly due to her that Oswald was so ill.

"It's beautiful, Oswald," she said huskily. "You never saw such a morning! The sky is as blue as a forget-me-not and the sun is so bright and lovely."

A ghost of a smile touched Oswald's haggard cheeks. He closed his eyes. "You never did get your mousebrass back," he murmured.

"Yes I did, for a short while. You were so brave, getting it for me amongst all those horrible rats."

"I don't think I shall ever get my . . . brass now," he continued mildly. "I wonder what it would . . . have been."

"The sign of utmost bravery," sobbed Audrey. She held her paw over her face.

"I'm so sorry Oswald," she cried. "This is all my fault."

"No, it had to be done . . . Jupiter had to be destroyed. Not your fault if . . . if I wasn't up to it."

"Don't, please! Just rest. Would you like some milk?" But Oswald had already fallen into a black swoon. Audrey cried silently.

A gentle, polite knock sounded. She dried her eyes and left the sickroom, pausing on the way to the main entrance to look in on Mrs Chitter who lay asleep in another room. Arabel's silvery head was old and shrivelled. It was startling to see it against the crisp whiteness of the pillows. But at least she was asleep and not fretting. Audrey crept away and made for the entrance.

"Oh, it's young Miss Audrey!" Sturdy Thomas Triton looked faintly surprised to see her when she drew the curtain back. "I was expectin' your mother, but if you aren't the very one anyway." The midshipmouse pulled off his hat and asked gravely, "How's the lad this morn?"

"No better, I'm afraid – we don't think he'll last much longer. Mother's resting just now: she and Twit have been up all night."

"Aye," muttered Thomas grimly, then he furrowed his spiky white brows and considered Audrey steadily with his wise, dark eyes. "'Tis a sore thing to bear – losing a friend," and an odd far-off expression stole over him, "specially if you think it's all your fault. That's a mighty burden, lass! Don't take it on yourself – guilt and grief aren't easy fellows to cart round with yer, believe you me."

Audrey turned away quickly. Thomas's insight was too unnerving and she cringed from it. "Would you like to see him?" she managed at last.

Thomas fidgeted with his hat, rolling it over in his strong paws. "Lead on, I'll look on the boy once more."

When they came to the sickroom he hesitated at the doorway and changed his mind. "Nay, I'll not enter. I've glimpsed the lad and that's enough. I've seen too many go down with fever to want to witness it again. He were a brave sort whatever he may have said to the contrary. A loss to us all. I see the father has not moved – is the mother still abed?" Audrey nodded. "That's bad! A whole family wiped out by sickness and grief. Well, how's little Twit bearing up?"

"Oh, you know Twit. He always tries to be bright and jolly. You never know what he's thinking deep down."

"Yes, you're right there. I like that fieldmouse – reminds me of someone I knew once – best friend I ever had. Twit's mighty fond of his cousin there – it'll be a tragic blow to his little heart."

A soft footfall behind them made them both turn sharply – but it was only Arthur.

"Hullo Mr Triton," he said politely. "Audrey, I've managed to put Mother to bed and she's asleep now, but I think Piccadilly's having trouble with Twit – he needs to rest, but won't settle. He can't stop worrying!"

"Right, I'll get him out of that," said Thomas firmly and he fixed his hat back on his head. "Come with me, miss, and you milladdo, stay here. I'll see to my young matey." The midshipmouse strode from the Chitter's home with Audrey following.

"Mr Triton," she said, catching up with him. "What did you mean before when you saw me and said I was the very one?"

"It wasn't just to see poor Oswald that I came," he explained as they entered the Brown's home, "but to see you as well."

"Me?" asked Audrey, puzzled. She had not spoken to the midshipmouse very much during the brief times that he had visited the Skirtings and she wondered what he was up to.

"Aye lass," he continued. "I've a message for you."

She looked blank as Thomas Triton charged into Arthur and Piccadilly's bedroom.

The city mouse was trying to get Twit to stay in bed. He had heated him some milk and honey but the fieldmouse would not rest. When Thomas

10

barged in Twit grinned in spite of himself.

"How do!" he said.

"Ahoy there matey," Thomas said sternly. "What you doin', lyin' in yer bunk on a day like this?" The midshipmouse winked a startled Piccadilly into silence. "Get up lad, there's folk to see!"

"But he's only just gone to bed" exclaimed Audrey.

Without turning round to look at her, Thomas said, "You, miss, had better make yourself presentable. What has happened to your hair?"

"I . . . I didn't put my ribbon in," stammered Audrey.

"Then chop chop lass. Go do whatever you do do to make a good impression. Someone wants to see you."

"Who's that then Thomas?" asked Twit, curiosity banishing the weary lines around his eyes.

The midshipmouse feigned astonishment. "Why, the Starwife lad – didn't I say?"

Twit's eyes shone with excitement. "What? Her that lives in Greenwich under those funny buildings I saw when the bats flew me over?"

"Aye matey. First thing this morning, when it was still dark, I had a message from herself delivered by one of her younger jumpy squirrels – took me a long time to calm him down. They are a watery lot! Well the gist of the story is," Thomas now turned to Audrey, "that the Starwife wants to see you, Miss Brown, and she won't be kept waitin'. I've come to fetch you, and milladdo here is welcome to join us."

For a second Twit's heart leapt, but when he thought of Oswald it sank down deeper and lower than ever. Sadly he shook his head. "I can't come Thomas. Oswald won't see the end of the day – my place is here."

The midshipmouse put his paw on Twit's

shoulder. "Lad, I promise you we'll be back for that time. If Oswald leaves us, I swear you'll be at his side."

Twit blinked. He trusted his seafaring friend so much, yet how could he be so certain? Thomas's eyes bore into him and under their solemn gaze the little fieldmouse felt sure that he was right.

"I'll just go an' have a quick swill," Twit said, running out of the bedroom.

Audrey stared at Thomas and began to say something when a stern command from him sent her dashing off to find her ribbon.

Thomas Triton sighed and smiled at Piccadilly. "I'll not keep them away long. The easiest bit's been done – I've got them to go. Your job's not as simple. Pray to the Green Mouse that the Chitter lad hangs on till we return!"

2

THE STARWIFE

Thomas Triton led a flustered Audrey and Twit across the hall. Through the cellar door they slipped and jumped down the stone steps beyond. Thomas strode through the cellar gloom to the Grill.

Wrought in iron with twirling leaf patterns this had always been an object of fear and dread. And indeed, when Jupiter the terrible God of the Rats had been alive it had possessed strange powers.

Now Audrey shivered as she stood before it, recalling how she had been dragged through the Grill by an evil band of rats. Twit backed away from it slightly. He remembered the horrible effect that the black enchantments had had upon Arthur. Only Thomas dared to touch the Grill.

With a hearty laugh he looked at the others. "Jupiter is dead," he reminded them. "Whatever forces were lurking in or beyond this grating are long gone." As if to prove it he banged an iron leaf with his fist. "The spells are as cold and lifeless as the mangy moggy who made them." The midshipmouse chuckled and squeezed himself through the rusted gap in the Grill.

"This is the quickest way to Greenwich," he said, popping up on the other side. Audrey and Twit still hesitated so Thomas pulled a silly face. It looked so ridiculous that they couldn't help laughing.

Perhaps the Grill was an ordinary metal grating after all. Audrey and Twit crawled through the gap and joined Thomas.

Down into the sewers they went. Although it was a hot summer day in the outside world here it was chill and damp. Audrey had forgotten how bleak it all was. So many ugly memories were kindled by everything around her; the musty, stale smell of the dark running water, the slippery slime on the ledges and the weird echoes which floated through the old air. Around every corner there was a dark memory.

Thomas sensed her unease and remarked casually, "I use the sewers quite a bit now. I never get lost, me. I can find my way home on a black foggy night with no moon and my hat over my eyes." Twit chuckled softly and Audrey was grateful to the midshipmouse; he took her mind off things.

"Now there ain't no more rats down 'ere," Twit piped up, "there's no danger of us gettin' peeled, is there Thomas?"

"'Sright matey."

"But won't others arrive and take over where Jupiter's rats left off?" Audrey asked, doubtfully looking over her shoulder.

"No, rats are mostly cowardly," answered Thomas. "Only the fear of Jupiter gave them a false sort of courage. Ask that city mouse – he'll tell you how cringey they are in the city. You just have to cuff 'em about the head if they start gettin' uppity."

Audrey felt relieved. Like Twit she found the midshipmouse to be a comforting figure. He was so sure of himself that it rubbed off onto everyone he was with. Audrey's thoughts returned to Oswald lying in his bed. She shook her head to dispel that image and tried to think of something else. "Tell me about the Starwife please Mr Triton," she asked.

"She'm the grand dame of the squirrels," put in Twit.

"Yes, but what can she want of me?" asked Audrey baffled. "I'd never heard of her before."

"Maybe," said Thomas, "but she's obviously heard of you. Somehow the name Audrey Brown has reached her ancient ears. Rumours spread quickly – she must have heard about Jupiter's downfall and wants to know all the details of it."

"Yes, but you were there as well Mr Triton. You could have told her, surely?"

"True, I was there on the altar when that old monster was sent to his watery grave – but you did the sendin' remember, and it was your mousebrass that toppled him."

"What shall I tell her then?" asked Audrey nervously.

Thomas whirled round. "Why the truth, lass and nothing but that! Don't go addin' bits or leavin' stuff out, or your ears'll ring for weeks after. It's plain speaking in the Starwife's drays and chambers – and that only when you're spoken to."

"Have you seen her then Mr Triton?" pressed Audrey, desperate to know as much as possible about the strange personage she was about to meet.

"That I have," he replied cautiously. "When I first came and settled round here I was summoned to meet her." Thomas grew grave and added, "There were matters which I needed to talk to her about." He stroked his white whiskers and cleared his throat. "I've been hurled around by tempests on angry, foaming seas and nearly got drowned twice, but I don't mind telling you that I've never been so skittish as when I went to her drays. And I was shakin' even worse when I came out of them!"

Twit whistled softly. He couldn't imagine sturdy Thomas being afraid of anything. What a creature this Starwife must be! "What did she do to you Thomas?" he asked wide-eyed.

"Well I went in there, knees-a-knockin'. I'd heard many a strange tale of the Greenwich Starwife, and only an idiot would go into her chambers unabashed. Well, down some tunnels I was took and there behind a fancy curtain was the Starwife. Oh, she saw right through me, knew everything about me – what I'd done, what I hoped to do – uncanny that was. I think I made a right tomfool of myself in front of her. She weren't impressed with her new neighbour at all. Still, I came away feeling better, but I ain't clapped eyes on her since."

"And this morning you got a message from her about me," added Audrey.

"Yes, that surprised me no end." Thomas paused and looked at Audrey. "In fact, it's so rare an occurrence that I'd be careful, if I were you, Miss Brown."

Audrey was worried. She imagined the Starwife to be as bad as the rats. Her thoughts must have showed plainly on her face, for Thomas added, "Oh she won't eat you, but the Starwife has motives of her own. She never does nothing for nothing. Sometimes she can be as subtle as Jupiter himself, and that's what I'm puzzled about. So I say again just watch yourself."

"You don't encourage me, Mr Triton. I'm not sure if I'm looking forward to this. I'd rather go back to the Skirtings."

"Too late for that, miss. Here we are now."

They had come to the end of the sewer journey and a small passage lay before them, at the end of which bright sunlight streamed through the holes in a grate.

Thomas led them down it and they followed him to the outside world.

The mice stood outside Greenwich Park. Before them the green lawns stretched away up to the observatory hill. The sweet scent of freshly mown grass tingled their noses.

Twit breathed it in deeply. "Oh," he sighed, "that do lighten me heart."

The fieldmouse leapt into the mounds of drying grass cuttings. Gurgling with delight he burrowed down into the soft damp darkness where the fragrances tugged at his memories and visions of home swam before him. Snug in the grass cave Twit's tiny eyes sparkled. The city was no place for him – he belonged to the open fields where corn swayed high above and ripened slowly in the sun until it burned with golden splendour.

The grass rustled above his head and the harsh dazzle of midday broke around him.

"Come on matey!" laughed Thomas parting the cuttings. "Not far to the Starwife now."

Twit scrambled out of the mound wiping his forehead with a clump of the sweetest, dampest grass. Audrey smiled at him as he rubbed it into his hair.

"Luvverly," he exclaimed, "I feel bright and breezy now." She had to agree: the fresh clean scent of the grass cleansed her nose of the smell of the sickroom.

"We better catch up with Mr Triton," Audrey suggested. "Just look how he's marching off."

"I'm thinkin' old Thomas ain't happy about meetin' that there Starwife again."

"Well I don't want to meet her a first time. She sounds like a right old battleaxe – I'm telling you Twit, no matter who she is I'm in no mood for a bad-tempered old squirrel."

"Oh I am," cried Twit, "anything to be out of those dark rooms for a while."

They ran after Thomas, skirting round the tangled roots of the large trees. Gradually the three mice made their way up the hill.

Thomas's brows were knitted together in concentration. They avoided the paths and kept on the grass, obeying their instincts of survival – out of sight, out of danger.

The further up the hill they went the more thoughtful and quiet Thomas became. By the time they were halfway up he was positively frowning and his tail switched to and fro irritably. Audrey caught his mood and stayed silent. Only Twit chirped up now and again, gasping at the view and remembering when the bats had flown him over this very hill.

Presently the Observatory buildings drew near. How high they were with their onion-shaped domes and solid walls! They sat proudly on top of the hill, fringed by railings and thick rhododendron bushes.

"Look," called Twit suddenly. "In those bushes there. No, it's gone now."

"What was it?" asked Audrey.

"A squirrel," explained the fieldmouse. "It were watchin' us – didn't half give me a shock. There it was a-starin' straight at me – grey as ash then poof! It darted away as speedy as anything."

"How long do you think it had been watching us?" asked Audrey, slightly unnerved. She had never seen a squirrel before.

Thomas glared into the bushes. "They've been keeping an eye on us ever since we stepped into the park. Thought they were being clever, but I spotted them a-spying and jumping from branch to branch over our heads. Let them scurry and keep her informed of our progress. Like a spider in a wide web she is, gathering news – you'd be surprised at what she hears," he added grimly.

Audrey twisted the lace of her skirt between her fingers. "Mr Triton," she began nervously. "I don't want to see her now. Please can we go back?"

"No lass," Thomas sighed, shaking his head. "She has summoned you and you've come this far. Don't let an old jaded rover like me frighten you now. Courtesy must be kept and you never know – maybe the old boot's mellowed since last I saw her."

Twit giggled at Thomas's description of the Starwife. "I can't wait," he babbled excitedly.

"Right ho matey," said Thomas, "let's take the cat by the whiskers." The midshipmouse ducked under a railing and scampered up the bush-covered bank. Audrey and Twit followed.

Thomas Triton stooped and sat down in the mossy shade of the dark-leaved rhododendrons.

"What are you doing?" asked Audrey in surprise, "I thought we were going to find the Starwife."

"We've come as far as we can on our own," said Thomas solemnly. "I'm waiting for our escort."

Twit blinked and peered around them. The shadows under the thick bushes were deep. "I don't see no-ones," he whispered. "Where is this escort, Thomas?"

"Oh they're here," replied the midshipmouse dryly. "I'm just waiting for them to find their guts and show themselves."

Above their heads amongst the leathery leaves nervous coughs were stifled.

Audrey glanced up. "What are they doing?" she murmured fearfully.

Thomas stretched and yawned, then he lay back and rested his head on the spongy moss. "This is where we have to wait till one of them plucks up enough nerve to come down and lead us further. Could be hours."

"But we can't wait too long, Thomas," urged Twit, thinking of Oswald.

The midshipmouse eyed Twit for a moment. "You're right matey. I'll not be idle while the Chitter lad's fadin' fast." He sprang to his feet, then in one swift movement snatched a small stone off the ground and flung it into the air.

Up shot the stone into the canopy of rhododendron. A surprised yell came from the leaves. Thomas jumped nimbly to one side and with a crash of twigs a grey lump dropped to the ground.

"Oh, oh!" cried the furry bundle in panic.

"Peace squire!" calmed Thomas. "We have no time for your formalities today. Forgive me for speeding up the proceedings."

Twit stared at the terrified squirrel before them. It was young and its tail was strong and bushy. The squirrel's face was small but his large black eyes seemed to be popping out of his head. He looked at the three mice in fright.

Thomas waited for him to find his voice, making no effort to conceal his impatience during the squirrel's stammerings.

"But . . . but . . ." the squirrel began, "three . . . there are three of you – we . . . I . . . thought there would be only two," he regarded Twit uneasily.

"This is my good young matey William Scuttle," Thomas roared in a voice that made the squirrel shrink away. "Where I go, he goes." He laid his paw firmly on the fieldmouse's shoulder.

"She won't like this . . . she won't like this – not at all, no."

"That's enough!" rapped Thomas. "I'll face whatever squalls she throws my way but we'll not sit here becalmed by your dithering. Lead us and have done."

"The . . . the girl first," instructed the squirrel

timidly. "The mouse-maiden is to follow me."

Audrey nearly laughed at the anxious grey figure which hesitated and twitched before her but she remembered her manners and tried to remain serious. She stepped in line behind her escort.

"Good . . . good," he muttered, and with a jerk of his tail he bounded through the bushes. The mice followed him as quickly as they could.

Into the leafy clumps they ran and there, in the shadows, were a dozen other squirrels all fluttering and trembling with fright. Their escort was laying into them as the mice approached.

"Why didn't you?" he scolded the others crossly. "Leaving me all alone to deal with them."

"Well we weren't to know," they answered meekly. "But you did so very well Piers," some added. "Sshh, here they are now." They fell back as the mice entered.

"Ermm . . . this way," the escort said shakily and he set off again.

The crowd of squirrels watched them leave and they turned to one another tut-tutting. "She won't like that will she? Three of them, I ask you. He ought to have said something. The look that little fellow gave you . . . little savages they are . . . makes me shiver all over. Who's going to tell her then? Don't be soft – you know she doesn't need us to tell her anything, she has her own ways of finding things out."

Audrey followed the escort's bushy tail as it bobbed before her. Through lanes of leaves it led her, under arches of twining roots and past startled squirrel sentries who disappeared in a flash of grey. The bushes grew thicker overhead and no daylight filtered down. Suddenly a great oak tree appeared at the end of the green tunnel and the escort vanished down a dark cleft in the trunk.

Audrey paused, wondering how far down the drop was. She braced herself and with her eyes closed tightly leapt into the black hole.

Down she plunged until she landed with a soft jolt on a bundle of dry leaves and ferns. Audrey rolled to one side as Twit came down, whistling and laughing.

"It smells in here," sniffed Audrey.

"Only oak wood and leaf mould," said Twit, staggering to his feet.

They were in the base of the old oak's trunk, hollowed out by years of squirrel labour. Small wooden bowls hung on the walls and these were filled with burning oils. The light they gave off was silver and flickering, illuminating the smooth worn oak with gentle, dancing waves.

"It's as cold as the sewers down here," shivered Audrey.

Twit sat beside her and brushed the leaves off her back. "I have heard some in my field at home as do call squirrels tree rats," he whispered.

A muffled crash and a mariner's curse announced Thomas's arrival.

"I'd forgotten about that drop," he muttered, rubbing his back. "Where's that nervy chap gone to now?"

"I don't know," said Audrey. "There are some openings over there – are they the roots of this tree?"

"Aye, we are in the heart of the squirrel domain and here the Starwife lives, but there were Starwives before this oak was an acorn and before this very hill was made. The Starwives go back a long way."

Just then the escort came bounding back. "What are you waiting for? Come, come," he implored, "she is impatient. Hurry now!" He scurried away down one of the openings.

Audrey and Twit set off after him. "I wish I'd brought some rum with me," murmured Thomas to himself.

Down the narrow passages the mice followed the squirrel. Deep into the earth they seemed to be going. After a short while Audrey noticed something other than the silver lights twinkling ahead. It was a richly embroidered banner hung across the width of the passage. The background was a dark blue and over it was stitched a field of twinkling stars that reflected the light of the lamps around them. As Audrey examined the stars more closely she saw that the silver thread of which they were made was in fact tarnished by great age.

The escort paused and bowed before the banner.

The three mice waited apprehensively. Audrey and Twit stared at one another and wondered what lay beyond this elaborate partition.

A strong, impatient voice snapped from the other side. "Bring them in Piers – stop dawdling boy!"

The squirrel jumped in fright. "Oh madam, forgive me!" He clutched one corner of the banner and popped his head through as he drew it aside. "By your leave, madam, may I introduce . . ."

"Show in the midshipmouse first!" commanded the voice.

The squirrel looked back at Thomas and said, "Come through when I announce you."

Thomas grinned at Twit. "Battle stations!" he remarked wryly, dragging the hat from his head.

"By your leave madam," the squirrel had begun again, "may I introduce to you, midshipmouse Thomas Triton."

"Triton," called the other, sharp voice, "come in here."

Thomas scowled as he straightened the red

kerchief around his neck and strode through the banner.

Audrey held on to Twit's paw as they waited for their turn.

With a rising dislike for the voice she presumed was the Starwife's Audrey tried to keep calm.

"So seafarer," said the voice on the other side of the banner. "It has been a long time since last I saw you in my chamber."

"Yes ma'am," came Thomas's awkward reply, "too long."

"The fly has kept away from the web as best he might. But now you could say that the old boot is on the other foot."

Audrey gasped. How did the Starwife know that Thomas had compared her to a spider and an old boot? Whatever her sources, it was unkind and downright rude of her to taunt Thomas with his own words. Audrey felt herself becoming angry.

The midshipmouse was coughing to cover his embarrassment. He was a mouse of action, not words, and the respect he had for the Starwife and his own code of honour would not allow him to answer back.

"I hear you've settled down in your retirement at last," the voice began once more. "No more nightmares to haunt you?"

"No ma'am, not since my last visit when you were kind enough to give me those powders. That particular ghost has been laid to rest."

"It should be so. Though wounds of the heart and mind are the hardest to heal. You seem to be on the right path at last."

"I have taken your advice ma'am and not taken to the water once in all these years."

"Let it be so always Thomas or . . ." the Starwife's voice dropped to a whisper and Audrey could not catch what she was saying. She considered all that she had heard. Evidently there was something in Thomas's past which he had not spoken about.

A loud sharp knock brought her up quickly. The escort peered around the banner.

"Bring in the fieldmouse," called the Starwife sternly. "I'll teach him to tag along when he's not invited."

Twit looked at Audrey in dismay. "She ain't magic is she?" he asked. "I don't want her to turn me into no frog or stuff like that."

"You stand up to her," Audrey told him. "Don't let her walk all over you."

"Master William Stutter!" announced the escort.

"Scuttle!" corrected Twit angrily as he pushed past. Audrey tried to glimpse what was beyond the banner but the escort pulled it across and tutted loudly.

"The very idea!" he said tersely.

"So, country mouse," greeted the Starwife coldly. "You have come to visit me have you?"

"If it pleases you, your ladyship," Twit's small voice piped up.

"It pleases me not at all," she snapped back. "Who are you to presume a welcome in my chamber? A lowly fieldmouse before the Starwife!"

"Now look 'ere missus," Twit protested.

Audrey was very angry. How dare that old battleaxe pick on little Twit like that? After all he had been through lately he deserved more than to be shouted at by that rude creature. She stood tight-lipped, her temper flaring.

"Please, ma'am," came Thomas's voice, "it's my fault. I brought the lad – he needed the break. Times are bad in the Skirtings."

"Silence Thomas," ordered the Starwife. "I know of the Chitters and their son. True the lad needed a rest from those dark rooms but what of you midshipmouse?"

"Ma'am?"

"I sense a strong bond has grown between you and young Scuttle. I find myself wondering why – a lone wanderer such as you taking friends on board at your time of life. Who do you see in him Thomas?"

"Ma'am please . . ."

"I see you walk a dangerous rope midshipmouse. Reality and memory ought never to entwine so closely! Beware your dreams and forget what has past."

"I try ma'am."

"Enough! Piers – fetch the girl." The loud knocking began again.

Audrey prepared herself and the escort pulled back the banner. "Follow me please," he said stiffly.

Audrey smoothed her lace collar and stepped into the Starwife's chamber.

After the cramped tunnel it was like walking out into the open for it was so spacious. Suspended from the ceiling above were hundreds of small shiny objects, coloured foils, metal lids, links from silver chains and polished pieces of glass. All were hung in a certain order and for a moment Audrey thought their pattern familiar but could not place it until she realised that, like the banner, they represented all the constellations of the heavens.

Below this dangling chart sat the Starwife.

"Miss Audrey Brown!" the escort pronounced.

"Come here girl. Where I can see you."

Audrey moved towards the Starwife. She was an ancient squirrel perched on a high oaken throne carved with images of twisting leaves and acorns. Audrey had never seen anyone like her before. Age seemed to smother the Starwife. It was a

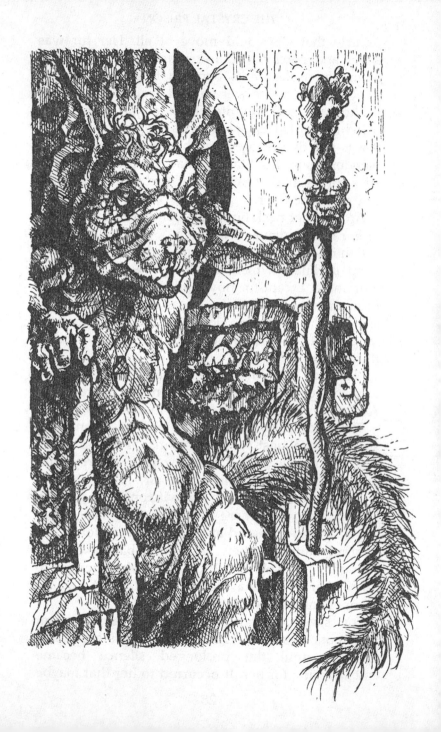

miracle that she could move at all. Her fur was silver and patchy, and her muscles were wasted, falling in useless rolls beneath fragile dry bones. The Starwife's eyes were a dull grey and over one of them was a thin white film like spilt milk.

In her gnarled, crippled paws she held a stick and it was this that Audrey had heard knocking on the wooden floor. The Starwife had sat there with that stick for so many years that it had worn a definite trough in the floor.

Around her neck hung a silver acorn, the symbol of her knowledge and wisdom.

Behind the throned figure Audrey could see a deep darkness which the lamps were unable to illuminate, except for now and again when a silver flash shone out brilliantly. It was curious, but before she had a chance to look further an impatient tapping of the stick brought her attention back to the Starwife.

"How do you do?" Audrey asked, dropping into a formal curtsey. The Starwife made no reply so Audrey repeated herself, a trifle louder than before.

The ancient squirrel shifted on her throne and sucked her almost toothless gums. "I'm half blind, girl, but not deaf yet." She gazed at Audrey with unblinking eyes and sniffed the air.

Audrey did not like the Starwife one little bit. She looked over to where Thomas and Twit were standing and grimaced at them. No way would this squirrel intimidate her. "Rude old battleaxe," she thought to herself. She didn't see why she had to be on her best behaviour if the Starwife had no manners of her own.

For several minutes Audrey remained silent and motionless under the continuing stare of the Starwife until the prolonged silence became embarrassing for her. It occurred to her that maybe the squirrel had nodded off like some old mice did in the Skirtings. Once more she thought of Oswald and felt that this was a waste of precious time.

"Excuse me," she began politely, "but we can't stay long I'm afraid."

The Starwife blinked and opened her mouth. She rose shakily in her throne and her joints cracked like twigs. The stick pounded the floor indignantly. Thomas put his hat over his face and the escort began to stammer idiotically.

The Starwife switched her stare from Audrey to him. "Piers!" she barked, "get out, you imbecile!" The escort looked around uncertainly, but at that moment the Starwife threw her stick at him. It struck him smartly on the nose and he fled howling from the chamber.

The Starwife eased herself gingerly back down onto her throne and gave a wicked chuckle. She relaxed and turned once more to Audrey. "You must think me a rude old battleaxe," she said calmly. Audrey flushed – it obviously wasn't safe to think in front of this creature. "I do have manners but it's so rare that I find anyone worth practising them on. You must forgive me child."

"Why did you send for me?" Audrey asked.

"There are two reasons Miss Brown. Firstly, I desired to speak to the one who sent Jupiter to his doom. Tell me all you know and all that happened on that glad day."

Audrey breathed deeply, not sure where to begin. Then she recounted all that had happened to her since One-Eyed Jake had dragged her through the Grill up to the time she had thrown her mousebrass at Jupiter. Throughout her tale the Starwife kept silent, nodding her head on occasion as if she understood more than Audrey about the events. When she had finished Audrey stepped back and waited for the other to comment.

"A dark story you have told, Miss Brown, with more horror than you know. There are certain things contained in your narrative which I had no knowledge of. Of course I knew all the time that Jupiter was a cat. I recognised the body he concealed in the darkness behind those burning eyes of his. A two-headed rat monster – rubbish, as I always maintained. But other things do surprise me. That episode in the pagan temple where Jake murdered Fletch, now that is disturbing – Mabb, Hobb and Bauchan are old gods and it frightens me to think they are but newly worshipped. Who can tell what folly will come of that?" The Starwife raised her head and gazed distractedly at the star maps.

"Your pardon ma'am," said Thomas softly. "You mentioned two reasons for wanting to see Miss Audrey – may we know the second?"

"Oh, I'm sorry Triton," she replied and it seemed to Audrey that the Starwife was just a harmless squirrel older than nature had ever intended her to be.

"Fetch me my stick will you lad," she motioned to Twit. The fieldmouse ran to retrieve it from the floor. He bowed as he presented it to her. The Starwife received it gratefully. "Thank you lad. It is more than a missile with which I bruise my subjects' stupid heads – I would not be able to walk without it."

"And now," she sighed, turning to Audrey once more, "you shall know the other reason why I brought you here." She banged the stick on the floor loudly and waited for the young squirrel to return.

"Ah there you are, Piers. Don't be afraid. I promise not to throw it any more today."

"Did you wish for anything madam?" asked the squirrel doubtfully.

The Starwife nodded and told him, "Bring in our guest."

Piers disappeared once more.

"It's over a week ago now," she began, "that our sentries spotted someone skulking in our park. The sight of this creature was fearful to behold and all fled before it. Nearer to my realm it drew. I could not get a word of sense from my guards – such a state they were in. "A gibbering ghost," they called it. I gave them a clip round the ear and told them they would be the gibbering ghosts if they didn't bring the creature to me." The Starwife allowed a slow smile to spread over her face.

"Did they bring the ghost?" asked Twit breathlessly.

"Oh yes they did right enough, but it was no ghost. They caught her in their nets and she was in a terrible state."

"She?" asked Audrey in surprise.

The Starwife narrowed her misty eyes. "Yes, her ribs were like roots poking through the soil and her belly was taut as a bark drum. She had not eaten for many days but she still managed to put up a hearty resistance. Seven of my sentries still have sore heads."

"So who was she?" Audrey broke in. "What did she want?"

"She wanted nothing, but I made her drink some milk and with that some life seemed to return to her dead eyes. I questioned her but could learn very little. In fact, Miss Brown, you have told me more about my guest than she has herself."

"*I* have?" Audrey could not believe it. Slowly a vague suspicion began to dawn on her.

"Yes, for she is known to you – can you not

guess? I see you suspect."

Audrey's heart was fluttering with apprehension and dread.

Behind the banner, coming down the passage she could hear Piers returning – his quick, nervous footsteps were unmistakable but alongside came a clumsy flapping of large ungainly feet and with them there was a voice.

"Go to see squirrel boss lady, oh yes."

Audrey's mouth fell open and she inhaled sharply.

The banner was thrust aside and Piers scampered into the chamber followed by . . . Madame Akkikuyu.

3

THE BARGAIN

Audrey backed away as Madame Akkikuyu entered.

Once she had been a beautiful rat maiden but her looks had faded with the cruel blows life had dealt her. When Audrey had first met her, Madame Akkikuyu had been a fortune-teller who also dabbled with poisonous love potions. But she had always craved genuine magical powers and that is how Jupiter had corrupted her into his service. It was Madame Akkikuyu who had delivered Audrey to him. Even then she had still been a striking figure – her fur a rich, sleek black and her eyes dark and fathomless.

Audrey pitied the fortune-teller now. As Madame Akkikuyu dragged her feet towards them they could plainly see that the rat had nearly starved to death in the past weeks. Her skin hung baggily off her frame and her fur was moulting away in ugly patches. Only the tattooed face on her ear looked the same. Around her shoulders she still wore the old spotted shawl, and strapped about her waist she carried her pouches of dried leaves and berries. In one large bag was her crystal ball.

Madame Akkikuyu stumbled up to those gathered around the throne and grinned sheepishly up at the Starwife. With a shock Audrey saw something terrible dancing in the rat's eyes – Madame Akkikuyu had lost her mind.

"Welcome Akkikuyu," said the Starwife warmly. "There are friends of yours here."

The rat gazed distractedly at the mice. She did not recognise the sturdy one with the red kerchief around his neck, but then she hardly knew anything any more. Her head was in such a muddle these days, ever since . . . no she could not remember when. There was a closed door in her head that she could not open and she knew that all the answers were locked behind it . . . and yet for some reason she was afraid to discover the truth.

Her memory was as patchy as her fur. She knew the crystal ball and the pouches of leaves were important to her but she did not know why. Since these nice squirrels had taken her in she had sat with the crystal in her hands many times and admired it – how the light curved over its perfect round surface and how it soothed her. She regarded it as her most precious belonging.

Occasionally a vivid image of some past time would flit over her eyes and she would snatch at it then hold it dear without knowing what it was. There was one scene where the sun beat down harshly and there was sand between her toes, and water all around. She felt as though she were travelling a great distance and when she looked down at her claws they were young.

Two other things she remembered. The first was a rat with one eye who faded into ash. Indeed, in with her herbs she had found an eyepatch. It was frustrating not to know what this meant and most nights Madame Akkikuyu wept long, bitter tears.

The last memory was the one that she feared the most. She was in a vast echoing chamber, and in front of her were two candles and, between them, an archway which she could not force herself to look into. This was the key to unlock that door but she was terrified to discover what lurked in there.

Madame Akkikuyu looked at Twit – the face of the little fieldmouse stirred nothing in the jumble of her memories. Finally she turned to Audrey.

The fortune-teller froze. Yes, she had seen that young mouse before, somewhere. A confused array of images crowded in. Audrey was standing before her but it seemed as though a ball of fire separated them. This was suddenly swept away and an overwhelming sense of guilt washed over her. As she continued to stare at the mouse her own voice spoke to her from the past.

"Mouselet. You, me – run away. Leave dark places, hide and be happy."

A tear rolled down Akkikuyu's sunken cheek – what had happened to that wonderful plan, she wondered? That was what she wanted now, to go away and have peace in a quiet spot where the sun shone. Swallowing the lump in her throat she said,

"Mouselet, Akkikuyu know you. Why did we not go to distant places and sleep in summer sunlight?"

Audrey felt uncomfortable. She knew why. The rat had been taking her to Jupiter when this idea had first gripped her. Akkikuyu had weighed up all the unhappiness she had suffered and would have escaped with her when Morgan, Jupiter's henchrat had interrupted them and Madame Akkikuyu had been forced to carry out her orders. Audrey had felt sorry for the rat even then but all the more so now. She could not answer her question.

The Starwife tapped her stick and all looked to her.

"Akkikuyu," she began, "you have been my guest for nine days now and are free to remain, yet I sense that there is a yearning in you and you feel you are

35

unable to stay here."

The fortune-teller bowed her head. "Oh wise boss lady, you see into Akkikuyu's heart." She closed her eyes and clasped her claws in front of her as though in prayer. "You so kind to Akkikuyu. You give food and shelter when others throw stones. Akkikuyu never forget you, sweet bushy one, but mouselet and me, we special – she and I promised. We go away together – we friends."

Audrey spluttered and lifted her head but the glitter she saw in the Starwife's eyes silenced any outcry she might have made.

Gently the old squirrel held out one arthritic paw to the fortune-teller.

The rat took it, careful not to hold too tightly. The Starwife bent down and patted the rat's claw.

"Peace, Akkikuyu," she said. "You shall go with your friend, but first you must make ready. The day after tomorrow you will leave. Go now to your room and prepare."

Madame Akkikuyu wept with joy and moved to embrace Audrey. The mouse backed away, horrified.

"Hurry, Akkikuyu," cut in the Starwife. "Run along now. There is much to do."

"Yes, yes, Akkikuyu go at once," chuckled the rat gleefully as she ran from the chamber.

When she had left, Audrey turned on the Starwife angrily. "That was the cruellest thing I've ever seen," she stormed. "Why did you build her hopes up like that?"

The Starwife sat back in the throne and heaved a sigh. "What is it I have done wrongly, girl? I merely told her a fact."

"But what will happen when she finds out that I'm not going anywhere with her?"

The stick began to tap the ground slowly. "She

will not find out any such thing, for one simple reason – you are going with her."

Audrey laughed. "Not on your life."

The stick crashed down. "Silence!" raged the Starwife. "I will not be spoken to in such a manner. I have told Akkikuyu, now I am telling you. You and she will depart the day after tomorrow."

Thomas Triton stepped up beside Audrey and put his paw on her arm. "Take care miss," he whispered. "She can make you do anything she wants."

Audrey glared at the old squirrel. Was this the real reason she had been summoned? Or was this a punishment for her rudeness before? One thing was certain however. Nothing would make her go anywhere with Madame Akkikuyu.

Thomas spoke to the old squirrel. "Ma'am," he began politely. "Where are they to go, the rat and this girl? And how are they to get there?"

The Starwife pointed her stick at Twit. "This lad does not belong round here," she said. "He knows it and was about to go home before his cousin fell ill. What better place for Akkikuyu than a remote field to spend the rest of her days in?"

"You have to be joking!" Audrey remarked, shaking her head in disbelief.

"Never was I more serious," the old squirrel replied, a deadly tone in her voice. "The day after tomorrow you, young Scuttle and Akkikuyu will leave."

Suddenly, Twit piped up, "But I can't go yet missus – poor Oswald . . ."

"The Chitter boy will die before this day is out," she said flatly.

The fieldmouse cried out in dismay.

"Silence!" the Starwife demanded. "You thought so yourself, remember. Late this afternoon the

Chitter lad will reach the crisis point and pass away."

Twit sobbed uncontrollably. "How do you know? He might not."

"This I have seen," snapped the Starwife irritably. "Look behind my throne. Behold the Starglass!"

The mice peered around the carved oak throne and there, as tall as three mice was a flat disc of black, polished glass set in a carved wooden frame. It was this that Audrey had glimpsed before. Over its surface silver flashes flickered and in its midnight depths swirled a multitude of vague and distant images.

"It is my life," explained the Starwife quietly, "and it has been the life of every Starwife before me. Our most precious and most powerful possession. With it I have looked into the heart of the rat Akkikuyu and found no evil. That is why she must be taken away from this place. She must not remember what happened in the sewers and never must you mention the name Jupiter to her – it would unhinge her totally. There is only this one chance of redemption for her – are you the one to deny her this, child?"

Audrey thought for a while. Finally she said, "I am truly sorry for her – but why must I go?"

"Because she will feel safe with you. Somewhere in her mind you have become linked with this notion of safety in the sun. Only you can lead her away. She will go with no-one else." The Starwife stared intently at Audrey as if willing her to accept the heavy burden she was offering.

Audrey looked at Thomas, but he was staring at his feet. She wondered what he was thinking. Had he known about this? No, he had suspected none of this – she was sure of that.

Twit was drying his eyes and saying, "Why must

we go so soon? We won't have time for . . ."

"I think one day is sufficient for the necessary arrangements to be made and undertaken," the Starwife replied coldly.

"What about Mr and Mrs Chitter?" pleaded Twit. "They'll need me to help them get over . . . it all."

An icy glint appeared in the old squirrel's eyes. "They will not need any comfort after tonight," she said darkly. Twit choked and buried his head in his hands.

Audrey felt cold. She stared grimly at the Starwife. How could anyone be so unfeeling? She put her arm around Twit's shoulder and spoke softly. "Don't you listen to her. I'm not going anywhere with that rat – no-one can make me do anything I don't want to." Thomas raised his eyes but said nothing.

"So, you still refuse," the Starwife remarked dryly.

"I do. There's no way I would ever do anything for you now."

The Starwife tapped her stick and called for Piers. The young squirrel had been waiting silently at the entrance of the chamber. Now he jumped to attention.

"Madam?" he asked eagerly.

"Fetch it Piers."

The young squirrel became agitated and flustered. "But my lady," he whined. "You know the consequences, my lady."

"I said fetch it!" she roared, the stick pounding on the floor. "There is more to this than you know."

Piers bowed and dashed off through the banner.

The Starwife tilted her head and smiled at Audrey triumphantly. "So, there is nothing I can do to make you take Akkikuyu away?" she almost chuckled as she said it.

"Nothing," answered Audrey firmly. She eyed the Starwife warily. Who could tell what she might try next?

Piers came bounding back. In his paws he carried a small cloth bag tied tightly at the neck. "I have it madam," he puffed.

The Starwife's smile disappeared and for a moment she looked sad and dejected. "Thank you Piers," she said as he handed it over. He stopped to kiss her paw. "Help me down now," she asked. "Mr Triton, could you take one arm and Piers the other?"

The midshipmouse rushed to help. Carefully they eased the Starwife off the great chair. Her face screwed up as her old bones creaked and the stiff, dry joints ground together noisily.

"Thank you," she said to both of them when finally she stood on the floor.

"I curse this old body of mine – it grows worse with every winter."

"That is because you do not sleep properly madam," said Piers unexpectedly.

"There is too much to attend to – how can I sleep? Now, the Starglass. Come along, young Scuttle, it needs the relative."

She hobbled slowly with her stick to the rear of the throne until she stood before the Starglass. There she leaned on the stick heavily and eyed Twit solemnly.

"Stand in front of me, lad," she told him, "and take this in your paws." She gave him the cloth bag and placed her own paws on his shoulders. "Now, hold your arms out straight – that's right."

"No, Twit," said Audrey violently. She had watched them curiously and now she was afraid of what the Starwife might do to him. "Don't trust her!"

"Ignore her, boy," rapped the Starwife crossly. "Do as you're told!"

Twit looked from Audrey to the Starwife. What was he to do? Was the old squirrel going to turn him into something dreadful after all? Audrey's face was anxious and frightened; the Starwife's was set and stern. But what about Thomas, his friend and hero, what did he think?

"What'll I do, Thomas?" asked the fieldmouse.

The midshipmouse gave him a smile and reassured him. "It'll be all right matey – I know what she's doin'. She won't hurt you."

"That's good enough fer me," said Twit, greatly relieved. "Don't worry Audrey, Thomas says there ain't nowt to fear." Audrey hoped he was right but then she noticed Piers turning away, a troubled look on his face.

"Go ahead missus," called Twit holding out his arms as straight as he could.

Before the Starglass stood the two figures, mouse and squirrel. The Starwife whispered under her breath and the silver lamps on the walls grew dim and went out. Only the flashes over the black glass lit the chamber now and as the Starwife chanted the light grew brighter.

Twit opened his eyes wide as he witnessed the strange squirrel magic happening before him.

From the depths of the dark glass he saw the night sky – only the stars shone a hundred times brighter. Presently the light from them gleamed stronger and the stars drew nearer. Twit gasped. It seemed as if the whole sky was about him now. In a blaze of blue and silver the stars leapt out of the glass and whirled all around. The chamber had vanished, and only he and the Starwife were left amid the burning heavens.

Twit heard the Starwife's voice calling into the

sky and felt her old paws on his shoulders. Suddenly the bag in his paws grew heavy and all the starlight seemed to be sucked down into it. At the same time he felt two sharp pains in his shoulders as the Starwife gripped too tightly.

Twit stifled a cry of surprise as a fierce tingling sensation shot down his arms, as if a thousand ants were crawling over them, stinging as they went. The tingle travelled to his paws and then seemed to enter the bag.

"Enough!" cried the Starwife. "It is done." She released Twit and blew on her paws as if to warm them. Then she groped for her stick.

Twit blinked. He was back in the chamber again and the lamps were lit once more, but the Starglass was dark and impenetrable. He shook himself and whistled softly.

Piers ran forward and took the Starwife by the arm. She seemed feebler than before, and older – if that was possible.

Audrey did not understand what had happened. She had heard the old squirrel mumbling strange words and seen Twit's face light up in awe, but then a bright flash had dazzled her. It seemed to have come from the bag but she was not sure. Now the Starwife was breathing hard and clinging onto Piers.

When she had regained her breath, the Starwife turned to Audrey and said, "Before, I told you to take Akkikuyu away to young Scuttle's field. Well, now I am asking you. Will you take her?" her voice was cracked and hoarse, she seemed to have no strength left in her at all.

Despite herself, Audrey felt sorry for her, but still she said, "I've told you, nothing will make me go."

"So you said – I remember. Well girl, what if the life of your friend Oswald depended on it?"

42

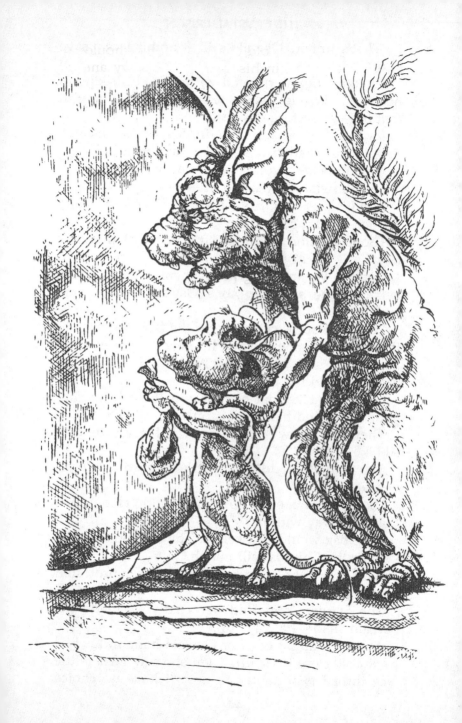

"That's unfair. Oswald's ill – nothing can save him."

The Starwife interrupted with a fierce striking of her stick. "Wrong!" she shouted. "What is now in that bag can restore his health."

Twit looked at the bag in his paws. "Really, missus?" a broad grin spread across his face.

"I don't believe you," said Audrey cautiously.

The Starwife sighed, too tired to reply.

"Oh it's perfectly true," Piers remarked, speaking for her, "and it costs dear."

Thomas Triton nodded. "It'll do what they say lass."

Audrey began to believe them. "That's marvellous," she said happily, "Oswald will be well again."

Piers had been trying to get the Starwife back to the throne but she pushed him away from her and pointed the stick furiously at Audrey. "If!" she cried.

Audrey did not understand.

"You may take that bag away with you and cure your friend and his parents only if . . ."

Then she knew. "You mean if I agree to take Akkikuyu away."

The Starwife nodded. The triumph was plain on her face.

"So if I said no, even now you wouldn't let us take that bag away with us?"

"The bag would be useless. The bargain must be kept or the Chitters will perish."

"But I made no such bargain," Audrey protested urgently.

The Starwife regarded her coldly. "I made the bargain child – I always do."

Audrey thought of poor Oswald lying in his bed perilously close to death. Then she saw Twit's little face turned expectantly to her. "I have no choice then," she said, "the day after tomorrow I will take Akkikuyu to Twit's field."

"I knew you would," replied the Starwife. "Piers show them out, the audience is at an end."

"But madam, let me help you into your throne first."

"Get out you fool – if I weren't so tired I'd throw this at you again," she snapped, waving the stick menacingly.

"This way please!" Piers called from the other side of the banner.

Thomas bowed before the Starwife. "May we meet again," he said to her.

"You stay in your ship and leave me alone," she answered shortly.

"Thank 'ee missus," laughed Twit when he stood before her. "This bag do make me so happy. I be fair burstin'."

"Get out, you country simpleton," said the Starwife. But she had a smile on her face as she said it.

When it was her turn to say goodbye Audrey looked at the old squirrel with intense resentment. She was glad to be leaving at last. Thomas had been right. The Starwife never did anything for nothing. She had known all along that Audrey would agree eventually. "Remember child," she said, "the bargain will keep. If you cure him this afternoon but later refuse to go with Akkikuyu then the fever will return and strike him down once more. This bargain is for life, girl. As long as Akkikuyu lives you must remain with her."

It was a chilling prospect and Audrey felt a cold dread grip her heart as she realised the doom that the Starwife had decreed for her. She shivered. "You are cruel," she said though wanting to say more. "Why is that fake fortune-teller so important to you? She's only a rat after all."

The Starwife looked steadily into her eyes. "And does that make a difference child?" she asked with scorn. "To me you are just a mouse – and a very rude mouse at that."

"Well . . ." Audrey stammered.

"Well nothing. Listen to me. I have seen in the Starglass an important future for Akkikuyu. Exactly what that may be I cannot be certain but I do know that she will make two choices in her life. Her decisions will undoubtedly affect us all. It may seem harsh to you but I want you to be with her all the time – good may come of it. I pray so anyway." She closed her eyes wearily and waved the mouse away from her. "Now leave me. I am too drained – you have been an expensive guest to entertain." The Starwife turned her back and laboriously limped to the great oak chair.

Audrey left the chamber deep in thought, but as the banner swept down behind her the Starwife raised an eyebrow and said softly to herself, "Can she be the one?"

In the passage Twit was asking Piers, "What does I do with this bag?"

"Steep it in hot water and when it is cool enough make him drink, then call his name three times. Remember, you must never open the bag."

"Oh I won't!" Twit was nearly back to his old self. Hope was filling his little chest and that was all that mattered.

Audrey caught up with them. "But Oswald can't bring himself to drink anything," she reminded Twit.

"He will drink this," said Piers haughtily. So saying, the young squirrel led them up through tunnels they had not seen before, along winding passages with the light of the silver lamps glimmering about them. Soon the soft lights became mingled with a brighter radiance. It was the sparkle of sunlight streaming through green leaves.

"There it is!" said Piers, halting suddenly. "I will go no further. Once you pass through those leaves you will find yourselves in the park once more. I presume you will be able to find your way from there?" he added sarcastically.

"Oh I think we can manage it," put in Thomas.

"Well, go straight back to your holes," retorted Piers pompously. "You will be watched."

"By your ferocious sentries, no doubt." Thomas arched his brows and a flicker of a smile wandered over his face.

"Indeed," said Piers, greatly agitated. "They are there to make sure you leave in an orderly fashion – we don't want riff-raff cluttering up our park."

Thomas laughed heartily. "And what would your brave lads do if we did leave in a disorderly fashion – pelt us with daisies?" Twit joined in the laughter.

The young squirrel pursed his lips and eyed them disdainfully. When he was able to be heard he loftily told Thomas, "When you have finished with the bag, you, midshipmouse must return it to us. Tonight at the latest. Now good day to you!" he dismissed them curtly.

The mice made their way to the opening and crawled out between the leaves. As Audrey stepped out into the sunlight, she turned to see Piers for one last time. For a moment she blinked blindly as her eyes adjusted to the brightness and then, through the leafy gateway, and partly hidden in the comparative darkness of the tunnel she saw the squirrel watching them intently. What a strange race they were, these bushy-tailed creatures, running around in a constant state of nervous fluster – all except the Starwife of course. Audrey shivered in spite of the afternoon heat as she thought of the old half-blind animal seated on her throne in the heart of the hill, weaving her cruel webs for everyone.

"He's making sure we go quietly," whispered Thomas in Audrey's ear. "Let's go back to the Skirtings and leave this hill far behind us."

Audrey continued to stare moodily through the leaves. "I hate squirrels," she decided and pulled such a grim face that Piers scurried further into the shade.

"Come lass," Thomas told her, "we've a pleasant task ahead of us."

"Yes," agreed Twit, "we're off to make Oswald well again."

Audrey finally tore herself away from the leaf-covered entrance but hesitated before following the others. She looked at how happy Twit was and felt guilty because she was unable to join him. It should have been a time of celebration for them all, but the Starwife had denied her that. The day after tomorrow she would have to leave with that awful Madame Akkikuyu and set off for a horrible field in the far away country.

"I don't want to leave Deptford!" she cried to herself.

4

A DRAUGHT
OF STARLIGHT

In the Skirtings, Oswald's condition was failing fast. His face had a deathly pallor and his temperature was soaring. Sweat beaded his forehead and ran glistening down his hollow cheeks.

Arthur watched him fearfully. "Go and rouse Mother," he told Piccadilly quickly. "I think this is it." The two mice exchanged hurried, meaningful glances then the grey city mouse dashed out of the sickroom.

Arthur knelt beside his stricken friend. "Oh Oswald," he sighed sadly. He took the albino's frail, hot paw in his own and waited.

Shortly, the muffled sound of hushed voices came to Arthur's ears. Evidently, curious mice anxious for news were gathering outside the Chitter's home. There was soon quite a commotion and Arthur could hear Piccadilly's voice above the clamouring queries.

"Put a lid on it and let Mrs Brown through there. I'm sorry we can't tell you more. Blimey!" Piccadilly's exasperated voice floundered amongst the good-natured and well-intentioned questions.

Arthur smiled grimly to himself at Piccadilly's

situation – coping with gossipy, fussing housemice was something he had not encountered in the city.

The outer curtain was drawn aside and Gwen Brown squeezed in. She had escaped the prying neighbours, although a covered bowl had been thrust into her arms. She shook herself and entered the sickroom.

"Piccadilly told me he's worse," she said, moving quickly to Oswald's bedside. She felt the albino's brow and studied his face. "Yes, this is the crisis," she sighed. Gwen turned to her son and drew him to her. "I'm afraid he hasn't the strength to fight it. This will be the end. How is Mr Chitter?"

They both looked at the figure asleep on the chair. Jacob Chitter was pale and weak – he appeared as ill as Oswald.

"I looked in on Mrs Chitter before," whispered Arthur. "She's as bad as he is."

"Yes," nodded Gwen. "The lives of this family are all tied together. As Oswald fades – so do they. It's so terrible." She laid the covered bowl which she had been carrying on the low table next to the pieces of raw onion.

"More ointment from Mrs Coltfoot?" guessed Arthur. "A bit late for that now."

"Let's not presume the end before it's come," breathed his mother. "We must continue as before. Audrey and I will see to Mrs Chitter, you see to . . ." She paused and puckered her brow as Arthur bit his lip. "Arthur?" she asked. "I haven't seen Audrey since I woke up . . . and Twit wasn't in his bed when I looked in on him. Where are they?"

Arthur gritted his teeth, then took a long deep breath whilst he shuffled his feet awkwardly.

"Arthur!" demanded his mother sternly.

"Well you had just gone to sleep so we didn't like to disturb you," he began earnestly.

"Who's we?"

"Well us and Mr Triton."

"Mr Triton!" Gwen Brown exclaimed. "What did he want?"

"He took Audrey and Twit to Greenwich," said Arthur nervously.

"To Greenwich? Oh Arthur, what's got into the old fool's head? And why did you let them go? I'm surprised at Twit – up and leaving like that."

Arthur waved his arms and tried to calm her down. "But it wasn't like that! He promised they'd be back in time and Twit needed to get away for a bit. Mr Triton can be very persuasive you know," he added lamely.

"Oh, I'm sorry I snapped, Arthur," smiled Gwen apologetically. "I do remember Mr Triton's way – he's a forceful one, there's no denying. I suppose they didn't have time to think what they were doing when he arrived. But why take Twit and Audrey to Greenwich? Audrey hardly knows him, for one thing and it isn't like her to be interested in boats and such."

"Oh didn't I say?" put in Arthur quickly. "Mr Triton brought a message from someone called the Starwife. She apparently wanted to speak with Audrey."

Gwen Brown was taken aback. "The Starwife! Let me see now . . . yes, I do seem to have heard of her. Oh dear – what can she want with our Audrey? I don't like it, Arthur. If I had been awake I would not have allowed her to go. Just wait till I see that midshipmouse – I'll bend his ear for him."

The afternoon crept by. The hot sun veered west and the evening clouds gathered lightly about the horizon.

In the hall of the old house many mice were gathered: Algy Coltfoot and his mother, the two

Raddle spinsters, flirty Miss Poot and many more had mustered together to see how the Chitters were faring. It was as if some instinct had told them that the end was near for that family. A dark shadow lay over all their hearts.

Poor Piccadilly was getting impatient with them all. They kept badgering him for information and they evidently considered his bulletins too few and scanty in detail. Just when the city mouse felt like punching a couple of stupid, nosey heads, Master Oldnose, disturbed by the row strode out of his rooms and waded through the crowd.

"Now then, now then!" He clapped his paws and looked round crossly.

Master Oldnose had been the tutor of most of the mice present and their memories of him with his ears white with anger awoke their old respect for him. Voices were hushed and silence fell.

Master Oldnose eyed everyone severely – even those mice who were older than him respected him and held their tongues. Besides his school duties, Master Oldnose was the mousebrass maker and that was a position of great honour.

Now he surveyed them all and waited until he was satisfied.

Piccadilly flicked the hair out of his eyes.

"Ta, mister, they were gettin' out of hand."

Master Oldnose bristled at being called "mister" by this uncouth and obviously ignorant city mouse but decided to pass over it. "You boy," he addressed Piccadilly. "What is the meaning of this riotous gathering? Explain yourself." He stood with his paws clasped firmly behind his back and rocked slightly on his heels awaiting a reply.

"It's the Chitters, mister. Oswald's in what Mrs Brown calls 'the crisis' and she an' Arthur are doin' their level best for 'em but this lot aren't happy with just knowin' that and won't shift."

"I see." Master Oldnose glared at the crowd as if they were children. "Go about your business – there is nothing more for you to learn here."

The mice stirred and mumbled feebly, and the two old maids fluttered shyly and hid their mouths behind nervous paws. Algy coughed and put on his most stubborn face. Nobody moved away.

"Tough luck, mister," grinned Piccadilly cheekily. "I thought you had 'em then."

"We only want to know how they are," said a small voice. It was Tom Cockle. "We owe the lad a lot, you see, and well – I've been stewin' all day, not knowin' how he was doin', so I come here and blow me if there wasn't a blessed crowd already."

"That's right," broke in Mrs Coltfoot. "Algy an' me were terrible restless – poor Oswald, I had an awful feeling about today." Murmurs of agreement ran through the crowd.

"We're not doin' any harm," continued Tom. "We're sorry if we were a bit rowdy but we're not budgin'."

Even the Raddle spinsters nodded. Master Oldnose sighed. He could see that today he would not be obeyed. Indeed, *he* had been sitting in his workroom unable to concentrate on the unfinished mousebrasses before him. He was quite prepared to remain with the others now and wait for news. Everyone expected the curtain to be pulled to one side at any moment and to see Gwen Brown's tearful face appear and relate grave, tragic words. All eyes were fixed on the curtain and even Piccadilly was forced to turn and stare at it glumly.

The evening drew closer. Outside, the day was still warm and the sun had not yet disappeared but no mouse took any notice.

Eventually, the mice on the Landings crept

down the stairway and stood, silent and depressed, with the Skirtings' folk. Time stole by – only the breathing of many mice disturbed the blanketing stillness.

All at once, confusion broke out. Cries of alarm rippled through the crowd. Piccadilly looked round. The Raddle spinsters, as usual, had the same expression on their faces. Even in panic they were identical. No one seemed to know what was happening. Master Oldnose scowled. The disturbance seemed to emanate from the back of the crowd near the cellar door. He gulped and wondered with dread what had crept out of that dark place. Something was forcing its way through the assembled mice. Master Oldnose drew back in fear.

"Out of my way!" shouted a gruff voice. "Let me through there!"

Piccadilly managed a smile – he knew that voice.

"Hey! Avast there." A blue woollen hat bobbed into view amongst the sea of startled mice.

Master Oldnose was relieved, but glowered as he saw Thomas Triton emerge from the crowd. "Mr Triton," he declared, "What means this rude interruption?"

Master Oldnose was not fond of the midshipmouse, for on the few occasions they had met, Thomas had flagrantly disregarded his authority.

"Evenin' Nosey!" greeted Thomas cheerily.

Master Oldnose's mouth dropped open as he watched the midshipmouse barge past him. Thomas ruffled Piccadilly's hair on his way then nipped behind the Chitter's curtain.

Excited whoops then came from the crowd. "How do Algy! Hello Algy's mum!" called a small but unmistakable voice. It was Twit, finding it more difficult to get through the crowd than the midshipmouse had done.

Master Oldnose came out of his sulk and looked up quickly.

"What you got in that bag, Twit?" asked Tom Cockle.

"Oh you'll see Tom, you'll see." Twit blundered out of the assembled mice carrying the Starwife's bag as high as his little arms could manage.

"Hello William," said Master Oldnose warmly. "Are you feelin' well boy?"

"The best I ever did!" And as if to prove it Twit burst into a fit of joyful laughter.

The crowd thought he had gone potty and sighed and tutted with disapproval. Audrey had been following Twit unnoticed by everyone, but now she stepped out and took his paw.

"He really is fine," she explained to them all, and hurried the still giggling fieldmouse into the Chitter's rooms.

"Audrey?" Piccadilly stopped her. "What *is* going on? Why were you so long and why is Twit acting so barmy?"

"He's just happy because Oswald is going to get well," she answered.

Piccadilly looked at her doubtfully. "Come off it," he whispered. "There's no way to save him now."

"Oh yes there is," said Audrey in a strange, sombre voice. "There's *one* way to save him." She turned suddenly and ran through the curtain.

The city mouse stared after her. He could have sworn he had seen tears in Audrey's eyes. But if Oswald was going to be cured, why was she so unhappy?

In Oswald's sickroom excitement charged the air. Thomas had told Gwen Brown about the Starwife's bag and she was already boiling some water.

Oswald lay still and silent on the bed like a

broken statue of cold marble. He was unaware of everyone around him. He felt so weak that even breathing seemed a dreadful labour. It was as if he had been falling down a deep black well: gradually the light at the top had grown fainter and more distant, until he accepted that there was no way out for him. Down he sank into the blackest night imaginable. He could hear nothing but the darkness filling his ears and closing in around him. How easy it was to sleep and forget everything, all he had known and all he had been – to be one with the rich velvet blackness.

Mrs Brown came into the sickroom carrying a bowl of hot steaming water. Twit was about to drop the bag in when he hesitated. Was this a cruel trick of the Starwife? He glanced round at his friends and at once drew heart from Thomas's wise, whiskered face. The bag plopped into the bowl.

At once the steam snaked higher and filled the sickroom completely. All who breathed it in felt refreshed and tingles ran all the way down their tails.

A silver light began to shine in the room. In his chair Jacob Chitter stirred in his sleep. Small stars gleamed through the steam and once again Twit felt as if he was swept up into the bright heavens. Only this time Oswald was next to him and there seemed to be music everywhere. As he looked at his cousin the fieldmouse gasped. For a moment it seemed as if he could see the Starwife lying in his place but the vision was snatched away and Twit could see that it was indeed Oswald lying there.

"The water is cooler now," said Gwen. "Twit dear, see if he will drink it."

Twit took the bowl from her and knelt beside Oswald. He used one paw to raise his cousin's head and tilted the bowl slightly with the other.

At first the water simply touched Oswald's lips and trickled down onto the pillows.

"Come on cuz," cried Twit urgently. "Drink it!"

Everyone held their breath and watched. More of the precious water spilled onto the pillows. The albino looked dead.

Twit's paw trembled as he feared they were too late. The pillow was very wet now and there was not much left in the bowl. Thomas lowered his eyes and removed his hat. Mrs Brown buried her face in her paws.

"Oh Oswald," the little fieldmouse cried. "Oswald, Oswald." Twit's little heart was breaking.

And then Oswald's lips moved.

"Look!" yelled Twit. "He be drinkin'." Oswald swallowed the liquid and then opened one eye feebly. He gazed at them all and managed a smile.

"Hooray!" shouted Twit skipping round the room. "Hooray!" he took Mrs Brown's paw and dragged her into the dance.

Thomas stepped up to Audrey and said softly to her, "I'll be off to Greenwich later to return the bag. No doubt I'll be told details of your departure. She won't leave anything to chance – everything will be planned and organised."

"Mr Triton, I have to go, don't I?" said Audrey. "I am the price of all this aren't I?"

He nodded regretfully. "Alas miss, I'm afraid you are. Forgive me for taking you to her. I am truly sorry."

Audrey smiled at him. "It isn't your fault Mr Triton – she would have done it with or without you."

They were interrupted by an impatient knocking on the wall. Everyone paused and listened.

"Where's my milk? What's all that noise? Can you hear me Jacob?" Mrs Chitter was in fine form by the sound of her.

Jacob Chitter jumped to attention in his chair. "Yes dear. Of course, dear, I . . ." he paused suddenly as he noticed his son smiling up at him. "Oh Oswald," he said, and burst into tears.

Gwen Brown led the others out of the sickroom. Thomas hung back and collected the small cloth bag.

On the way out to the hall Gwen looked in on Mrs Chitter. She was sitting up in bed fussing with her hair. "Oh Gwen what is going on in there?" she asked. "What does my husband think he's doing, the old fool?"

"Arabel," cried Mrs Brown. "Oswald is better! It's all over now."

Mrs Chitter dabbed her eyes and gave thanks to the Green Mouse. "Well if that isn't the best news I've ever heard," she sobbed. "You see Gwen, I told you those pieces of onion would do the trick."

In the hall, Thomas was telling an awestruck crowd about Oswald's recovery. For a short time they simply blinked at the midshipmouse – not sure if they had heard him properly and then with one voice they cheered.

"My word!" exclaimed Master Oldnose.

"Let's celebrate," called Tom Cockle.

Audrey felt miserable and dragged her feet back home. Arthur was munching away in the kitchen and getting crumbs everywhere.

"Isn't it terrific?" he mumbled, with his mouth full.

"Oh yes Arthur, I couldn't be happier for the Chitters." Her voice fell and she sat down heavily.

Arthur swallowed and licked the crumbs round his mouth, forgetting the ones clinging to his whiskers. "What's the matter?" he asked seriously, sensing his sister's mood.

"Didn't Mr Triton tell you?" she asked wearily.

Arthur sat down beside her and said fearfully, "Tell us what? You're all right aren't you? You're not coming down with what Oswald had are you?"

"Oh no Arthur – nothing like that. My fate's much worse than that," she said morosely. "It's the miracle cure of the Starwife."

"That was amazing wasn't it – really magic stuff that was."

Audrey stared at him steadily. "It had . . . conditions, Arthur. We could only take the cure *if* I agreed to go with Twit to his field the day after tomorrow *and* . . . take Madame Akkikuyu with me."

"Audrey! That's terrible. I thought that rat woman was dead." Arthur thought deeply for a moment then brightened. "But Oswald is cured now – they can't make you go if you back out now can they?"

"I'm afraid so. Oswald and his family will fall sick again if I don't stick to it."

Arthur put his arm around her. "Don't worry Sis," he soothed. "I'll come with you. I promise. How long do you think it will take to get there and back?"

"But that's just it," wept Audrey. "I shan't be coming back – I've got to stay with Akkikuyu for ever."

Arthur gasped. "But that's dreadful. Oh how shall we tell Mother?"

"I don't know," sobbed Audrey.

"My dears!" Mrs Brown was standing in the doorway, tears falling down her cheeks – she had heard it all.

She wrapped her arms around Audrey and kissed her. "There must be a way," she whimpered. "Oh what would your father do if he were here?"

An apologetic cough sounded behind them. "Forgive me good lady," said Thomas self-consciously. "I came to tell you about the party the rest of your Skirtings folk are arranging but I see you are busy. Excuse me."

"No wait please," called Gwen desperately. "Mr Triton, you seem to know this Starwife better than us. Is there any way she would release Audrey from this horrible bargain?"

Thomas's eyes were grave beneath his frosty white brows. "No ma'am. I'm sorry, but the Starwife clings to a bargain like a limpet to a stone. She does not make idle threats either: that family will surely perish if Miss Audrey does not go." The midshipmouse fumbled with the cloth bag in his paws. "I must leave now," he said, tugging the edge of his hat. "I have to return this, you see. No doubt you will see me in the morning if I guess rightly about the messages I'll find waiting for me." He turned and left the Skirtings and began the journey back to Greenwich.

"If it's all right with you Mother," ventured Arthur, "I'd like to go with Audrey to make sure she's safe."

"I don't need looking after," said Audrey indignantly. "Just you stay here with Mother!"

"Listen silly," argued her brother crossly. "I can go with you, make sure you settle in, then come back and tell Mother how you're doing."

"Oh," said Audrey – she could see the sense in that.

So could Mrs Brown. "That's a very good idea Arthur," she said and hugged them both tightly.

Meanwhile, Algy Coltfoot and Tom Cockle had brought out their instruments – whisker fiddle and bark drum – and soon the strains of a melody came floating in through the hall.

Gwen Brown made her children wash the tear stains from their faces. "It may sound silly of me," she said, "but I don't feel as though you'll be away too long. Let's regard this evening as a sort of grand going-away party. We'll all be together again soon, you see."

Audrey and Arthur agreed – for her sake – though in their own hearts they doubted her. Audrey went to fetch her tail bells, which she had not worn for weeks. She felt that tonight was a good occasion to wear them once more.

In the hall the other mice had not been idle. To celebrate the Chitters' return to health, food had been brought out and decorations festooned the walls. Algy and Tom played "The Summer Jig" and their audience danced and clapped heartily. Between tunes Mr Cockle slipped out a bowl of his own berrybrew and quaffed it down happily, hoping his wife wouldn't see. Mrs Coltfoot was being congratulated on the success of her ointment and the Raddle spinsters were tittering on the stairs as usual.

Into this mirth came Twit. He was immediately grabbed and hauled into the dancing – until someone called for him to play on his reed pipe. The fieldmouse darted away to fetch it.

It was a joyful chaos of noise and laughter. Soon the tensions of the last weeks were forgotten – forgotten by everyone except Audrey.

"Perhaps this is the last time I shall wear bells on my tail or have a ribbon in my hair," she thought. "With a rat for company I shan't need to look nice."

"Come on Audrey," said Arthur, suddenly interrupting her thoughts. "There's some terrific food here. Mrs Cockle and Mrs Coltfoot have been busy." Arthur dragged his sister over to a crowded area where a cloth had been spread on the floor and laid with biscuits, cheeses, soft grain buns, jam rings and a large bowl of Mrs Coltfoot's own speciality – Hawthorn Blossom Cup. Gwen Brown was chatting mildly to Biddy Cockle.

"Here she is," Arthur told his mother. "I found her over there all dreamy and sorry for herself."

Gwen linked her arm in her daughter's. "Try to be happy, my love," she said. "It'll be all right, you'll see!"

"Where's Piccadilly?" asked Audrey suddenly. It occurred to her that he knew nothing of the bargain. Perhaps he would come with them to Twit's field – it might not be so bad after all if the cheeky city mouse came too.

"Piccadilly was over there before with the dancers," said Mrs Brown, relieved that Audrey had snapped out of herself.

Audrey left her mother behind and went in search of the grey mouse. The musicians were now playing "Cowslips Folly", a lively dance in which a ring of boy mice rushed round a central circle of girl mice and chose a partner from them. Audrey hovered at the edge of the dancing. She saw Piccadilly choose Nel Poot three times. Miss Poot was evidently enjoying all the attention and she was brazen enough to wave at Audrey!

At first Audrey was amused – everyone knew how dotty Nel Poot was. But when Piccadilly chose her a fourth time the smile twitched off Audrey's face and her foot began to tap bad temperedly. What did Piccadilly think he was doing?

"Cowslips Folly" ceased and the musical trio went to see if there was any food left. Audrey watched the dancers break up, but before she could turn away Piccadilly caught her glance, excused himself from Nel and sauntered over.

"Did you want summat?" he asked her. "Only

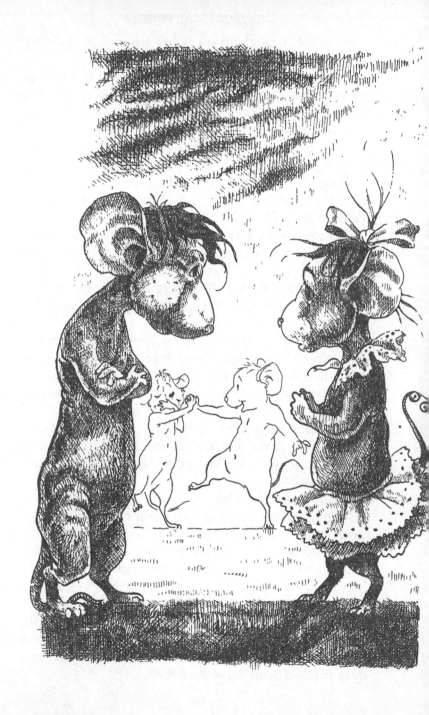

Miss Poot thought you were trying to get my attention."

Audrey answered casually. "Yes, I did as a matter of fact. I just wanted to say goodbye to you and take this opportunity to thank you for all you have done for me and my family."

"You gone soft in the head?" laughed Piccadilly. "What you on about?"

"I'm leaving," said Audrey, enjoying the moment. "Arthur and I are going with Twit to his field on a visit."

Piccadilly's face fell and his shoulders drooped sadly. Audrey bit her lip and cursed her stupid tongue.

"I see," he managed, "I hope you have a nice time," he muttered, staring at the ground miserably. "When was all this decided?"

"Oh we decided as soon as Oswald got better," she said. "We're going the day after tomorrow. You can come and wave us off if you like." How could she be so cruel, she wondered. Had the Starwife put a spell on her too?

Piccadilly raised his head as if stung. He stared at Audrey incredulously, then, with anger said, "Sorry ducks but I'm goin' back to the city tomorrow."

"Oh," gasped Audrey.

"Well, Whitey's better now, ain't he and there's nowt to keep me here is there?"

"I suppose not," said Audrey in a small voice. She wanted to tell him of the terrible bargain that she had to keep – surely he would not think she was cruel then. "Piccadilly . . ." she began.

"Listen to that," he said cocking one ear to the band. "That's the Suitors' Dance and I promised Miss Poot." The city mouse left her and Audrey's eyes pricked with wretched tears.

The rest of the evening swept by merrily. Nobody noticed Audrey slipping away to her room with her paws over her eyes.

Slowly the party broke up. Those from the Landings yawned and made their way up the stairs. The Raddle sisters tittered at Tom Cockle who was sound asleep and snoring loudly with an empty bowl of berrybrew at his side. Biddy Cockle scolded and shook him, then with some help from Algy, Tom Cockle staggered home singing at the top of his voice about a mouse called Gertie. Biddy was not amused and made him sleep in the spare room for three days afterwards.

Eventually, Piccadilly was left alone in the hall. "I must go tomorrow," he told himself miserably. "Back to the grit and grime of the city." He bowed his head and wept silently beneath the crescent summer moon.

5

A MEETING AT MIDNIGHT

It was not yet dawn. The greyness of night lingered reluctantly in corners and doorways. Somewhere, behind the tall tower blocks and council estates the sun rose slowly over the hidden horizon and the night shadows shrank deep into the earth for the rest of the day.

Piccadilly quietly rose from his bed and put on his belt. He checked everything was where it should be: small knife – yes that was there, mousebrass – yes the belt was looped through it securely, and finally, biscuit supply – well the leather pouch was there but it was empty. He wondered if Mrs Brown would mind if he took some of her biscuits. It might take a long time to walk back to the city. Piccadilly frowned – it would seem like stealing to take without asking, but he wanted to slip away without any fuss – maybe he ought to leave a note. He crept into the Browns' kitchen.

The biscuits were next to the crackers, so Piccadilly took two of each, broke them into small pieces and slipped them into his pouch. He looked around for a bit of paper to write on. Then he wondered what he could put – it needed a long explanation to tell Mrs Brown why he was going but how could he put into words all that he felt?

In the end, Piccadilly simply wrote: *"Have gon back to the city. Thank you for having me. Have took some biskitts hope you don't mind – Piccadilly."*

He was not very good at writing. Long ago he had neglected his schooling for more exciting adventures. Now he regarded his handiwork with some doubt. Would anyone read his note? His handwriting was unsteady and he had pressed too hard with the pencil. He pulled a wry face. "I bet Audrey can read an' write perfect," he grumbled to himself.

Outside the house a sparrow began to sing to the new day. Piccadilly looked up quickly. It had taken longer than he had intended to write that note. Now he had no time to spare. He propped the piece of paper on the table, tiptoed out of the Brown's home and passed through the cellar doorway. Quickly he scrambled down the cellar steps and through the Grill into the sewers.

The morning stretched and shook itself. The clouds were few and wispy – it was going to be another blazing June day.

When Audrey woke, her mother handed the note to her. She read it quietly and with dismay. "Has he really gone?" she asked.

"Yes love," said her mother. "Arthur has looked everywhere."

"Oh, it's all my fault," was all Audrey was able to say.

She ate her breakfast dismally as she thought about Piccadilly. Her heart told her that she was the reason he had gone off without a word. When Arthur came in she avoided his accusing eyes and went to start her packing.

Arthur was unhappy too. He had begun to consider Piccadilly as his best friend and he guessed that Audrey had something to do with his abrupt departure. It was about time she stopped playing games with everyone. Ever since poor old Piccadilly had arrived she had used him, made him feel guilty for surviving the horrors of the rats when their father had not. She had sent him into peril with Oswald down into the rat-infested sewers to look for her mousebrass and had never really apologised for that. She really was a silly lump. To cheer himself up Arthur went with his mother to see the Chitters.

In the sickroom even the air felt healthier. The sickly smell had gone completely. Oswald was propped up in bed with a great smile on his face as Twit told him funny stories. Mrs Chitter was up and about, chiding and tutting, finding dust where there was none and rearranging all her ornaments. She herded Gwen Brown into the kitchen where she demanded to know all the latest doings of everyone in the Skirtings.

Arthur sat himself on the end of the bed next to Twit and waited for a tale to end. Idly he looked about the room. Something was missing, something which had seemed such a fixture that now it was gone he couldn't think what it could be. Oswald saw his puzzled expression and laughed.

"Father's gone to bed finally," he said. "It does seem odd without him in here doesn't it? I wanted to get up today but Mother wouldn't let me. She says I'll be here for at least two weeks – or until she's satisfied with my health."

"You'm in bed forever then," giggled Twit, holding his feet and rocking backwards.

"Twit says he's going home tomorrow and that you and Audrey are going too – I'm so jealous Arthur. I wish I could go too."

Arthur caught a quick, cautionary glance from

the fieldmouse and understood that Oswald had not been told about the Starwife's bargain.

"Still . . ." continued the albino. "I suppose my hayfever would have driven me crazy in the country. I can't wait for you to come back and tell me all your adventures."

"I will," said Arthur.

"Of course we shall all miss cousin Twit but he says he might come visiting again. I'm going to be terribly bored all alone here, but I suppose I should count myself lucky really."

A knock sounded outside and the patter of Mrs Chitter's feet accompanied by the clucking of her tongue came to them as she went to see who it was. There were some muffled words which the three friends were unable to catch but presently Arthur's mother popped her head into the sickroom.

"Arthur dear and Twit, could you step out here for a moment please?"

Soon Oswald was left alone to stare at the table covered in raw onion.

Outside Twit and Arthur found Thomas Triton. He grinned warmly at the fieldmouse and began.

"I've come from the Starwife," he said. "Plans are slightly changed. You leave tonight – seems the old dame can't get none of her folk to escort the rat woman down to the river in the daylight so tonight it is."

"Oh dear," sighed Mrs Brown. "Arthur, fetch Audrey – she has to hear this."

"Wait lad, I already told the lass. I went there first y'see, thinkin' you'd all be there like," the midship-mouse explained. "Seems there's a merchant chappy the Starwife's persuaded to take you to my young matey's field."

"A merchant mouse?" asked Twit.

"Aye lad, he's a sort of pedlar – sells and trades

things. Well, it seems he knows everywhere along the river, stocks up in Greenwich then takes his goods round to out of the way places."

"Well, I ain't never seen him afore in my field," said Twit.

Mrs Brown had been frowning deeply. Now she suddenly said, "Would this pedlar be Mr Kempe?"

Thomas looked surprised. "Why yes ma'am that it is – how do you know of him?"

"Why he comes here in the autumn to see Master Oldnose on mousebrass business. Yes he seems respectable enough . . . I think I'll feel a lot happier knowing my children are in his paws."

Thomas agreed. "Just so ma'am. Well, as for tonight I shall lead milladdo here and your two children down to Greenwich Pier where Kempe will meet us. There we shall all wait until the rat arrives with those fidgety squirrels."

"About what time will this be Mr Triton?" asked Gwen.

"Midnight, if it pleases you ma'am."

"Oh Mr Triton it does not please me – not at all. Still there is much to be done. Arthur come with me. Are you packed yet Twit?"

"Bless me. I clean forgot about that," admitted the fieldmouse.

*   *   *

The rippling river was dark, and cool air drifted lazily up from its shimmering surface. It was a clear, clean night pricked all over by brilliant stars. Greenwich Pier huddled over the lapping water like a tired old lady. Its timbers were creaky, its ironwork rusted and yellow paint flaked and fell from it like tears. Daily trips departed from the pier to see the landmarks of London from the river and in the summer many crowded the benches and ice cream stands. But now it was still and dark, its gates were closed and the visitors had all deserted the pier for gaudier delights.

The only sound was the water breaking gently against the supports and slopping round a broken wooden jetty nearby.

There were no lights on the pier at night, all was dim and grey – a place of alarming shadow.

Audrey held on to her mother's paw. They had come through the sewers once more, led again by the midshipmouse. She watched Arthur and Twit run ahead to explore the deep pools of darkness and shuddered. She was cold, but her mother had knitted her a yellow shawl and she pulled it tightly over her shoulders.

All the mice were carrying bags, packed with provisions, blankets and personal treasures. Audrey's arms ached with the weight of hers and she was glad when Thomas said it was not much further. Somewhere, in amongst the folded clothes was a dried hawthorn blossom. Oswald had given it to her when she said goodbye to him that evening – it was one of those he had saved from the Spring festival.

Gwen Brown was savouring every moment with her children, storing up the sound of their voices for when she was alone.

Twit and Arthur ran ahead once more, swinging their baggage happily. After some moments they came rushing back, their faces aglow with excitement.

"Thomas," squealed Twit eagerly, "there be summat up there. We done heard it."

"Yes," joined in Arthur. "Someone's singing."

The little group of mice edged forward cautiously. In the shade ahead nothing could be seen, but gradually a voice floated to them on the night air.

It was a merry, hearty sound, first singing now humming.

> Poor Rosie! Poor Rosie!
> I'll tell you of poor Rosie,
> The tragedy that was Rosie
> And why she died so lonely
>
> Coz for all her looks her armpits stank,
> The suitors came, but away they shrank
> Far away from Rosie,
> With their paws tight on their nosey.

Twit spluttered and laughed helplessly as the song continued. Gwen Brown gave Thomas a doubtful look. The midshipmouse shrugged and hid a smile.

"Who is it, Mother?" asked Audrey.

"That is Mr Kempe," Gwen replied dryly.

Thomas coughed and shouted. "Ahoy Mr Kempe! Come out so we may see you! And before your verses become too colourful, remember there are tender ears here."

From the shadows a great clanking noise replaced the song, as if some metal monster had been roused from sleep. Audrey waited with wide eyes wondering what this Mr Kempe would be like.

"Are you the party bound for Fennywolde?" came the hearty voice.

"That's right," Twit piped up, "that be the name o' my field."

"Why that sounds like a fieldmouse."

"I be 'un."

The clanking drew nearer and into the dim light stepped one of the strangest figures Audrey had ever seen.

There was a mass of bags, pans, straps and

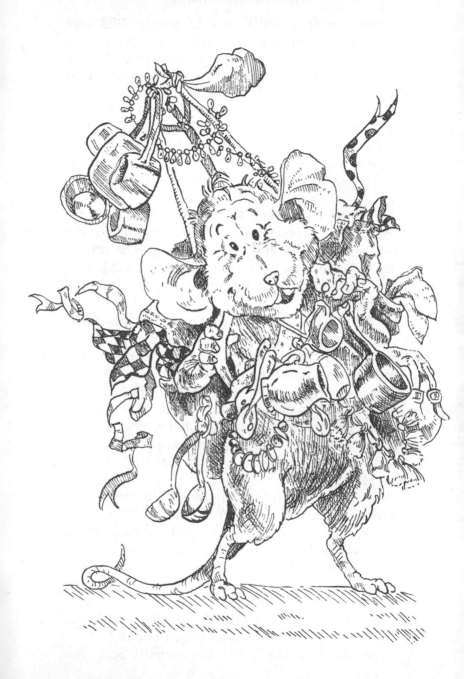

buckles mounted on a pair of sturdy legs and somewhere amongst all this madness was a furry round face and two small bead-like eyes. It was friendly and welcoming, and Audrey warmed to Kempe immediately – especially as he said,

"Bless my goods, two beautiful ladies and I knew nought of it. A curse on my palsied tongue that you should hear it yammering away like that. But 'tis the lot of the lone traveller to sing when he's on his tod. Forgive my verses dear ladies." The clanking began again as he attempted to bow.

Gwen Brown smiled as she accepted his apology. "You just keep your songs tucked away while my daughter travels with you, Mr Kempe," she said.

"Oh please," he protested, "there's no 'Mister', plain Kempe I am – no titles no end pieces! Kempe and that's all."

Audrey was staring in fascination at his bags. Poking through the sides there were glimpses of fine silks and silver lace and strung round the handles of his pans and around his own neck were beads of every type and variety. Pear-shaped droplets done in gold, green leaf patterns threaded on a single hair from a pony's mane, little charms worked in wood and hung on a copper wire and chains of fine links from which dangled tears of blue glass.

"I'll trade anything for anything," he continued, catching Audrey's eye. "Well, young lady – see anything that tickles you? I see you like fine things, with your ribbon and all that lace. Why I've got such an array of ribbons in here – enough to make rainbows jealous. Take your pick, and all I ask are those wee bells on your tail."

"But these bells are silver!" Audrey exclaimed. "They're worth more than all your ribbons."

"Alas for sensible girls," he sighed. "Still, you

can't blame a mouse for trying."

Thomas chuckled and introduced everyone to the traveller.

"What a fine party we'll be making to be sure, sailing up the river together, leaving the fume of the city behind us. A pity you'll not be joinin' us Mrs Brown, but have no fear. I'll keep one eye on my goods and the other on my charges." He turned to Thomas. "And you Mr Triton sir, sorry I am not to have your stout company on board, I bet you know many a worthy tale."

"That I do," replied Thomas, "though not all are comfortable to listen to."

"Still, I'll wager we'd not get bored with you on hand."

"Oh I don't think you need worry on that score Kempe my boy," smiled Thomas. "Have you met your other travelling companion yet?"

"Why no, that's the truth of it, but I had word from herself what lives up yon hill – the batty old squirrel."

"What did she tell you exactly?" asked Thomas smiling.

"To be here tonight, at this hour, to guide certain parties to Fennywolde – they being your own good selves and one other, a special lady." He turned to Gwen Brown and confessed. "To be honest I thought my luck was in and you were she – alas it seems not." He clapped his paws together. "So where is this other of our jolly group?"

Thomas considered Kempe for a moment and said, "Has the Starwife promised you anything for your services?"

"Why no sir," he seemed surprised. "Why 'tis only a simple task and I'll have the pleasure of it, such fine young fellows a trader never had to journey with! I'd do it for nought . . . but now you mention it, herself made me give my traveller's oath not to change my mind – ain't that funny now?"

"Not really," said Mrs Brown, "not when you know who this lady is. The Starwife has used you like she has used my daughter – deviously."

Kempe looked at the mice before him and grew concerned at the expressions on their faces. "Why there you go worrying a body – kindly tell me who this lady is."

But even as he spoke they all heard voices, one loud, the other timid.

Madame Akkikuyu strode onto the pier followed by two squirrels.

"Mouslings!" cried the rat, dropping her many bags and flinging her arms open.

Kempe's face sagged and it seemed as if all his goods drooped as well. Audrey ducked quickly behind her mother, avoiding Akkikuyu's attention.

"We travel at last," the fortune-teller exclaimed triumphantly. "Off to sun and rest – together forever."

"Why the batty old she-divil," bellowed Kempe, cursing the Starwife and shaking his fist at the two terrified squirrels. "My traveller's oath an' all – for this, this . . . lump of a rat. I be conned outright."

One of the squirrels braved a reply. "The bargain with you must stand," he said, dodging a blow from a pan. "If not, all the river will know of your falseness."

The trader stood still, but his face looked as though it would burst. "A traveller depends on his reputation and the good will of others – why if his traveller's oath is doubted he goes out of business."

"Just so," replied the squirrel smartly.

"A plague on you," called Kempe angrily.

Thomas intervened. "Now look squire," he said

to Akkikuyu's escort. "You've done your delivery, now tell your mistress it's all working well for her. Get you gone before this chap cracks you both one."

The squirrel stroked his tail smugly and glanced casually round for his silent comrade – but he had already run away. That was enough. The squirrel jumped in the air and dashed after him.

"They sure are watery, Thomas," said Twit.

"So," said Kempe sourly, "here we are with that baggage to join us. A pretty lot we are, to be sure."

"Yes," said Thomas briskly. "And if I'm going to get some kip tonight I've got to take Mrs Brown home first. Make your farewells please – it's time to go."

Gwen held Audrey in a desperate embrace. "You will come back, Audrey my love – I know it."

"I hope so Mother, I wish I was as sure as you." She tried not to cry, but her eyes were already raw and swollen from Piccadilly's departure.

Gwen turned to her son. "Now Arthur," she said, "you look after your sister and come home when you can." She hugged and kissed him, much to his embarrassment.

Thomas Triton turned to Twit. "Well matey," he said awkwardly, "there's no denyin' I'll miss your cheerful face round here. Ever since you dropped on my ship we've got on famous." He fumbled with a flask that was slung over his shoulder and thrust it into the fieldmouse's paws.

"What is it, Thomas?" asked Twit.

"Just a little something for your journey – and to remember our first meeting by."

"Will you come visitin' one day Thomas?"

The midshipmouse shook his head. "No Woodget – not by water, you know I can't go that way again."

"What did you call me then Thomas? It's me –

Twit, remember."

The midshipmouse looked flustered and apologised for getting muddled. Twit laughed and said it didn't matter. "I reckon I'll be poppin' this way again some time," said Twit. "I bet there's a bundle of stories you've still to tell me."

"Maybe, matey, maybe."

Then Madame Akkikuyu, who up till then had been gazing earnestly up at the stars, hugged Mrs Brown. Gwen gasped but found nothing to say.

"Oh mother of my friend, goodbye," Akkikuyu breathed with feeling. "And you old salty mouseling farewell also."

Thomas cleared his throat and hurriedly waved "Cheerio" before she had a chance to hug him. Then he led Gwen Brown away from the pier.

The three young mice sadly watched them go. "Well," began Kempe. "I'll show you our trusty vessel."

"Are we to leave tonight?" asked Audrey.

"No missey," said Kempe above the jangle of his goods. "The boat sets off in the morning but we've got to settle down."

"I shall be near my mousey friend," declared Madame Akkikuyu, stooping to collect her things. Audrey looked at Arthur and grimaced.

Kempe took them further along the pier to where the river splashed through the planks under their feet. A large tourist cruiser was moored at the edge and it bobbed gently up and down bumping against the pier.

"There she is," said Kempe. "Our transport – well one of them anyway. Now up this rope here and we'll be on deck."

"Easy," cried Twit and scampered up the mooring rope in a twinkling.

"Akkikuyu do that also." The fortune-teller

hauled herself onto the rope bridge and clumsily made her way along with her thick tail flicking behind her.

"That's right missus," grinned Kempe. "Don't go fallin' in now – we wouldn't want to lose you!"

It was Arthur's turn next; he stared at the rope warily. "I'm not usually very good at balancing," he admitted. "I can climb but . . ." he looked despondently at the sloshing water below – it seemed green and cold, and he did not want to land in there.

"Come on now laddie, just don't look down."

From the boat Twit watched them and laughed, "Come on Arthur. If you spend any time in my field you'll have to learn to climb stalks. But I suppose you'd have to lose some weight first."

"I'm not fat," protested Arthur.

"Course not – you great puddin'."

That settled it. Arthur virtually ran up the rope and began scuffling with the fieldmouse who was helpless with giggling.

Now it was Audrey's turn, but she stepped onto the rope nimbly and was soon aboard – straight into the welcoming arms of Akkikuyu.

"Clever mouselet. Akkikuyu knew mouselet could do it."

Whistling a quick tune Kempe ambled up to them, balancing with perfect poise on the rope, his many goods not affecting him whatsoever.

"Now follow me, fellow travellers," he said once he was on deck. They strode over the boards and between wooden benches to where a steep flight of wooden steps plunged darkly down into an invisible blackness.

"Down here," called Kempe briskly jumping onto the first step.

Silently they all descended. Twit followed

Kempe, then Arthur, followed by Audrey and Madame Akkikuyu brought up the rear.

Audrey tried to hurry down the steps as quickly as she could. Close above she could hear the rat's claws clicking as they caught on the steps and Akkikuyu's croaky muttering breaths. Once the fortune-teller's tail brushed against Audrey's face in the dark and the mouse cried out in alarm, nearly falling off the steps altogether.

"Hush mouselet," the rat cooed, "only the tail of Akkikuyu – fright not."

When they were all at the bottom of the steps Kempe lit a small candle and they looked around them.

It was a storage hold. Oil drums and tarpaulins surrounded them, thick black rope snaked across the floor and a stack of folded wooden chairs was piled precariously in one corner. It smelt strongly of the river and of stagnant, neglected pools.

"This is where we bunk tonight," said Kempe brightly as though he was used to much worse accommodation. "And tomorrow we'll hide here under the tarpaulin out of the way – until we change boats."

"Change boats?" repeated Arthur. "Why? Doesn't this one take us to Twit's field?"

"Bless you laddy no. Whatever made you think it did? I'm sure I said. Never mind. No, three vessels will bear us on our way. That's the joy of the traveller, hopping from boat to boat. Knowing which one goes where and when. Why I know the sailing time of everything along the whole great stretch of Grand Daddy Thames, from the biggest ship to the smallest barge."

They put their bags down and Kempe disentangled himself from his rattling goods. Without them he seemed a much smaller figure.

Madame Akkikuyu hugged her knees and muttered happily to herself.

Audrey did not like the hold: it was stuffy and more like a prison than anything she could imagine. The small flickering candle flame brought no cheer to the gloomy place and the rocking of the boat made her feel sick.

Arthur and Twit sat near Kempe each lost in their own thoughts. The fieldmouse delved into his little bag and brought out his reed pipe. He put it to his lips and blew absentmindedly. He was thinking of his home and wondering if it had changed in all the months he had been away.

Arthur listened wistfully to the slow, solemn notes from the pipe. He too was thinking of Twit's home. What had Kempe called it – Fennywolde? Strange how Twit had never called it by that name before – it was always "my field" or just simply "back home". Arthur wondered what he and Audrey would find there.

The haunting music stopped and after a short while Twit's little voice gurgled with pleasure. "Good old Thomas!" he cried. He had remembered the little flask which the midshipmouse had given to him and pulled the cork out. The exotic smell of rum met his twitching nose.

Kempe was sorting through one of his bags, pulling out scraps of material and stuffing them back again. He hummed quietly to himself – it had been a busy week for the travelling mouse, deals had been made, a good bit of trading done down Tilbury way, and in Greenwich itself earlier that evening he had done a nice little deal with a Norwegian mouse from a ship docked near that old power station. Seven little wooden charms he had got in return for two spoons and a length of buttercup yellow satin. It was these small charms that Kempe was looking for – he was sure he had put them in this bag. Ah – yes there they were. Kempe fished them out and examined them in the candlelight.

"Oooh," admired Twit, "they'm pretty. Can I see 'em proper?" Kempe inspected the fieldmouse's paws for dirt, then, when he was satisfied, handed the little carvings to him one by one.

All were figures of mice delicately done in box wood. Every detail was correct down to the suggestion of fur. There were running mice, old wise-looking mice, pretty damsel mice curtseying and dancing and an angry mouse with a sword in his paw.

"They're terrific," said Arthur peering over Twit's shoulder.

"To be sure they're right dandy little things," nodded Kempe. "Chap I traded with says he got them from a holy mouse what lived up in some mountain or other – not that I believed him like, probably knocked them up himself but I took a fancy to 'em."

"I ain't never seen so neat a bit o' carvin'," said Twit, handing them back. "We never had nowt like that in my field."

Kempe raised his eyebrows and shrugged. "In Fennywolde – I'm not a bit surprised. I never go there."

"Why not?" asked Arthur.

"Got chased out only time I did go," Kempe replied, shaking his head. "Some pious feller it was, babbling about frippery and vanity."

"What do you mean?" pressed Arthur. "What's wrong with what you sell?"

"Why nothing! I have the finest selection on all the river. But you see – and begging your pardon youngster," he said to Twit, "there are some in this world who think we come into it empty-handed and should leave that way, with no decoration or little luxury to cheer us along. And they don't like those of us who deal in these indulgences."

"But I still don't understand why," said Arthur confused. "What harm can your wares do?"

Kempe raised his hands in a gesture that showed he too had asked that question many times.

It was Twit who answered. Slowly he said, "Because they go against the design of the Green Mouse." He spoke the words as though he was repeating something he had heard many times.

"Twit!" exclaimed Arthur in surprise.

"Staunch Green Mousers," put in Kempe darkly, "fanatics too busy livin' in fear of the Almighty to enjoy his bounty."

Arthur stared at the fieldmouse, "But you never said," he stammered, "I thought your field was a happy place."

"Oh it is," Twit assured him quickly. "Most of us don't think and reckon things like that. It's only a few what's hot against 'owt different an' such."

"Really?" Arthur was slightly annoyed. "What do you think that few will make of Audrey with her bells and lace?"

"Oh they won't take to her," agreed Kempe. "Specially that pious feller what chased me – if he's still there."

"Oh he be there all right," confirmed Twit glumly. "Old Isaac still goes into a fume and temper when it comes to the Green Mouse design."

"What do you make of this, Audrey?" asked Arthur turning round. But his sister was not there – nor was Madame Akkikuyu.

*   *   *

The night breeze had made Audrey feel better. She hated being cooped up in that dreary, musty hold.

She had left everyone engrossed and climbed the steps once more. Audrey leant against one of the railings along the deck and gazed up at the bright stars. The sloshing of the water and the motion of the boat lulled her senses and the rich green smell of the river was brought to her on the breeze. She closed her eyes and a calm descended on her.

"Mouselet."

Audrey jumped at the sound of that voice behind her. Akkikuyu had followed her from the hold. The rat's black eyes were gleaming.

"The night – she is beautiful. See the stars – how they burn." She raised her claws to the heavens and spun round. "Oh mouselet," she cried. "Finally we are together and we shall never be parted."

Once more Audrey felt a wave of compassion flow over her. Madame Akkikuyu was really a creature to be pitied. Audrey decided that the Starwife must be right – all the rat's wicked memories had indeed been forgotten. Madame Akkikuyu was little more than a harmless mouse child dressed in a rat's skin.

From the other side of the river a dog howled, breaking the peace of the night.

Akkikuyu traced a wide circle in the air with her claws and drew her breath.

"Wolf sees death and gives warning," she muttered. "Akkikuyu must not linger in dark places – listen to the wolf voice, 'Beware', he says, 'old Mr Death walk near'." She pulled her spotted shawl tighter and kissed her dog tooth pendant. Whatever else she may have forgotten, Akkikuyu's instinctive belief in the supernatural remained.

Turning to Audrey the rat added, "Akkikuyu have many treasures, mouselet. Things she not understand, powders in pouches, leaf and herb in bundles, secret packets that do smell most strange and a terrible trophy of a kitty head." She frowned as she looked into the swirling water as if all her answers lay there. "What they all about? Why for Akkikuyu keep such grislys? Was she doctor to have bowl for pounding and mixing? A darkness is behind Akkikuyu – too black to see." Her voice trailed off as she sighed with regret.

On impulse Audrey said, "Don't worry, leave the past alone – look to the future, Madame Akkikuyu. There will be answers enough for you there."

"Oh mousey, how good it is for you to be such a friend." The fortune-teller grabbed Audrey and because the mouse pitied her she did not struggle as the other hugged her tightly. Large rat tears ran down Audrey's neck.

Arthur, Twit and Kempe peered over the top of the steps.

"We've a tidy way to go before we get to Fennywolde," said the traveller slowly. "We had better keep an eye on that Madame there, bad business to be sure. You can wash a rat and comb a rat but it will still be a rat. You can't trust 'em!"

"We know that," said Arthur.

"What I says is," continued Kempe, "nourish a rat and one day it will bite your head off. Just you watch her when you get to your field young laddie – rats is always trouble."

*　　　*　　　*

It was much later that night when they had all bedded down in the hold that it really began.

The mice were sleeping soundly. Arthur's soft snores rose and fell with a steady rhythm. Kempe twitched his whiskers as he dreamed of pearls and silks flowing through his trader's paws. Twit, as always, was curled up in a circle, looking for all the world like an addition to Kempe's wooden carvings. Audrey had untied her ribbon and her hair spread around her like a fine network of fairy webs.

Nearby, Akkikuyu grunted as she wandered through her own dark dreams. She was sprawled amongst her bags and sacks, and occasionally her face would screw itself up into an expression of pain and her tail would beat the tarpaulin with heavy, agitated smacks. She rolled over and over, shaking her great head and mumbling to herself.

From somewhere in her dreams a voice seemed to be calling to her: "Akkikuyu! Akkikuyu – are you there?"

In her sleep Madame Akkikuyu groaned aloud. "Yes I am here," she muttered, as if in answer to the unseen thing of her dreams. "What do you want? Who is it? Leave me alone."

For the rest of the journey along the river the night was to become a time of dread for Madame Akkikuyu – a time when the nameless voice invaded her sleep to call her name unceasingly.

6

FENNYWOLDE

The sunlight spread across the growing corn and cast deep charcoal shadows under the elm trees. The field was a large one – a mass of green, rippling like the ocean as the wind played over its surface and murmuring with lovers' whispers as the breeze sighed through it. The corn soaked up the sun, drank its gold and grew tall.

The field was bordered on one side by a deep ditch that fed a pool at the far end where the hawthorn grew thick and impenetrable. But now the ditch was dry and the mud at the bottom was cracked and studded with sharp stones. Along the side grew the tall elms and one solitary yew, dark giants rearing high over the swaying grasses and stretching into the fierce blue.

To the left of the ditch was a meadow. Too small and difficult to plough, the meadow was rich in the glossy show of buttercups and flowering grasses. An enchanted scent hung over the place – a perfect blending of wild perfumes, so strong that you could almost taste them. Beyond the meadow was a great clump of oaks, fully in leaf, like green clouds come to rest on the earth.

This small land was what the fieldmice called "Fennywolde" or "the land of Fenny" – he being the first mouse to have lived there many years ago.

It provided them with everything they needed: an abundant supply of corn, berries from the hawthorn, water from the pool and brambles for autumn brewing. In the winter the steep banks of the ditch provided excellent shelter, and there were numerous tunnels and passages under the roots of the elms, which had been dug a long time ago by venerable ancestors. Secret holes to hide from the bitter winds and escape the midwinter death, places to spend chill dark days and spacious halls to store supplies.

During the summer it was usual for the fieldmice to move out of their tunnels and take up residence in the field – to delight in climbing the tall stems and nibble the ripening corn. So far, however, the inhabitants of Fennywolde had remained in their winter quarters. Only during the day would they dare venture into the field and woe betide any mouse not safe in the tunnels at dusk. A terror was hunting in the night.

*   *   *

Alison sauntered through the meadow lazily. She was a beautiful country mouse, her strawberry blonde hair hung in two creamy pony tails behind her ears. Her fur, like the fur of all fieldmice was reddish gold but Alison's held a secret glint that dazzled when it caught the sun. She was a curvy young mouse maid with an impish pout and large brown eyes. Her skirt was of simple cotton stitched around with humble rustic embroidery. At her breast a mousebrass dangled – a sickle moon with a tiny brass bell – the sign of grace and beauty. And this was the trouble. Alison had received the charm a year ago and it had gone straight to her head.

She flirted with the boys, flicking back her hair and flashing her eyes at them, promising sweetness. They had all fallen for her: Todkin,

Hodge, Young Whortle and even skinny Samuel had been victims of her careless, dangerous glances. Those slight tosses of her head and devastating grins had been practised and scrutinised in the mirror of the still pool where she spent most of her days preening and rehearsing her powers.

The warm afternoon, mingled with the dry rustle of the grasses, was a potent drug. Alison slumped on the ground, face upturned. The seeding grass heads bobbing overhead seemed to be bowing before her beauty. She fanned herself with a buttercup allowing its rich buttery aura to wrap around her.

"Poor Dimsel," mused Alison in a throaty whisper. "Face like a cow's behind and wit to match." She laughed softly and stretched. "Dear Iris, legs like a redshank and not a curl in her hair." She passed her paw through her own crowning glory and made a mock appeal to the world in general. "But friends, let us not forget Lily Clover, she has the grace of a swan – but she do stink like a fresh steaming dung hill." They were the names of Alison's rivals and she spoke of them with casual disregard, because today she had decided she had surpassed them all. It was clear in her mind now that she had no equal anywhere.

A bee droned in and out of the clear patch of blue above. "Old Bumble knows," laughed Alison and her voice rose high and flutey. "He do know it! Bees go to honey and I be the sweetest thing by far." She rolled over and spied a forget-me-not pricking through the grass stems. Reaching out she plucked it mercilessly. After weaving it into her hair she paraded up and down for her invisible audience. She contemplated whether she should return to the pool to assess the impact of the flower but then her mouth curled and she set off purposefully.

* * *

Jenkin kicked the hard ground and scratched his head. He was carrying a large bundle of dry wood and felt like throwing it all into the ditch. His friends, Hodge and Todkin were in the field practising their stalk climbing whilst Samuel and Young Whortle had gone off to quest the oaks beyond the meadow.

Jenkin was tired and fed up – his father made him work hard. "Waste not the hours the good Green gives" was just one of the rules drummed into him.

Suddenly his mousebrass reflected the sun full into his downcast eyes. He dropped the sticks and rubbed them. For a moment he was blinded. It was a brass of life and hope – a sun sign. His father, the local mousebrass maker, had forged it specially with him in mind and was gravely pleased when Jenkin managed to choose it from the sack two springs ago.

"Ho there! Jolly Jenkin!" came a clear voice suddenly. "Why for you rubbin' your eyes? Do I dazzle so much?"

Jenkin blinked. As his eyes readjusted through the misty haze of light he could just see Alison strolling towards him out of the meadow. Her fur was a fiery gold and there was buttercup dust glittering on her face. In her eyes there were dancing lights.

"Is that you, Alison Sedge?" he ventured, doubting his vision.

"Might be," she answered, staying just within the fringes of the meadow grass. "Then again I might be the goddess come down from the moon to torment you with my beauty."

Jenkin snorted. "Pah!" You don't half talk addled sometimes, Alison Sedge. Just you mind my dad don't hear you goin' on like that. He'll tell your folks he will."

"Pooh." She stepped out onto the hard ground.

Jenkin eyed her again. She had certainly changed in the past year – why before she had been given that mousebrass they had been firm friends. He had even thought that perhaps ... He saw her eyebrows arch in that infuriating way of hers. She had guessed what he was thinking about and tossed her head.

"Like my flower?" she asked huskily.

"Look better in the ground," Jenkin replied shyly, turning away from those eyes which held those dangerous lights. "Why don't you go show Hodge?"

"I may," Alison answered mildly. It amused her to flirt with the boys and see how she set them at odds with one another. How easily they could be confounded by a sideways glance or a sweet smile. It was Jenkin though, whom she enjoyed teasing most. He was so serious and po-faced and when he was with his father she revelled in disconcerting him. In fact, if her pride and vanity had not swelled so much she would quite happily have married Jenkin. He was by far the most handsome mouse in Fennywolde. Now though she enjoyed dangling him on a string with all the others, tempting and rejecting with soft, mocking laughter.

An impatient voice rang out over the field. "Jenkin! Where are thee lad?"

He jumped up and hastily retrieved the bundle of sticks. "That be my dad callin' for me." Jenkin began to run to the ditch, past the bare stony stretch and up to the cool shade of the elms.

Isaac Nettle stood stiff and stern outside one of the entrances to the winter quarters. He scowled as his son came panting up to him. He was a lean mouse whose face was always grim and forbidding – no-one had heard him laugh since his wife had died. His eyes were steely and humourless, set deep beneath wiry brows in a sour face.

"Where did thee get to?" he snapped. "Idling again, I'll warrant. Come here boy."

Jenkin set the wood down before his father, watching him warily.

"What's this!" bellowed Isaac. "The wood is green. How am I to burn that! We should choke on smoke!" He grabbed his son by the neck and raised his hard paws to him. "I'll beat sense into thee yet boy and with the Green's help I'll cure thee of thine idleness."

Jenkin knew better than to protest. He gritted his teeth and screwed up his face. His father's paw came viciously down on him. Jenkin gasped as he opened his eyes; the blow had been a severe one. The blood pounded in his head and the side of his face throbbed with pain.

Isaac raised his paw again and smacked his son across the head once more. He spared no effort, so that Jenkin sobbed this time. "Thou must learn," exulted his father. He hit him one more time to emphasise his words.

Jenkin staggered on his feet when Isaac had finished. His head was reeling and already he felt a swelling around his eye. In his mouth he tasted the tang of iron and knew that his lip was bleeding. Soon the shock would wear off and he would be left with a dull ache and painful stinging.

"Now what have thee to say?" rumbled Isaac.

"I . . . I thank thee Father," stammered Jenkin holding his sore lip.

"We shall pray together," intoned Isaac to his son. "Midsummer scarce a week away and still we live in winter holes. 'Tis a judgement on us all. The

Green is angry. There are those in our midst who have offended thee Lord. Heathen loutishness creeps in. Give your servants strength to drive out the vain pride which you despise. Let us walk free at night once more." He dragged Jenkin inside.

From a safe distance Alison had watched it all. She had flinched as she saw Jenkin suffer those three terrible blows. Everyone in Fennywolde feared Mr Nettle. His temper was dreadful but he commanded the authority and respect due to the mousebrass maker. Several times Jenkin had carried the bruises given to him by his father and no-one dared do anything about it – indeed Mr Nettle was not the only staunch Green Mouser in Fennywolde.

Alison walked up to the ditch. She knew that Isaac classed her as one of the offenders in the field. He sermonised at her whenever he saw her. She thought of the miserable night which lay before Jenkin: he would have to kneel on a painfully hard floor next to his father for hours praying to the Green Mouse for deliverance and forgiveness. Alison sighed and told herself that she must make sure to be kind to Jenkin the next time she met him – why she might even let him kiss her. She chuckled at the notion and looked about her.

The evening was growing old, and clouds of gnats were spinning over the barren stretch of ditch. It was time for her to go home.

She turned on her heel and made for one of the other entrances to the winter quarters.

"Alison Sedge," came a distraught voice. She looked up quickly and noticed a group of six worried mice. A plump harassed mouse bustled over.

"Hello Mrs Gorse," greeted Alison politely.

The mouse brushed a long wisp of hair out of her

red-rimmed eyes and asked, "Have you seen our Samuel?"

Alison shook her head. "Why no, Mrs Gorse. I think he went off with Young Whortle this morning."

"Oh dear," murmured Mrs Gorse. "I was hoping you might know where they were. Mr and Mrs Nep are asking everyone in the shelters. If they don't come back soon . . ."

Alison turned towards the meadow and stared at the grasses intently. It was getting dark and no mouse was safe above ground then.

*   *   *

Samuel Gorse was close to tears. He held on tightly to his friend and tried to pull himself further under the oak root.

It had been a magnificent day. The morning had been so fine that he and Young Whortle Nep had decided against joining Todkin and Hodge in the field and planned an adventure.

"Warty" as Samuel was fond of calling his friend was always full of terrific ideas. Last year he had built a raft and together they had sailed it along the ditch, fending off imaginary pirates and monsters from the deep. This year though, the ditch had dried up and they had been forbidden to sail the raft on the still pool as it was too deep.

Young Whortle was older than Samuel though not as tall. "Right Sammy," he had said that morning. "If Jenkin's too busy an' Todders an' Hodge are set on climbin' today then it be up to us to take what thrills the day has to offer."

So they sat down and thought seriously about what they could do. They had already explored the field this year and the ditch promised little in the way of adventure in its parched state. They had been to the pool once or twice but Alison Sedge was always there teasing them. Alison Sedge had been declared dangerous territory by them both so the pool was out of the question, with or without the raft.

Whilst the two friends contemplated the day's destination Young Whortle had raised his head and seen the oaks in the hazy distance.

"Aha!" he cried, jumping to his feet and assuming a triumphant pose. "The oaks, Sammy. We shall quest the oaks and see what secrets they keep." So off they went, passing a dejected Jenkin and waving cheerily to him as they entered the meadow.

Now Samuel shivered. Fear chilled him and his teeth began to chatter.

"Sshh!" whispered Young Whortle close by. "It'll hear you."

What a situation they had landed themselves in. All had been going wonderfully. They had charged through the piles of last year's leaves which still filled the hollows near the oaks and had played hide and seek behind the roots; then Young Whortle had suggested that they attempt a climb.

"Don't go frettin', Sammy," he had said. "We won't pick a difficult tree and we won't go too high – promise."

"But Warty," Samuel had protested, "shouldn't we be getting along now?"

"Bags of time yet! Sun ain't low enough to think on going back. Come on, give us a leg up."

So up an oak tree they had climbed. It was gnarled, knobbly and ideal to climb. Footholds were plentiful and there were lots of low branches to run along and swing from.

Then Samuel had noticed the hole.

"What's that up there?" he had asked, pointing higher up the tree trunk. "Looks like some sort of big gap in the bark."

Higher they had clambered. Samuel had been determined not to look down and had kept his eyes strictly on his paws. Eventually, Young Whortle had drawn near to the hole.

"Seems like the tree's hollow here," he had called down.

"Wait for me!" Samuel had pulled himself up to his friend's side. Together they had peeped over the brink of the hole.

Inside all had been dark . . . but their sharp eyes had picked out something in the gloom. Something terrible . . .

Samuel shrieked and nearly fell off the tree. Young Whortle's eyes opened very wide and he gave a funny sort of yelp. Here, in the oak, was the frightful thing which had kept the fieldmice below ground this year – a large and very fearsome barn owl.

It was fast asleep amongst some old straw but it stirred when the mice gasped in fright. Lazily it opened one eye and puffed out its soft feathery chest.

Quickly Young Whortle and Samuel ran down the tree. They slid and slithered, scraped their knees and broke the skin on their paws scurrying down it.

As Young Whortle jumped from the lowest branch a great shadow fell on him. Quickly he yanked Samuel to the ground and ducked under one of the roots.

Seconds later sharp talons scored the ground where they had been.

Now here they were, two small frightened field-mice cowering in terror from a dreadful enemy.

"Be it still up there?" asked Samuel in a tiny voice.

"Aye Sammy, prob'ly sat on one o' them low

branches just a-waitin' for us to make a move."

"Oh Warty, I'm whacked," whimpered Samuel. "It's gettin' so dark now an' I haven't eaten for ages: just listen to my belly!"

"I hear it an' so can the owl most like. Put your paws over it or summat."

"I can't! I be starved."

"So be yon owl, Sammy an' I don't want to be no bird's breakfast."

Samuel tried to control the growls and rumbles coming from his stomach. He was a thin mouse, "too thin" some said. The likes of Alison even called him "skinny Samuel". His mother was most perturbed by his weight, but no matter how much he ate he never got any fatter. "'Tis his age," Old Todmore said of him. "Too much energy – he'll plump out afore he's wed." Now the thought that he would make a poor breakfast brought Samuel no comfort at all.

"We can't stay here," he said softly.

Young Whortle patted his friend on the shoulder. "Right," he said decisively. "I got me an idea."

"Smashin'!" Samuel brightened instantly. "I knowed you'd think o' summat. What be the plan?"

"Well," Young Whortle kept his voice low in case the owl was listening, "if I throws a stone yonder," he pointed behind them to a patch of ferns and bracken, "it just might fool Hooty up there an' distract him long enough for us to make a dash for them hollows full o' leaves."

"You're barmy!" exclaimed Samuel. "No way will that work. He's crafty he is. He'll spot that trick for sure an' we'll be runnin' straight down his gizzards."

Young Whortle said nothing. Instead he picked up a good paw-sized pebble and threw it for all he was worth. The ferns rustled and swayed as it crashed through them.

"Now!" he hissed grabbing Samuel by the arm.

The fieldmice darted from under the root. Samuel ran as fast as he could, too terrified to look up in case he saw the owl rushing down to meet them – talons outstretched.

And then they were at the edge of the hollows and with one leap they dived into the heaps of dry leaves.

"It worked!" Samuel cried. His heart was racing and his ears flushed with excitement.

"I told 'ee we'd have adventures today," said Young Whortle. "Now we'll have to be careful. He won't have liked that trick and it might make him anxious to get us."

"So what now?"

"We tunnel through these here leaves till we're at the point closest to the meadow. Then you just run like crazy."

Samuel gulped nervously, but their first success at owl-foxing heartened him. "Lead on then," he said.

In the leaves it was easy to believe that it was autumn again. The smell of the dry decay was the very essence of that season. The leaves crackled over and beneath them as they pushed their way through. The sound filled their ears, like the noise of a greedy consuming fire. The mice moved quickly. Like moles they scooped the leaves out of the way with their paws and kicked them backwards with their feet. Through the leafy ceiling the owl could be heard hooting irritably. It froze their hearts and made them move faster than ever.

Suddenly there was an explosion of leaves and twilight shone down on them.

"He's dive-bombing us," wailed Samuel. He looked up and could see the owl soaring above, gaining height for the next dive.

"We'll have to zig-zag and hope he misses us," shouted Young Whortle, burying himself in the leaves once more.

Samuel jumped in after him, and they madly dashed from side to side.

The owl tore into the leaves close by and gave an angry hoot at finding his talons empty. "Hooo mooouses, I'll get yooooou!" he bellowed furiously. The owl beat his great wings fiercely and rose high above the treetops. He stared with his great round eyes at the leafy hollow and glided on the night airs, silent as a ghost. There – a movement.

He dropped like a stone. With murderous intent he descended. He'd show them! How dare they wake him then hide and play silly tricks.

The owl skimmed the surface of the hollow with his talons, churning up leaves and twigs in the chaos of his wake.

Samuel and Young Whortle had managed to dodge that onslaught – but only just. Samuel lost the tip of his tail and the pain was terrible. Blood poured out of it and made him feel sick.

Young Whortle was near to panic himself. Both mice were tired now but the owl had been asleep all day. Young Whortle wished they had stayed under that oak root after all. Even in the dim light he saw how pale Samuel had become, and in horror he noticed his friend's wounded tail. He knew then that they would not survive the next attack; they were exposed and too tired to move fast enough.

An insane idea gripped him suddenly and in a wild frenzy Young Whortle scrabbled amongst the muck of the floor until he found a stout twig.

Samuel was too groggy and near to fainting to question his friend. He watched Young Whortle bite the twig and strip away the bark with his teeth, gnawing like a demented demon. Then high above he saw the dark sinister shape of the owl plummeting towards them.

The owl had licked the blood from his talons and was cackling to himself, eager for the kill. The blood was warm and it tasted wonderful. The first mouse of the night was always the best and he had been unable to find any for months. But now, oho! Two lovely mice for him to swallow.

The cool night air streamed over his flat face as he hurtled down, legs stiff and talons glinting under the light of the first stars.

He had them in his sights – wise of them to stop running. "Ooooh mooouses," he chuckled licking his beak in anticipation.

"FENNY!" bawled a voice. The owl blinked and as he bore down on the mice one of them jumped up and drove something sharp into his left leg.

"Ooooww!" screeched the owl, floundering in the air with the shock. He rose up, shaking his head in disbelief. How dare they! The audacity of it! The owl was really furious now. Screaming with rage he plucked the twig from his leg with one deft movement, spat it out and glared down. This was serious; insult and injury – that had never happened to him before and he was deadly in his wrath.

"Mooouses!" he cried in a bitter cold voice. "Mahooot will find yoooou!"

Young Whortle had wasted no time. As soon as he had wounded the owl he had dragged the wilting Samuel out of the hollow and pulled him towards the meadow.

How they managed he never knew. Samuel had lost a lot of blood and kept swooning. But fear kept them going and suddenly they were in.

Tall grasses surrounded them. Young Whortle

knew however that it would take more protection than the meadow afforded to save them from a determined owl.

Samuel panted heavily. He felt very weak and his legs were like water. He tried to focus his eyes but everything was blurred. Young Whortle's voice came to him urgently, calling his name.

"Sammy! Come on, we've made it to the meadow but Hooty's still after us."

As if in agreement a frightful screech came down out of the night sky.

Samuel felt himself tugged at roughly. "Leave me, Warty," he mumbled. "Too tired, you go."

"Shut up!" Young Whortle gripped his friend none too gently and shoved him further into the meadow.

They stumbled and staggered along, flinging themselves to the ground when they felt a shadow pass overhead.

"What's he doing?" Young Whortle asked himself. "Why doesn't he strike? He must know where we are. Why doesn't he get it over with?"

A wicked cackle told him the reason. The owl was tormenting them, letting them know the full meaning of fear before the kill.

"Mooouses," he called, "Mahooot sees yooou." A dark wing swept over the tops of the grass.

Young Whortle bowed his head in defeat. He could run no more and even if he could the owl would snatch him before he made it to the ditch. The dark wing soared over again; this time battering down the grass.

"Next time," thought Young Whortle desperately. "This is it Sammy," he said, "I'm sorry this adventure has ended so badly."

Samuel shook his head feebly. "Not your fault Warty." He held out a thin, trembling paw and

Young Whortle clasped it tightly. Together they waited for the end.

Down came Mahooot the owl. He smashed through the grass and landed in front of the fieldmice.

"Ohooo mooouses!" he said wickedly – narrowing his baleful, round, tawny eyes into evil slits. "Piece by piece will yooou slide dooown." He stepped nearer and opened his sharp beak. "Mahooot learn yooou tooo behave."

The owl shot out a talon and grasped Young Whortle by the shoulder. The small mouse squealed in pain as Mahooot drew him near to his waiting beak.

Samuel felt his friend's paw being dragged out of his own but he was too far gone to be frightened of the sinister night bird about to feast on them.

Young Whortle saw through his tears the ghastly beak open. He felt the iron grip of the talons squeeze even tighter. The musty breath of the bird swept over him and he swooned. Mahooot sniggered. He was about to pop the fieldmouse's head into his beak when . . .

"Aiee! Aiee!" screamed a strange voice. "Aiee!"

Mahooot blinked and glanced up. Who was that disturbing his breakfast? The owl swivelled his face around but could see nothing. He grunted irritably and turned his attention back to the mouse.

"Aiee!" A stone came flying out of nowhere and stung Mahooot right on the beak.

"Whoooo? Whooo?" he began ferociously. He unfurled his wings but kept a tight hold on Young Whortle.

Great clumping footsteps came rushing towards them. Mahooot twitched with uncertainty – he would take to the air and see who this intruder was. His wings opened out and he began to flap them.

He decided to leave the thin mouse behind, this one would do, he could eat it at his leisure in the oak tree.

"Aiee, beaky hooter!" came the voice. "Put down the mouselet!" Into view, crashing through the meadow, came a large ratwoman with a shawl around her shoulders and a bone in her hair. It was Madame Akkikuyu.

Mahooot eyed her doubtfully and rose into the air; he didn't like rats.

"Help!" squeaked Young Whortle dangling from his talons.

The rat leapt up and grabbed the owl's other leg, bringing him sprawling to the ground with an astounded screech.

Madame Akkikuyu hopped onto Mahooot's back and dealt him a great thump with the bone from her hair. "Let go feathery one, free mouselet."

The owl twisted under her and scrabbled at the ground in a bewildered frenzy. Another "thwack" hit his head. "Oooow!" he roared.

Madame Akkikuyu laughed out loud, then thrust the bone back in her hair and proceeded to pluck the owl.

Mahooot's screeches were deafening and he turned his head to snap at the rat.

"Oh no fowl one," she laughed, giving the slashing beak a swift smack with her claws.

Clouds of soft, pale feathers floated into the air as the raw bare patch on Mahooot's neck grew larger. Madame Akkikuyu began to hoot herself, mocking him as she tore out large clumps of feathers and threw them before the owl for him to see.

Suddenly Young Whortle was free. The talons opened and he staggered over to Samuel where he fell unconscious.

Mahooot writhed and managed to scramble upright. Madame Akkikuyu clenched her claw and gave him a powerful punch. He staggered backwards and she flung her arms around his neck and bit deeply into his shoulder.

That was enough for him. The owl let out one last hoot of pain, shook the rat off his back and rose shakily off the ground – but not before a hail of stones and twigs battered him as Madame Akkikuyu jumped up and down with glee below.

"Scardee Birdee!" she shouted, sticking out her tongue at the receding dark shape in the sky. The fortune-teller smiled then rushed over to the fieldmice and inspected their wounds. "Poor mouseys," she cooed sadly, "very bad they are." She fumbled in one of the pouches which hung round her waist and brought out a broad-leafed herb. With it she dabbed Young Whortle's punctured shoulder and then with some more, bound Samuel's mutilated tail.

Madame Akkikuyu stepped back and sat down with a bump. How had she known what to do? She looked into her pouches and knew the properties of all the herbs in it – most of them were deadly. "Oh Akkikuyu," she gasped breathlessly. "What memories are you waking?" She looked at Samuel's tail and it seemed to dissolve away and its place was a rough rat's tail, stumpy and with an old rag tied at the end. From out of the past a coarse voice said, "Just don't get in my way, witch!"

Madame Akkikuyu shuddered and all her instincts told her not to delve into her past too deeply. Yet she began to wonder, just who was she and why did she carry all these weird objects and powders around with her?

A sound from the real world reached her ears and she broke out of her brooding. The others were

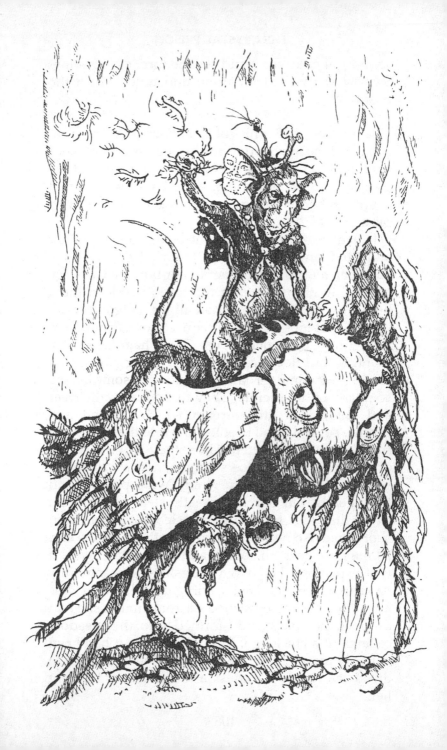

coming; already she could see the torches flickering. Silently she waited for them and reflected on the past days.

* * *

The journey to Fennywolde had been uneventful but it had been so wonderful to be with her friend Audrey, to know that they were going somewhere pleasant in the sunshine. She had not stopped counting her blessings and hugged herself with pleasure.

It had taken three different boats to get this far and Mr Kempe had guided them all the way. He had been a little standoffish to her but she was very grateful to him for taking the trouble to lead them here. This afternoon they had all waved goodbye to him and set foot on dry land once more. From there that funny little fieldmouse Twit had led them, pointing out local features and telling amusing stories. Madame Akkikuyu had revelled in the company of her friends. They turned from the river and followed a little stream which divided and became several small brooks. The one they followed soon became a dry ditch. There they found a crowd of worried-looking mice staring across a meadow.

Someone had gone to fetch Twit's parents and they nearly hugged the breath clear out of him when they saw him. But the celebration had been short-lived. An owl screeched over the meadow and all the mice gasped; some had tears in their eyes. It was explained that two youngsters were missing. Akkikuyu saw the owl circling and knew it was about to strike. To everyone's astonishment she had dropped her bags and stormed into the meadow calling out a challenge. Yes, what a day it had been – if only the nights were as good. She had come to dread the empty darkness and the fear it brought her.

*   *   *

"Over here!" came the babble of voices. Madame Akkikuyu wrenched herself back to the present and got to her feet.

The meadow was lit by little burning torches carried by a host of fieldmice. They hurried towards her and she threw open her arms in welcome. The mice came and stared at the scene before them with open mouths.

There were the two youngsters lying, dead for all they knew, on the ground, and the peculiar ratwoman was boldly waving her arms about. Covering everything was a layer of downy feathers like a light fall of snow. They gazed at Madame Akkikuyu dumbly, not knowing what to do.

Mrs Gorse pushed her way to the front and ran to her son's side. She wept over his damaged tail and kissed his forehead.

"He need rest," advised the fortune-teller. "I make broth to heal tomorrow."

Young Whortle's parents came squeezing out of the crowd and knelt beside their son. Slowly his eyes opened and he managed a weak smile for them. Then he lifted a finger and pointed at the rat.

"She saved us, Dad." he said. "Saved us from the owl she did."

"Thank you," said Mr Nep gratefully to Madame Akkikuyu.

The crowd cheered until she flushed with pleasure. Then to her great surprise and enduring delight they picked her up and carried her on their shoulders, although it took eight of the strongest husbands to manage this feat. Others helped to take Young Whortle and Samuel back to the winter quarters.

Arthur and Audrey could not believe their eyes. Here they were, newly arrived in Fennywolde and

Madame Akkikuyu was being fêted as a heroine. Everything was happening so quickly. They hadn't had a chance to meet Twit's parents yet.

Arthur stood amongst the feathers and shrugged. "I'd never have believed it," he said flatly.

"She is remarkable," said a voice behind them. They turned round and saw a fieldmouse sticking a feather in his hair. "Even my father approved of her," he added. "Oh, sorry, my name's Jenkin. You're the ones who came back with Twit aren't you?"

"Yes," replied Audrey. She liked the look of this mouse and he had been the first one in Fennywolde to speak to them so far. "I'm Audrey and this is my brother Arthur. What's been going on here?"

"Oh an owl's kept us in our winter quarters all year. We daredn't go out at night coz he'd catch us an' eat us. But it looks like we've done seen the last of him for a while." Jenkin beamed at them and Audrey noticed an ugly bruise on his ear and that his lip was badly swollen.

"You've been in a fight," she said to him.

Jenkin turned quickly away and said, "We better get goin' – the others are nearly home now." The rows of bobbing torches had dwindled in the distance. "Follow me," he told them, and set off back to the ditch.

"You embarrassed him," Arthur hissed at Audrey, "Why can't you mind your own business?"

"Why should it have embarrassed him?" protested Audrey. "I shouldn't think he's trying to keep the fact a secret. Did you see the state of his bruises?"

"Yes I did, but I've had worse. Anyway we must follow him now, I don't want to spend our first night here tramping through the fields lost. Come on."

At the ditch, the fieldmice put Madame Akkikuyu down and the husbands wiped their brows wearily. The fortune-teller gazed about her enraptured. She could not remember ever feeling like this before – she wanted to burst with joy.

By the time Arthur and Audrey arrived she was speaking: "Owly not come back in hurry, if he do – Akkikuyu bite him again."

There was thunderous applause and some mice cried, "We can move into the field at last!" and "Hooray for the rat lady!" Then other voices called,

"Where be Mr Woodruffe? He's got to declare the field open." The mice looked at one another and muttered agreement. Hastily a young mouse ran into the shelters to fetch him.

At the Spring Ceremony every year the fieldmice elected a "King of the Field". This year the honour had gone to Mr Abraham Woodruffe – a well-liked and respected mouse who so far had been unable to enjoy his high office, being stuck in the winter quarters all the time.

The mice waited for him and excited expectation charged the cool night air. Audrey and Arthur sensed their mood and they too grew impatient. Audrey began to fidget and started to look around at the fieldmice. It was the first chance she had had so far to view them properly. There were fat mice, thin mice, some tiny ones with large pink ears and long twitchy tails but no tall mice. Except perhaps . . . yes on the far side of the crowd Audrey saw a lofty mouse. She stared at him curiously: what a grim face he had! It seemed as if his face never saw a smile. Idly she wondered who he was and then, next to him, she noticed Jenkin, who to her surprise and lasting embarrassment was looking straight at her. Audrey coughed and turned quickly away. She felt her ears burn with her blushes and hoped it would not show under the torchlight.

Audrey tried to compose herself and gazed fixedly ahead, hoping that her ribbon was tied properly. However, she could not resist having a crafty peep round to see if Jenkin was still looking at her.

As casually as she could manage, Audrey turned, but Jenkin was speaking with that tall mouse now. She was amused to find that she was disappointed and smiled broadly at herself until she saw something that made her cough and turn away again.

A girl mouse was glaring at her – glaring with real hatred in her eyes. Audrey could feel them boring into the back of her neck. She could not think who the girl was and asked herself if she had done anything to deserve it.

"Oh what the heck!" she said to herself in a low determined whisper and looked back at the girl. Alison Sedge was still eyeing Audrey with a face like thunder. Their eyes met and Miss Brown gave her her most insolent, pretty smile then turned away.

Suddenly a hush fell on the gathered fieldmice as Mr Woodruffe stepped out of the winter quarters. He was a jovial mouse and seemed quite ordinary except that on his brow he wore a crown of plaited corn. Mr Woodruffe raised his paws and began solemnly.

"May the field be blessed and may the goodwill of the Green Mouse follow us therein."

"Amen to that!" called out Isaac Nettle, but he was drowned out by the frantic cheers of everyone else.

Mr Woodruffe waved his arms for silence and continued. "I have been told of the daring bravery shown 'ere by our guest." He bowed to Madame

Akkikuyu. She pointed her foot and managed a curtsey back. "And as 'King of the Field'," he went on, "it is my pleasure to offer her the freedom of Fennywolde, for surely she is a messenger of the Green Mouse come in our most desperate hour."

There were shouts of agreement from the fieldmice. Arthur and Audrey stared at one another. Isaac Nettle nodded his head gravely.

"And now," shouted Mr Woodruffe, "you may all enter the field!" He stood aside and the fieldmice scurried past him.

"Make the Hall," they yelled happily.

Soon only Mr Woodruffe, Madame Akkikuyu, Audrey and Arthur were left standing by the ditch and the field was filled was joyous calls and mysterious sounds.

Mr Woodruffe looked at the Deptford mice and smiled. "So you are Twit's companions. Come, he is below with his folks. I think we can interrupt them now. You look like you could do with a good sleep. The field is no place for you tonight. The work would keep you awake."

"Please sir," Arthur asked, "what work?"

"Hah, you'll see tomorrow lad." Mr Woodruffe turned to Madame Akkikuyu and raised his eyebrows. "Will you join us below ma'am? We would be most honoured."

The fortune-teller grinned at him and came over to give Audrey a big hug.

"Yes Akkikuyu come, she not leave her friend. First Akkikuyu find bags. You go, I follow."

The three mice left the rat to find her things and entered the winter quarters.

Madame Akkikuyu was left alone in the dark. In her mind she relived the thrilling moments of glory, and the thrill that those cheers gave her. What undreamt wonders there were in the world and how her heart swelled with pride to think that all these mice honoured her!

As a tear fell from her furry cheek, Madame Akkikuyu knew that she had never been so happy before. Tonight, she thought, would be a good time to die, whilst she was happiest. The fortune-teller sniffed. No, with her friend there would be many more times such as this – if not greater. Madame Akkikuyu blew her nose on her shawl then cast about for her bags.

It was too dark to see them. The sky had clouded over and the moon was hidden. She stooped down and groped for her things. It was so quiet. The noise of the mice in the field had died down or they had moved further away out of earshot.

"Akkikuyu!"

Madame Akkikuyu paused and tilted her head to one side.

"Akkikuyu!"

There it was again. A distant, echoing voice calling her name. It had troubled her on the river but no-one else seemed to have heard it. Madame Akkikuyu despaired. Tearing at her hair she shook her head violently. "Leave me!" she wailed. "Go away. Akkikuyu not listen!" And she ran up the side of the ditch and down into the shelters.

7

THE HALL OF CORN

The sun brimmed over the tops of the oak trees and its dazzling, early rays moved slowly over the meadow, pushing back the grey dawn and creeping towards the field. The corn seemed to stir at the sun's warm touch and stretched as high as it could. Fennywolde awoke.

Audrey rubbed her eyes and gazed sleepily at the low, rough ceiling. She was in a small room in the winter quarters, that part lived in by the Scuttles. The room was bare – there was no decoration on the lumpy earth walls, no flowers, drawings, ornaments – nothing. Only a small tallow candle flickered miserably in one corner and Audrey looked at it thoughtfully. She was sure she had blown that out before she had gone to sleep. Someone must have been in to relight it. Yes, on the floor near her bed was a bowl of water for her to wash in. That was a kind thought and one which Audrey felt she needed.

She dragged herself out of bed and began splashing the drowsiness and grime of the past few days away.

"Is that you awake now Audrey?" came a friendly voice just outside the room. "Well breakfast's ready when you are."

Audrey finished dressing and smoothed the

creases out of her lace. She tied a new ribbon in her hair – a parting gift from Kempe, then she slipped her bells onto her tail and went into the breakfast room.

Again it was bleak and bare with only a table in the centre and three stools around it. Mrs Scuttle pattered in carrying a bowl of porridge.

Audrey and Arthur had been surprised when they first saw Mrs Chitter's sister. She wasn't a bit like that gossipy old fusspot. Gladwin Scuttle was a brown house mouse as they were. She was slender with short, chestnut hair, greying at the crown and a thin, delicate face. Around her neck she wore a prim starched collar. Audrey thought that she must have been quite lovely when she was younger.

"Where's my brother and Twit?" asked Audrey between mouthfuls.

"Gone out with Elijah," replied Mrs Scuttle settling down on a stool and beaming warmly. "Oh and your . . . er . . . friend, Madame – what was it?"

"Akkikuyu," prompted Audrey, "but she's not exactly my friend, you know."

"Well, I did wonder. I came from Deptford too, remember and I know how horrible the rats were there. I'd watch her if I were you, wouldn't trust her an inch despite her doings last night."

Audrey wondered about that. "That's what Kempe said, but you know I really do think she's changed. She really is trying her best."

"Hmm," Mrs Scuttle sounded doubtful. "Still, I suppose I shouldn't judge her too harshly. My William's been telling me all about you and her and . . ." here she lowered her voice to a faint whisper, " . . . Jupiter."

"Please," begged Audrey, "you mustn't mention that name to Madame Akkikuyu. She can't remember a thing and it might just be too much for her."

"Oh quite dear . . . I can keep mum. I don't suppose my sister has learned how yet – no your smile gives that away. So, Arabel's not changed a bit, I thought William was being too polite when I asked him about her. Still it was good of her to look after him all this time."

Audrey finished her breakfast and then said, "You never did tell me where Madame Akkikuyu had gone."

"Oh yes, why there I go again – forgetting things. I tell you dear my head's like a sieve these days. Oh . . . where was I?"

"Madame Akkikuyu."

"Yes, such an odd name. Well you should have seen how much she ate this morning, and I'm sorry but her table manners are dreadful. Anyway, after making a right mess she ups and goes outside hauling one of those big bags with her. What does she keep in them, do you know?"

Audrey nodded. "They're her herbs, powders, mixing tins and other stuff like that."

"Well. William did tell me how she's supposed to be a fortune-teller, I didn't like to ask her myself – I find that sort of thing very frightening."

"Oh it's all right," assured Audrey. "She doesn't do any of that any more. I think she just carries that junk around with her out of habit. You don't have to worry, she's not likely to start brewing up spells now."

Mrs Scuttle put her paws on the table and stared at Audrey. "But my dear! That's precisely what she is doing. That's where everyone's gone. She's making a healing broth, so she says, – for Young Whortle Nep and Samuel Gorse."

"What!" spluttered Audrey aghast. "But she

doesn't know how. She'll probably poison them with what's in those bags of hers." She jumped up from the table and ran out of the Scuttle's rooms.

The winter quarters were a series of drab tunnels with family rooms leading off the main passages. There was no decoration anywhere, just the dismal tallow candles flickering on the walls. Up the tunnel Audrey hurried and sped out into the fresh air.

She followed the sound of voices and ran along the top of the ditch overlooking the bare stony stretch. There were all the fieldmice and in the centre was Madame Akkikuyu.

Her brewing pot was over a crackling fire and she stirred the bubbling contents with the bone from her hair. Occasionally she delved into one of her pouches and threw some leaves in the boiling mixture.

The fieldmice watched her with keen interest and admiration. Audrey spotted Arthur and Twit and pushed past the others to reach them.

"Mornin' Audrey," greeted Twit brightly.

"Hello," she mumbled. "Arthur what do you think you're doing letting her do this? It's bound to be poisonous."

"What am I supposed to do?" asked Arthur crossly. "She'd already started by the time we got here."

"But she might poison one of those boys," Audrey said. "I can't let her carry on." She forced her way through the fieldmice to the front.

"My," whistled Twit, "your Audrey ain't one for standin' by."

"That's what worries me," said Arthur.

Audrey went to the fortune-teller's side and tugged her elbow fiercely.

"Mouselet!" cried the rat gleefully. "You sleep well, yes? Akkikuyu look in on you before she go.

You sleep like twig." She put her arm around the mouse and Audrey squirmed.

"What are you doing?" she asked. "You don't know what those herbs and powders are for."

Madame Akkikuyu gave a deep fruity laugh. "But my mouselet. Akkikuyu remember now – leaves make you better, heal wounds. They strong nature magic."

"But they're poisonous," hissed Audrey.

"No, no," tutted the fortune-teller, "some leaves bad yes, Akkikuyu chuck them, she knows those that heal." She gave the potion one last stir and declared to the fieldmice, "Is ready, come – take to the poorly little ones."

Mrs Gorse stepped forward and looked apprehensively at the steaming thick broth bubbling away in the pot.

"Come, come," encouraged the rat, beckoning with her claws.

Mrs Gorse held out a wooden bowl and Madame Akkikuyu scooped some of the potion into it.

"Take to boy, make him drink all. He get better soon."

Audrey rushed over to Mrs Gorse. "Don't take it to him," she implored and a murmur of surprise rippled through the fieldmice. "Madame Akkikuyu isn't well herself. She doesn't know what she's put in there, it might make your son worse."

Mrs Gorse blinked and regarded the bowl with suspicion. The crowd muttered and stirred uneasily.

"Mouselet!" exclaimed the fortune-teller in a shocked tone. "Why you say such fibs? Akkikuyu knows – she not moon calf. Potion good – take to boy," she insisted.

"Well," began Mrs Gorse uncertainly.

"See," cried Madame Akkikuyu and she took the

bowl from her and drank down the whole lot.

The crowd fell silent and stared at her wide-eyed.

Madame Akkikuyu swilled some of the potion around in her mouth before swallowing. She knitted her brows and Audrey looked up at her, fearfully expecting the rat to keel over or for her claws to drop out. The fortune-teller licked her lips and simply said, "Need salt." She sprinkled some into the pot.

That was enough for the fieldmice. They broke out into a peal of applause.

"But that doesn't prove anything," Audrey tried to make herself heard.

Mrs Gorse took the bowl again and filled it herself. "Listen young lady," she said to Audrey, "This Madame Akkikookoo saved my Samuel last night and that's good enough for me. It's wicked of you to say such things about her."

Audrey was speechless. It was no use. Mr Nep came forward and took a bowl for Young Whortle, giving her a very disagreeable look in the process.

"This potion keep," shouted Madame Akkikuyu: "If mouseys seal it in jar, potion last till spring."

"My Nelly's got jars," said Mr Nep. "You come with me, missuss, we'll see to our boy then root some out for 'ee."

The crowd cheered as Madame Akkikuyu followed Mr Nep to the shelters. The rat waved regally as she passed by. As the fieldmice dispersed and went into the field, Arthur and Twit came over to Audrey. Arthur was shaking his head.

"A right idiot you made of yourself there, you soft lump," he said. "I've never seen anyone make such an ass of themselves before."

"Stow it, Arthur." Audrey was in no mood for brotherly criticism.

"Never mind," piped up Twit. "Maybe Young

Whortle and Sammy will get better."

"I wouldn't bet on it," said Audrey. "They can't say I didn't try and warn them, can they?"

"Aye," laughed Twit, "but you made a right pig's ear of it."

Audrey could never be angry with Twit and she sighed loudly. "Oh you're right, both of you. What a fool I must have looked to them." She laughed at the thought of it. "Oh well, what shall we do now?"

"There's the Hall to see," Twit said. "They've been at it all night – me dad's gone to see it already."

"The Hall?" asked Audrey mildly. "What's that?"

"Oh you'll see soon enough," chuckled Twit, leading them away from the edge of the ditch and into the field.

*   *   *

Jenkin held tightly to the corn stalk. He could see Todkin a little further away and behind he heard Figgy humming to himself. Jenkin waved at Todkin and a little paw was raised in answer.

"Jenkin," a familiar voice called up to him. He looked down and on the ground below, Alison Sedge was peering up at him with a paw shielding her eyes from the sun.

"What you wantin?" he shouted down to her.

"To talk to 'ee," she answered. "Come down – me neck's startin' to ache."

"Darn her," grumbled Jenkin as he nimbly descended the stalk. It was the only free day he had had for weeks. His father had told him to celebrate the Green Mouse's bounty in the field and he was only too happy to do so. He did not want to waste his time with Alison Sedge.

She waited patiently at the base of the stalk for him and twisted her hair coyly. Suddenly Jenkin was at her side. "Mornin'," she said.

119

"Don't tell me that's all you wanted to say, Alison Sedge," he puffed.

"No, just bein' p'lite that's all," she told him sniffily. "'Ere, what you got that feather in your hair for, Jenkin Nettle?" She reached over to pull it out. "Let me put it in mine – suit me better."

He stepped quickly aside. "You go pick yourself another flower," he said irritated. "This is my good luck charm this is."

"Luck is it?" she asked in surprise. "What does your dad say to that?"

"Nowt, cause I ain't told him and don't you either." He licked his sore lip and Alison had enough tact to change the subject.

"What I really come to tell 'ee is about the ratwoman and that girl what came with her."

"Oh yes?" Jenkin tried to disguise his interest.

"Had a right old ding-dong they just did. There was that Mrs Akky Yakky a-makin' a potion to heal Young Whortle and Skinny Samuel when that girl comes bargin' up and rants on about it bein' poison."

"Was it?"

"No, she's barmy," Alison sniggered. "That rat up an' drank some an' she didn't snuff it. Made that town mouse look real daft she did."

Jenkin looked past her, and curious, Alison turned round. Towards them came Arthur, Twit and Audrey. "Well here she is herself," said Jenkin. "Shall I ask her if she is potty for you?"

"Pah," said Alison tossing her head. "I ain't stayin' to talk to no loony. I'm goin' to meet Hodge – see if he wants to come to the meadow with me."

"Suit yourself," Jenkin grinned as she hastily departed.

Arthur and Audrey had never been in a corn field before. They gazed about them with great interest.

It was like a thick, dense wood of stalks. If the fieldmice had not made pathways they would have had to struggle and fight their way through like explorers in a jungle. They craned their necks to see the tops of the stems where the young ears waved gently in the breeze. Bright red poppies were tangled in the field and Audrey gaped in wonder at the gorgeous flaming flowers. It was a more beautiful place than she had expected.

"Look," said Twit presently, "there's Jenkin. Hoy there Jolly Jenkin!"

"How do," he said shyly with his eyes on the ground. "Where you goin' then Twit?"

"Arthur and Audrey ain't seen the Hall yet," Twit replied. "I was jus' takin' em there. You on sentry Jenkin?"

"Sentry?" asked Arthur.

"We don't leave the field unguarded once the Hall's been done," said Twit. "There's a girt ring of lads circling the Hall keepin' a look out for enemies."

"Where?" put in Audrey. "I haven't seen anyone so far."

"Hah miss," laughed Jenkin, "you ain't been lookin' proper." He pointed upwards. "How's things, Figgy?"

"Fine so far!" came an answering call from above.

"There's someone up there!" gasped Arthur. "He's at the very top of the stalk."

"Where else would you sentry from?" asked Jenkin, highly amused.

"I'd love to do that," Arthur said as he stared upwards.

"Have a go then," urged Jenkin.

"Old Arthur won't make it," tittered Twit, "not with his tummy."

"Huh!" snorted Arthur, stepping up to the

nearest stalk. He hesitated. Now that he had to climb it the stalk did seem very high.

"Go on then," encouraged Jenkin, "ignore Twit."

Arthur frowned and breathed deeply. Then with a loud grunt he jumped up and grasped the stem with his paws. He dangled in the air like a caught fish, winning another giggle from Twit. Arthur tried to climb, passing paw over paw. The stalk wobbled and swayed treacherously.

"Wrap your tail round it," advised Jenkin.

Arthur tried but once his tail had gripped the stalk it refused to budge anymore.

"I'm stuck," he cried, and with a thud he fell to the ground.

Twit rolled around, his sides aching. Even Audrey laughed and Arthur glared at them both – after he had shaken some of the dust out of his fur.

"Shall we show you how it's done," offered Jenkin. "Twit?"

Twit wiped the tears from his eyes and stood beneath the stalk Arthur had tried to climb. "Ready?" he asked Jenkin.

Jenkin, standing under another stalk nodded. "First to the top," he said. "Say when, Miss."

Audrey counted them down. "Three two one – go."

The fieldmice shot up the corn as if they had wings. Their legs and paws were a blur and their tails spiralled around the stems faster than anything had seen. It was Jenkin who won – just a second before Twit.

"Beat you at last," he waved triumphantly.

"I be out of practice," panted Twit, "this time next week I'll leave you standin'."

Arthur regarded them enviously, wishing he could do half as well. Jenkin slid down quickly, eyed Audrey bashfully then said to Arthur,

"Don't worry – you'll soon learn. Come see me after you've been to the Hall if you're willin' an' we'll get you up a stalk afore the end of the day."

"If only I could," Arthur sighed in disbelief.

"Anyway, you best get goin'," said Jenkin, "soonest there sooner you can come back." He looked up, Twit was still enjoying being at the top of the corn. "Been a long time since he sat up on sentry," murmured Jenkin. "Thought he were dead you know – we all did. He's a good bloke, but a bit simple."

"He doesn't get into fights," remarked Audrey sternly, "and I bet he's done more in his life than you ever will."

"Never said he hadn't!" Jenkin refused to be provoked. "All I'm sayin' is, there's some in Fennywolde who don't respect the Scuttles – say Twit's a dimmy and more besides. Not me – I like him. I reckon he's too good-natured though. Folk take advantage and think he's daft. That's all."

"I think," said Arthur breaking in, "that one day Twit might get pressed too hard, and he may surprise a few round here if that kind nature of his snaps."

Twit slid down the stalk. "Oooh that did me good," he said beaming from ear to ear. "Ain't nowt like it for blowin' the cobwebs away. You ready to see the Hall now? Come on then."

They left Jenkin behind and he flashed up his stalk and resumed his sentry duty.

Deeper into the field went the three friends until the dense corn around them began to thin out more considerably and appeared to form a corridor, the ceiling of which was made by twisting together the ears of corn from opposite "walls". It began to look very grand and imposing.

"This be the main way to the Hall," Twit

informed them in a hushed, reverent tone. "This be what they all were doin' last night."

"It's very clever," remarked Arthur.

Twit chuckled, "Just you wait."

"What's that ahead?" asked Audrey as they turned a corner.

"The great doors," Twit answered.

At the end of the corridor there were two large doors made completely from tightly woven corn stems. They reached up as high as the growing corn itself and on either side of them were two fieldmice who carried themselves importantly – they were the door guards.

"Mornin' Twit," greeted one of them.

"Hello Grommel, how've you been keepin'? Your back still playin' you up?"

"Somethin' chronic, Twit lad. These your town friends?"

"Right enough. This here's Audrey Brown and this be her brother Arthur. I be takin' 'em to see the Hall."

"Then pass friends," said the door guard and he stood aside, pushing open one of the large doors.

Audrey and Arthur stepped through and blinked.

The Hall of Corn was immense. It was wide and long, and clumps of corn had been left standing at regular intervals giving the impression of mighty pillars – but the Hall was open to the sky. At the far end, on a wickerwork throne, sat Mr Woodruffe – able at last to take up his plaited sceptre and govern the Hall as every King of the Field had done since the time of Fenny.

Many fieldmice were bustling about, building large spherical structures halfway up the corn stems.

"What are they doing?" asked Arthur.

"They be our summer quarters," replied Twit

gleefully. "You never slept till you spent a night in a fieldmouse's nest – not on the ground, but halfway in the sky," he added dreamily.

It certainly was very grand. Audrey was overcome by the industriousness of the Fennywolders. All this had taken only one night to accomplish. She was amazed.

"There's me dad," said Twit suddenly and he ran over to where Elijah Scuttle was working. He had built a good, large nest for him and Mrs Scuttle and was in the process of completing a slightly smaller one.

"How do Willum," he nodded to his son. "Thought 'ee an' Master Brown could share a nest."

"Terrific!" said Arthur.

"Don't be doin' it too high though Dad," laughed Twit. "Old Arthur can't climb too good."

"Now now Willum," chided his father softly. "You knows I do make your mam a straw ladder every year – I'll do 'un for Master Brown too."

Mr Scuttle was a pleasant fieldmouse. He looked like an older version of his son, except there were creamy whiskers fringing his chops and on his shoulders there were two white scars where no fur would grow. He did however, have the same mischievous twinkle in his eye.

"And what about you, missey?" Elijah addressed Audrey. "I'm not sure if you want to kip with your ratty friend."

"Oh no, Mr Scuttle," gasped Audrey, horrified, until she realised he was teasing her. He grinned and said, "I'll make 'ee a real pirty nest for one so she can't squeeze in."

"Thank you," said Audrey greatly relieved. The thought of having to share a nest with Madame Akkikuyu was too terrible even to joke about.

"Look," began Arthur. "I better go back and find

that Jenkin chap – I'm not going to be the only boy using a ladder – what would everyone say?"

"I'll come with you Arthur," said Twit. "I got me some practisin' to do." So the two boys went off, laughing and jostling each other.

Audrey decided not to join them. "Is there anything I can do, Mr Scuttle?" she asked.

Elijah looked surprised, then pleased. "Aye, missey," he said delighted. "See you over there," he pointed to a pile of moss and soft grass picked early that morning by a robust group of mouse wives. "That there," he continued, "is what we do line our nests with – 'featherin' we calls it. Makes 'em real comfy and soft it do – you could fetch some if you're willin'."

"Certainly," said Audrey. She made her way over to the heap of feathering – although she could see no feathers in it whatsoever.

She passed beneath half-made nests where husbands not as deft as Mr Scuttle cursed as the weave fell apart. She wanted to learn more of the families who shouted cheerfully to one another from nest to nest and drew the very young children up on straw ropes. Some stout wives who refused to be parted from the bed linen were taking sheets and pillows into the nests with them. Audrey walked by one group of children who were all sitting down, listening with eyes agog and breaths held to an old mouse brindled white with age telling them stories. It was Old Todmore – the storyteller of the field, and today he had a new tale to tell. Most of the children had been in bed the night before so had missed the excitement of Madame Akkikuyu and the owl and were now listening to the story, thrilled and captivated.

"Well, there's poor Young Whortle Nep with this girt deadly owl about to chew off his bonce when crashin' through the meader comes the answer to our prayers – Madame Ak ... Akky .." Old Todmore was finding it difficult to get his tongue around the fortune-teller's name.

"Stop a-doin' that Abel Madder!" he said vexed. "Now where was I? Oh aye, well, crashin' through the meader comes the answer to our prayers – Madame Ratlady."

Audrey did not know whether to be amused or alarmed at how the fieldmice considered Madame Akkikuyu to be their saviour. She wondered how those two young mice were faring after drinking that potion.

Finally she reached the heap of feathering and gathered some spongy moss in her arms. Three other girl mice were there doing the same. They smiled at her nervously.

"Hello," said Audrey.

They nodded their heads in reply.

"I'm Audrey Brown," she persisted.

One of the girls who had a mass of coarse, straight red hair said, "You be Twit's friend."

"That's right."

"Saw you last night with another towny."

"That's my brother Arthur."

"Arthur is it?" cooed one of the others.

"Aye Dimsel, and only a brother," said the first.

"Tush you," cried the one called Dimsel nudging her friend.

The girl who had not yet spoken pushed the others aside and said, "How do Audrey. I be Lily Clover. This one with the nose of a Hogpry be Iris Crowfoot."

"Hogpry yourself," shoved Iris.

"And this be Dimsel Bottom, she's mad keen on your Arthur."

"Oh Lily!"

"It's true ain't it?"

"Well!"

Audrey laughed. She liked these three and she wished Dimsel the best of luck concerning her brother. For a while they chatted amiably then Iris said, "We best be goin', our mams'll take on so if we don't 'ave the featherin' done soon."

As they left Lily turned and asked Audrey.

"You met Alison Sedge yet?"

"No – I don't think so."

"Well you just mind when you do – got claws has our Alison." Lily cast a lazy, lingering eye over Audrey's ribbon and lace before she said, "Aye, you watch out, me dear." And with that she left.

Audrey wandered back to Mr Scuttle. He had started work on her nest now and he called down to her.

"Leave it down there missey if'n you're not sure of your stalk paws yet."

Audrey waved to him then fetched some more.

The morning turned into lunch time and merry wives brought out cheese and hot, fresh bread for their hardworking husbands.

Gladwin Scuttle appeared with her arms laden and Arthur and Twit were following eagerly. They sat down and munched happily, Mr Scuttle swilling down the bread which stuck in his throat with some blackberry ferment and telling his wife how he was progressing. It was hot work and he was glad of the rest. He sat with his back to a stalk, his ears beetroot red.

Mrs Scuttle passed a critical eye over her bedroom for the summer and nodded satisfactorily, then told her husband to help some of the others she had seen whose attempts at nest building were pitiful.

"Ah," said Elijah, "Josiah Down won't never

learn if'n I always do it fer 'im. Never has patience with the framework, that's what does it."

"Well," tutted Gladwin, "I passed Mrs Down just now and she did ask me to mention it to you."

"Reckon I'll pop over later on," he promised.

All around the light, happy sound of fieldmice talking, relaxing, eating and laughing filled the air. Audrey lay on her side and watched the inhabitants of Fennywolde content in their element. The Hall of Corn was near to completion. Nearly all the nests were finished and it was interesting to see the different styles. Some were perfectly round, others egg-shaped; there were small ones and those large enough to need supporting by many stalks. Yes, the Hall was a marvellous place and Audrey could not wait to sleep in her nest and see the stars shining through the small entrance.

The midday sun glittered on the dust from the straw which swirled in a fine mist over their heads. It made everything look hazy and unreal.

Twit saw her gazing round and said, "You should see it when the corn is really ripe, then it looks as if the entire Hall is made of gold."

"It is marvellous," she sighed. "Grand yet simple as well." She wondered if the fieldmice would decorate the Hall properly with garlands of flowers and chains of daisies. In a small way it reminded her of the chamber of spring and summer that she had entered in Deptford when she had received her mousebrass. As she thought of it an idea came to her.

Just then their lunch was disturbed by a cheer from some of the families and calls of, "Hooray."

Audrey strained to see. There was Jenkin coming through the doors and with him was Young Whortle.

The families rushed up to him to see if he was

really all right. But apart from some nasty bruises and a bandage over his shoulder he seemed fine.

"It was that potion," he said. "Didn't taste too good but made me sit up and take notice. Sammy's gettin' better too – that ratlady reckons he'll be up an' about in a few days."

The crowd murmured in wonder and praised Madame Akkikuyu's skill in healing.

"Where be she now?" asked one of them.

"Why she's with my mam a-bottlin' that stuff to keep for next time someone gets ill," replied Young Whortle.

"That's a turn-up for the books," whistled Arthur when all the commotion had died down. "Who'd have thought that goo actually worked?"

"Well I didn't, for one," said Audrey. "I look an even bigger idiot now, don't I? Oh well, rather that than have one of those two get poisoned."

Lunch was over and Elijah climbed up to the nest again taking some feathering with him. Mrs Scuttle tidied up and went to the still pool to wash the bowls. Twit scurried up and helped his father.

Arthur was eating the last bit of cheese absently. Then forgetting to wipe his whiskers, as usual, he pulled Audrey to one side and told her.

"Look, Twit's been telling me about Jenkin – you really mustn't tease him anymore about those bruises you know."

"Why ever not?" demanded his sister curiously.

"Because his dad gave them to him. Apparently, Mr Nettle often hits Jenkin – thinks it's good for him."

"Oh," stammered Audrey, "I feel terrible now. Why doesn't his mother do something?"

"Because she's dead – died when he was born apparently and no-one else likes to interfere with Mr Nettle – he's the mousebrass maker you see."

"Poor Jenkin."

"Yes – so just be a bit nicer next time, eh?"

"Of course, Arthur."

"Well," Arthur said, changing the subject, "this afternoon I'm going to crack climbing one of those dratted stalks if it kills me. What are you going to do?"

"Oh I've had an idea to make something for the Hall."

Arthur regarded her doubtfully. "What sort of 'something'?" he asked.

"A corn dolly. You know, like the ones at home in the chambers of summer in the spring ceremony. I'm surprised they haven't already got some here."

"Maybe they don't know how – I didn't know you did either."

Audrey shrugged. "Easy, I watched the Raddle sisters once."

Arthur considered the idea for a moment then said, "Yes, that sounds nice, you could present it to Mr Woodruffe when you've finished and let him decide where to hang it." He looked around to see if any crumbs had fallen on the floor, but was disappointed, so he went off to talk to Jenkin again about his climbing.

Audrey picked up some thin straws and began to plait them together.

It was more difficult than she had thought. The plaits were impossible to keep even and free from ugly gaps. However, eventually Audrey became more adept with the straw and her confidence grew.

She intended to make something simple to begin with – a bell shape perhaps, but as the straw flicked between her fingers her ambitions for it soared.

Audrey decided that the figure of a girl would be best, with corn ears for arms and a dress of bunched stalks.

The afternoon wore on. The dolly grew larger under her fingers, far larger than she had intended. Some mouse children who had been running around playing chase stopped and watched her. They had never seen anything like it before and Audrey talked to them happily as she made it.

Alison Sedge wandered into the Hall. Hodge had walked with her to the meadow but she was in such a sulk that he had left her and gone to join Todkin on sentry.

Alison was thinking about Jenkin and the look that he had on his face when he saw that town-mouse. It was uncomfortably hot and Alison was in a bad mood with the world. She decided to go to the still pool to bathe and admire her reflection. She had just been gathering some wild rosemary to rinse her hair with when she decided to see how the Hall was coming along and if her father had finished her own nest.

It was as she crossed the Hall that she noticed a small crowd of children near the Scuttle's nests. And there, in the centre of all the attention was that town mouse! Curious and irritated Alison tossed her head and strode nearer.

The dolly was now taller than Audrey, its head was a loop of plaited straw and she was busily straightening it as at the moment the whole thing had an amusing drunken air about it.

The children were watching everything Audrey did keenly. Alison quietly drew close and observed the scene acidly. She looked at the town mouse's silver bells tinkling on her tail and noted with envy the lace dress. Alison glanced down at her own, simple frock which seemed shabbier by comparison and pursed her full lips.

The dolly was getting better every minute and Alison saw the admiring looks Audrey was getting

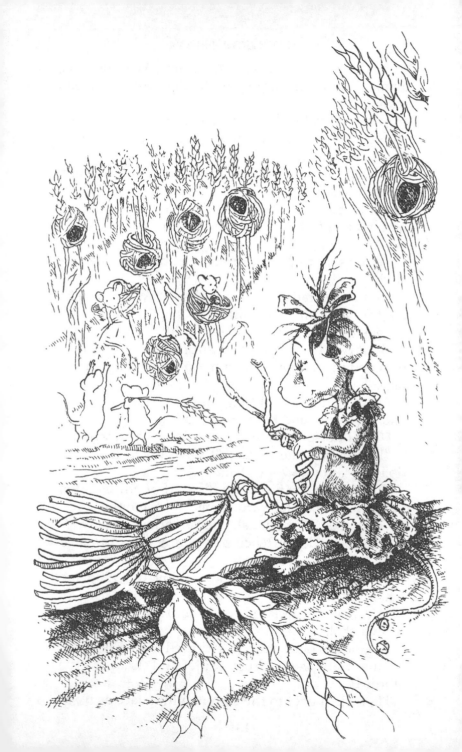

from the boys who went by. Young Whortle was leaning out of the large Nep family nest positively ogling.

Alison regarded Audrey coldly, then a slow smile curled over her mouth and she spun on her heel and ran out of the Hall.

There, the dolly was finished. Audrey was very pleased with the final result even though it was much larger than she had anticipated. The plaiting had worked well and only the Raddle sisters would be able to criticise it – but they were not there.

"What's it for?" ventured one of the children shyly.

"It's a decoration," said Audrey. "Will you help me take it to Mr Woodruffe?"

Eagerly small paws helped her lift the corn dolly and carry it to the wicker throne. Mr Woodruffe watched them approach with a puzzled look on his face.

Audrey and the children put the corn dolly down and curtseyed and bowed before him.

"Can I do something for you, lass?" he asked.

"Please sir," she began, "I have made this corn dolly to decorate your Hall."

The King of the Field laid his staff of office on his knee and leaned forward to inspect the dolly.

"It is most . . . unusual," he remarked jovially. "I wonder, could you teach our young ones to make such things?"

"Why yes sir, they seem to enjoy watching me making this."

"Very well," declared Mr Woodruffe, "you Miss Brown shall . . ."

A sudden commotion interrupted him. The doors of the Hall were thrust aside and Isaac Nettle stormed in.

He rushed over to the throne with a face as black

as thunder and no-one stood in his way – they had seen that mood before.

Isaac pointed a shaking finger at the King of the Field and cried, "What heresy is this? What sin have thee welcomed, Woodruffe?" He flung his arms open wide and yelled to the sky. "Forgive thy subject Almighty that he should have fallen into such folly."

"Isaac!" muttered Mr Woodruffe sternly. "What's all this about?"

Mr Nettle glared round at Audrey. "Pagan idolatry! Brought hither by this unclean creature."

Audrey was astounded at his passion. She had never seen anyone so angry before and some of the children began to cry.

"It's only a decoration," she protested.

"Silence, fiend of the deep cold," ranted Isaac. "Thy craft speaks for itself. It is a blasphemous effigy and mocks the design of the Green Mouse. Oh Great One, do not let us pay for the misguided deeds of the ignorant. She is the scum of the vile cities, the cream of the sinners – not one of your true servants. Punish us not for her wrong doing."

"Now look here!" fumed Audrey, her astonishment boiling to anger. But he would not listen to her.

"Shun the image maker," he cried to the mice who were gathering to see what was going on. "See how she wears her vanities!" he flicked her ribbon with contempt.

"Don't you touch me!" she shouted, outraged.

By now everyone in the Hall was watching them. Twit dropped his feathering and slid down the stalk.

"Beware the maker of dolls. Repent ye or the vengeance of the Green shall smite ye down." Isaac moved nearer to the corn dolly and raised his fists to smash it.

"Don't you dare!" cried Audrey, pushing herself between him and the figure of straw.

"Away profane one!" roared Isaac shoving her roughly. Audrey stumbled and fell backwards.

Twit reached Isaac before he had a chance to smash the dolly and stood glaring up at him, his eyes smouldering with a frightening fire that none had seen before.

"Get thee gone," warned Mr Nettle harshly.

Twit was breathing hard. No-one had ever known this mood in the little fieldmouse and the crowd gasped and wondered at the outcome. Twit's teeth flashed as he bared them and put up his fist.

"You oughtn't to have done that," he shouted, trembling with emotion. "Try it again an' I'll do fer you."

Isaac stared at Twit and bawled, "See how the heathens taint your subjects Lord. Out of my way simpleton."

Twit stood his ground and an alarming, unpleasant growl came from his throat.

Arthur and Jenkin came running into the Hall. Word had spread round the sentries about what was happening.

They saw Isaac raise his hard paw to Twit. "Father!" shouted Jenkin, "No, you mustn't."

Arthur sped over to Audrey and helped her up whilst Jenkin swung on his father's arm.

"Nettle!" bellowed Mr Woodruffe. "That is enough. I will not allow you to spoil the Hall of Corn."

Isaac threw him a foul glance, but he persisted.

"Listen to me. I am your King! I am the law here."

Isaac faltered and put his arm down slowly, all the while staring steadily into the level eyes of Mr Woodruffe.

"I cannot allow this behaviour," continued the King of the Field.

"I do but honour the Green and keep His laws."

"Maybe, but you offend me!"

"Then I shall not enter here again," Isaac roared. He whirled round, snatched up the corn dolly and strode off crying, "This abomination has stunk before the Green Mouse long enough." And he carried it out through the doors before anyone could stop him.

"Consider yourself banished from the Hall till your temper cools," the King called after him.

All the fieldmice relaxed and muttered, shaking their heads. Then mothers came and fetched their children away from Audrey.

Elijah Scuttle came puffing up red-eared and worried for his son. Twit though had calmed down.

"You all right?" he asked Audrey. She nodded and thanked him. Twit let out a great sigh of relief.

"I'm so sorry," stuttered Jenkin to both of them. He was dreadfully ashamed of his father.

"Oh Jolly Jenkin," Twit brushed the incident away as his humour returned, "thank'ee for comin' quick – I nearly let fly then."

"Oh dear," Audrey said to Arthur, "I seem to be getting on the wrong side of everyone here, don't I?"

He tried to reassure her. "But it wasn't your fault, I'm sorry about your corn dolly – you spent such a long time on it."

"That doesn't matter," she said, "I'm just glad no-one got hurt. That could have been very nasty then. Twit really took everyone by surprise, didn't he?"

"Maybe," remarked Arthur thoughtfully, "I suppose it's this terrible heat as well." He frowned suddenly.

"What is it?" asked his sister.

"Just this," he began slowly. "How did Mr Nettle know you were making a dolly. He passed below us in the field and he was angry before he got here."

"That is strange," agreed Audrey.

From her nest, Alison Sedge watched them with a satisfied smile on her pretty face.

8

THE VOICE

Arthur made it to the top of a stalk at last, to the cheers of Twit and Jenkin. He could barely see them as night was falling and already its shadows were gathering about Fennywolde.

Arthur gazed over the top of the field. The silver light of dusk played over the rippling corn ears so that it really did look like a shimmering sea and he, Arthur, was floating on it. It was a bizarre feeling. Now he began to understand the love that fieldmice have for climbing.

"Come on Art," called up Twit. "I don't want to stay down here all night – I wants me bed."

Arthur tried to slide down as he had seen his friends do but he scraped his paws and bloodied his heels, then landed with an undignified "bump" on the hard ground.

"Did 'ee like it?" inquired Jenkin.

"It's just wonderful up there," enthused Arthur, scrabbling off the ground. "Could I be a sentry do you think?"

"Wait till tomorrow Arthur," yawned Twit.

"I'd best be off now," said Jenkin. "I'd like to stay with Figgy and the others on sentry but my dad wouldn't like that."

"Will those mice be on sentry all night?" asked Arthur, surprised.

"Course," replied Jenkin. "No good havin' sentries if they go home at night."

"Well, shouldn't we stay?" Arthur addressed Twit.

Twit yawned again. "Oh come on Art," he said sleepily. "If I do sentry tonight like as not I'll drop clear off and bash me head in – I was up all hours last night a-talkin' to my folks. Let me have one good night's sleep an' we'll do a ghoster tomorrow."

"Well," Jenkin began, "if I don't go now I'll be for it. 'Night lads."

"Hope your dad's calmed down now," Twit ventured.

Jenkin licked his sore lip and nodded. "So do I. Oh well, I'll probably have a lot of praying to do when I get back, that's all. See you tomorrow hopefully." He ran off out of the field.

Arthur watched him go until the night swallowed him. "Will he really be okay do you think?"

"Should be," Twit answered. "It's not him Isaac's mad at. Now, we gonna get some shut-eye tonight?" They made their way through the corridor to the great doors.

*   *   *

In the Hall of Corn all was calm. Nearly all the mice had gone to bed to try out their new nests and here and there orange lights showed through the openings as they settled down. Some fieldmice were talking, enjoying the refreshing change of a night spent under the sky without having to dread an owl attack. The hum of their chatter mingled with the quiet snores of sleepers which in turn blended with the rustle of the corn.

The summer stars shone down onto Audrey's face. Her nest was snug and warm, and the moss which lined it was soft and scented. She nuzzled down into the cool fragrant feathering which smelt of the green earth and shady forests. It was at times like these, when the peace and beauty of Fennywolde were overpowering, that she thought it might not be so bad to spend the rest of her days there.

She closed her eyes and, breathing heavily, sunk deeper into her bed.

Suddenly the world seemed to quake. The nest shook violently from side to side. Audrey was jolted out of her short velvet sleep and hurled about. What was happening? She tried to cling on to the round walls of the nest and staggered to and fro, unable to keep her balance. The bells which she had removed from her tail jangled and rattled round the nest like beads in a baby's rattle.

A claw appeared over the opening and then everything went dark.

"Mouselet?" Madame Akkikuyu squeezed her huge head through the tiny hole, blocking out the light. She looked at Audrey. "Why mouselet in here?" she asked curiously. "No room for Akkikuyu to kip – come down mouselet and we sleep on ground together."

"No!" answered Audrey sharply. "This is my bedroom now and it's not big enough for two."

Madame Akkikuyu insisted. "But mouselet – little friend, Akkikuyu not like be alone in dark. Night has voices they speak to her," the rat whimpered. "Besides, Akkikuyu not well – she need friend, need mouselet to help."

"What's wrong with you?" demanded Audrey sternly.

"Akkikuyu's ear – it aches and pounds."

"Why don't you go and make yourself some potion or other," Audrey suggested.

"Have tried, mouselet," assured the fortune-teller. "Akkikuyu has rubbed on bramble leaves and said the charm, she has made the paste of the camomile flower but still it hurts. I am frightened mouselet."

"Look," said Audrey, too tired to continue. "Why don't you get some sleep. It might be better in the morning and you could ask Mr Scuttle to build you a nest tomorrow next to this one."

But Madame Akkikuyu merely stared back at her with the eyes of a scolded dog, hurt and confused. "Come down," she asked one last time, "for Akkikuyu sake."

"No," Audrey said and she hated herself immediately.

The fortune-teller looked crestfallen. She stuck out her bottom lip and said sullenly. "Akkikuyu go – she sleep on ground alone, poor Akkikuyu." She pulled her head out of the nest and began to climb down again.

Audrey leant out and saw the diminishing bulky figure reach the ground. In the darkness of the Hall floor she could just make out the spots on the rat's red shawl and they quickly bobbed away.

"Oh she can please herself," mumbled Audrey. "I never promised to stay with her all day and night did I?"

She remained leaning out of her nest for some time. Fennywolde was cooling after a hot day. The wind had dropped to a whispering breeze which brought sweet fragrances out of the meadow.

Presently the muffled sound of voices drifted up to her. It was Twit and Arthur returning at last. Their nest was above hers and slightly to the left. She waited for them to climb up.

Out of the gloom appeared two little paws and then Twit's head popped up.

"Hello Audrey," he said, drawing level with her.

"You comfy in there?"

"Yes it's lovely, your father's very clever."

"Reckon he is – oh!" two plumper paws had emerged and grabbed Twit's tail tightly.

"Shove up!" shouted Arthur.

Twit giggled, then said goodnight to Audrey before vanishing into his nest.

Arthur came into view, climbing the stalk determinedly. His tongue was sticking out as it always did when he was concentrating.

"Arthur," said Audrey when it looked as if he would continue up without noticing her.

Arthur flinched in surprise. "Hello sis," he said, startled. "You still awake then?"

"Yes – I had a visit from Madame Akkikuyu."

"Didn't try to get in did she?"

"Yes but it was too small. I sent her away in a sulk and I wish I hadn't."

"Oh blow," said Arthur. "If she goes running off at the slightest thing, well . . ."

Audrey interrupted him. "But Arthur she said she wasn't well and she mentioned that voice of hers again."

Arthur scoffed. "She's going batty – none of us heard that voice on the boat, did we? Yet she swore blind she had. I wouldn't worry about it Sis, really. Now look, I'm sorry, but I've got to go – my paws are killin' me, hanging on like this. See you in the morning."

"Goodnight," Audrey called after him as he wriggled into the nest above. She withdrew into her own bed and sank into a deep, untroubled sleep.

*   *   *

Madame Akkikuyu wandered through the field miserably. Her right ear ached terribly and her best friend had not done anything to help. She kicked stones belligerently and felt sorry for herself.

The field was soon left behind and she walked along the edge of the ditch, cursing her ear and rubbing it vigorously. How it pained her. A constant dull throb pulsed inside like the worst tooth ache imaginable. It was almost bad enough for her to want to run to the lonely yew tree and chew on its deadly poisonous bark.

Bit by bit the pain increased.

"Oooh," whimpered the fortune-teller despairingly.

Madame Akkikuyu sat down at the stony stretch of ditch and buried her head in her claws moaning to herself. The pain had only begun when the sun set and as the night became darker and cooler it grew more intense.

"Akkikuyu."

The rat looked up quickly. She could see no-one – only the ghost-like moths fluttering overhead.

"Akkikuyu!" repeated the voice.

The fortune-teller wailed loudly. It was that voice again – the one that had haunted her from Greenwich.

"Leave me!" she cried.

"Akkikuyu," the voice persisted. It was stronger than it had been on those previous occasions. It was a strange, sickly sweet voice which made her shudder.

"Listen to me," it said softly.

"No," snapped the rat. "Never, Akkikuyu not want to go round bend. Leave me."

"Listen to me, let me help you."

"No, you not real – Akkikuyu barmy, she hear voice when nobody there."

"But I am real, Akkikuyu."

"Who are you then?"

"My name is – Nicodemus," whispered the voice, "I am your friend."

"Then why you hide?" asked Akkikuyu, glaring suspiciously at the shadows which seemed to have closed round her. She rubbed her head. She had seen something out of the corner of her eye and thought it was a spider dangling from her hair.

"I do not hide, Akkikuyu," crooned the voice of Nicodemus. "I am here."

And to her everlasting horror Madame Akkikuyu saw who it was that spoke to her.

"Aaaghh!" she screamed, getting to her feet in panic. But there was nowhere to run. On her right ear the tattooed face was moving and talking. The old ink lips were opening and closing and the drawn eyes were staring straight at her.

"*Aaghh!*" she screamed again. She thought she had finally gone out of her mind. "Akkikuyu is cracked! Oh poor Akkikuyu," she sobbed.

"Listen to me Akkikuyu," Nicodemus ordered, "trust me, you are not mad."

"Stop, stop," whined the rat. "Stop, or Akkikuyu murder herself. This cannot be. Inky faces do not talk – they are doodles on skin, not real peoples."

The face on her ear began again. "Akkikuyu listen, I am merely using this tattoo to talk to you. It is a channel through which you are able to hear me. I am really far, far away."

The fortune-teller ceased her sobs. "What are you?" she asked slowly.

"I am a spirit of the fields," said the tattoo smiling. "I am the essence of the harvest, the sunlight on a distant hill, the splendour of a golden meadow, the heady perfume of the hawthorn in bloom."

"Why you speak to Akkikuyu? Spirits not supposed to talk to feather or fur."

"Because, dearest lady, I am trapped. Caught in a void – a horrible limbo where nightmare spirits of darkness dwell. I must escape. You must help me, I must return to the fields ere I perish for eternity."

"How you get trapped?" asked the fortune-teller doubtfully.

"That is a long and frightening tale which I cannot relate. Help me Akkikuyu – give me sweet liberty."

She considered his entreaty then shook her head. "No," she answered plainly. "Akkikuyu is mad – you not there – she imagine all this, so shut up."

"What proof do you need, woman?" demanded Nicodemus sternly and in his impatience his voice faltered and became ugly. "You must release me."

"So you say," said Madame Akkikuyu, "but how is this to be? Akkikuyu have no great magicks to work for you. She know only herbs and medicines to make mouselings better."

The voice shouted, "But I can teach you Akkikuyu. All the forces of nature are mine to command. You could learn from me secret knowledge known to none of your kind – just think of it." The voice lulled and coaxed most invitingly.

Madame Akkikuyu thought hard. A yearning awoke inside her – it seemed to be a very old feeling nudged to the surface by Nicodemus's promises. Magical power, he would give her that! The hunger for it which welled up inside her felt so new, yet also strangely familiar. Nicodemus's voice began again.

"You could be a queen Akkikuyu," the tattoo went on, "mighty above all others."

Madame Akkikuyu seemed to come out of the illusions he was weaving about her.

"Tach!" she snorted. "Akkikuyu not believe in magic. Power of herb yes, and rule of fate yes, but not magic. Tricks and tomfool nonsense."

The face on her ear screwed itself up with impatience. "Do you want a demonstration? Very well. I shall show you what can be done and what powers can be yours."

"What you do?" inquired the fortune-teller expectantly.

"Look down there!" said Nicodemus. "At the bottom of the ditch!"

There, lying on the stones where Mr Nettle had thrown it were the remains of Audrey's corn dolly.

"Go down there," instructed Nicodemus. The fortune-teller did as she was bid and made her way down the side of the ditch, hanging on to the tufts of coarse grass which grew up its steep banks.

The dolly was in four pieces, testaments to Mr Nettle's passion. The head and arms had been torn from the dress section.

Madame Akkikuyu tutted to see the damage. She had heard of Audrey's corn dolly from Young Whortle.

"Straw lady bust," she said aloud.

"Then join it together, Akkikuyu," said Nicodemus craftily. "Put back the head and fix in the arms."

"No," said the rat, "Straw ripped. She not go back together now."

"Then put the pieces where they belong and I shall do the rest," beamed the face.

Madame Akkikuyu arranged the arms and head around the body in their correct positions and stepped aside.

"Now," said Nicodemus, "with the bone from your hair draw a triangle around it. Good, now throw open your arms to the night and repeat after me – only make sure you do it exactly."

They began the invocation to the unseen spirits of the world.

"Come Brud. By slaughterous cold and searing ice I call thee. Come out of the shadows, awake from your empty tomb and walk amongst us. I entreat thee, make whole again your effigy."

Madame Akkikuyu repeated all the words and watched the corn dolly in fascinated silence.

All around them the grasses and leaves began to stir and rustle, beating against each other like applause. Inside the triangle the moss that grew over the stones writhed like clusters of angry maggots and burst open new shoots like green fireworks. Everything living within that area grew and bloomed a thousand times faster than normal. Then, as Madame Akkikuyu stared in disbelief, the severed stems of the corn dolly's grain arms twisted and coiled into the body section. The plaited head put out a tentative wiry tendril like a bather testing the water then rooted itself onto the shoulders.

"Aha," squealed Madame Akkikuyu, "dummy repaired."

"Quite," said the tattoo matter of factly. "Are you convinced now, Akkikuyu?"

The rat nodded quickly, "Oh yes Nicodemus my friend – you real, Akkikuyu not bonkers." She hugged herself as she gazed at the completed figure of straw.

Nicodemus continued. "Would you like to see more?"

"More?" repeated the rat. "How so?"

"This has been a mere child's trick, Akkikuyu, compared with what you could achieve under my learned guidance."

"Tell me more," said the fortune-teller, eager to see other wonders. "Akkikuyu want to see more."

"Very well," the voice muttered softly, "step nearer to the straw maiden. Enough – do not touch the triangle. Now we need blood."

Madame Akkikuyu backed away. She did not like the sound of that. "Blood?" she queried cautiously.

"Why for you want blood and where from?"

"To give the doll life," announced Nicodemus. "Blood is a symbol of that. Just three drops are needed. I daresay you could nick your thumb and squeeze some out."

"Give doll life!" exclaimed the rat wondrously. "You can do such? You are very strong in magicks, field spirit. Quickly show Akkikuyu."

She took out her small knife and made a tiny cut in her thumb.

"The blood must fall on the straw," Nicodemus told her, as three crimson drops were forced out onto the corn dress.

"Now stand back," commanded the voice.

Madame Akkikuyu did so and felt a thrill of fear tingle its way along her spine and down to the tip of her tail.

"Hear me, oh Brud!" called out Nicodemus. "Give this image life – let sap be as the blood on the straw. Pour breath into its empty breast and let stems be as sinew."

A deathly silence descended over the whole of Fennywolde. The fieldmice shifted uncomfortably in their soft nests as a shadow passed over the sky. Birds shrank into their feathers as they roosted in the tops of the elms and feared the worst. A hedgehog in his den of old, dry leaves felt the charged atmosphere and curled himself into a tight ball of spikes. Down came the shadow, thundering from the empty night on the back of the wind. The tree tops swayed and the leaves whipped round. The grass in the meadow parted as the force fell upon it and travelled wildly through, flattening and battering everything in its path. It rushed towards the ditch and went howling down into it.

Madame Akkikuyu stood her ground as the unseen fury tore at her hair and pulled her shawl till it choked her.

And then all was still.

The fortune-teller lowered the claws she had raised against the ravaging gale and looked down at the dolly.

"Command it," said Nicodemus.

"I . . . I?" she stammered.

"Who else? It will obey none but you."

Madame Akkikuyu swept back the hair which had blown over her face and peered again at the corn dolly. "Up," she ordered meekly.

One of the grain arms gave a sudden twitch and the rat drew her breath sharply.

"Up!" she said again with more force.

The straw figure flipped itself over, rustling and crackling. It leant on its arm and jolted itself up until it stood before her.

The fortune-teller took some steps around the dolly and waved her arms over it just in case someone was tricking her with cotton threads. But no, the corn dolly was alive!

"Instruct it to bow before you," suggested Nicodemus.

"Bow," said the rat.

With a snapping and splintering the corn dolly bent over and bowed.

"Hee hee," cackled Madame Akkikuyu joyfully jumping up and down, her tail waving around like an angry snake. "It moves, it moves," she called. "And only for Akkikuyu, for she alone. See how it dances."

She pointed to the figure and jerkily it moved from the confines of the triangle, making odd jarring movements. Its dress swept over the stone floor like the twigs of a broom as it pranced in a peculiar waltz. The arms quivered in mockery of life and the loop head twisted from time to time as

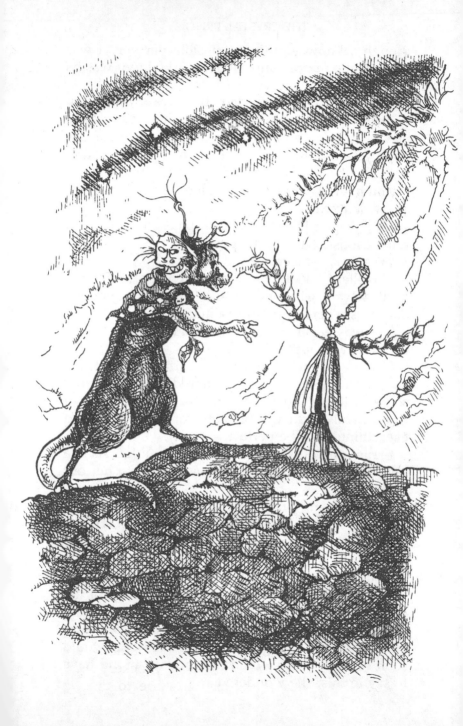

though acknowledging an invisible partner. It was a grotesque puppet and Madame Akkikuyu was its master.

The corn dolly tottered this way and that, buckling occasionally in a spasm that might have been a curtsey and shaking its dress with a dry papery sound. Madame Akkikuyu capered around with it, beckoning and following, teasing and pushing until finally she panted "Stop!" and the straw dancer became motionless.

"So," began Nicodemus in a pleased tone, "you must choose, will you help me?"

"Yes, yes," she crowed gladly.

"Excellent Akkikuyu. We must prepare for the spell which will release me from this endless darkness where I am imprisoned."

She was eager to learn more and asked, "What do we need Nico? I fetch, I get."

"Hah!" laughed the tattoo. "First I must teach you, and there are many ingredients to find – some will not be easy, others will. There is a ritual involved in the breaking of my bonds and everything must be perfect."

"Trust me, oh spirit. Akkikuyu no fluff." As she said it she thought her own voice came to her out of the past.

"Come then, let us talk away from this ditch. Only the hours of night are afforded to me. That is the only time I may speak with you Akkikuyu, so spend your days wisely and make no exertion that may tire you out ere night falls."

She agreed and promised to rest for most of the daytime from then on. As she climbed up the bank the fortune-teller glanced back at the corn dolly and grinned as she thought of the powers that would soon be hers. What would her mousey friend have to say to this, she wondered.

9

MOULD TO MOULD

It was another baking hot day. Audrey awoke to a blazing blue sky empty of cloud. She rubbed the sleep from her eyes and peeped out of the nest.

The Hall of Corn was glowing with light. The sun shone down on the stems and those stout wives who had insisted on taking their sheets were shaking them vigorously outside the nests, waving them like dazzling flags of surrender.

Old Todmore passed below, swaggering on his bowed legs and nibbling a straw. He took up his usual position in the Hall and watched the world hurry by.

"Bless the Green for morns like this," he sighed, stroking his whiskers.

Tired sentries came into the Hall blinking and yawning whilst those newly awake ran to take their places.

"Where's our Hodge?" a small mouse woman asked Figgy.

"Haven't seen him," was the sleepy reply.

"Well, I'm not takin' his breakfast to him. Sentry, sentry – that's all that boy thinks about."

Arthur poked his head out of his nest. He was covered in bits of grass and moss. "Mornin' Sis!" he said brightly. "Breakfast's ready – didn't you hear Mrs Scuttle calling?"

"No," replied Audrey, "but I'll be down in a minute." She retreated back into her nest, but after breathing the fresh air of the outside world the atmosphere in her bedroom seemed stifling. She decided that nests were lovely places to spend a night but in the daytime they were like ovens.

As soon as she had dressed and brushed away some stray bits of straw she clambered out and descended the ladder Mr Scuttle had made for her.

On the ground below, Gladwin Scuttle had spread a clean cloth and laid out the breakfast things. Arthur was well into his third helping when Audrey arrived.

"Mornin' Missey," greeted Elijah. "And how did you sleep last night?"

"Very well, Mr Scuttle, thank you."

Mrs Scuttle patted the cloth by her side and said, "You sit down here, dear, and tell me what you think you'll be doing today."

"I think I'd better find Madame Akkikuyu," Audrey answered glumly. "I was a bit nasty to her last night."

"Hey Sis," Arthur butted in, "I'm going to be a sentry today. Twit's going to present me to Mr Woodruffe and they do a little ceremony or something," he added with his mouth full.

"That's right," agreed Elijah, "you'll be made to swear an oath of allegiance to Fennywolde for the rest of your days."

"But Arthur," Audrey pointed out, "you can't promise that. What about Mother? You said you'd go back."

· Arthur looked ashamed. "You're right. Do you know, I hadn't thought about home since I've been here – aren't I awful?"

"Never you mind," consoled Elijah. "I'll pop an' have a word or three with Mr Woodruffe – we'll see if'n we can't bend the rules a tiny bit." He got to his feet and set off in the direction of the throne.

The doors of the Hall opened and in came Madame Akkikuyu. She looked tired and she trudged along with heavy limbs. The families of fieldmice waved and nodded to her as though she were a dear old friend and Mr Nep bowed politely as she walked by.

"Here comes trouble," observed Arthur dryly.

"Good morning, Madame Akkikuyu," called Audrey, trying to be as nice as possible. "Did you sleep well – how's your ear today?"

The fortune-teller gave her a weary glance and mumbled. "Akkikuyu not sleep – she busy all night finding root and herb for mousling potions." She showed them her claws, which were caked in soil and dirt. "Ear better," she added grudgingly.

"Sit down and have something to eat Madame er . . ." offered Gladwin kindly.

Madame Akkikuyu grabbed a whole loaf and shook her head. "Akkikuyu not sit – she off to sleep."

"Oh," said Mrs Scuttle. "Well, when my Elijah gets back I'm sure he'll make you a nest of your own."

"No," the rat declined sharply. "Akkikuyu no like mousey house. She go find place to kip."

"Akkikuyu," said Audrey, "if you like we can go for a walk or something later."

The rat regarded Audrey for a moment and shrugged. "Maybe," she replied and stalked away, tearing the bread into great chunks and gulping them down as she went.

"Oh dear," said Gladwin.

"She ain't happy with us mouselets," remarked Twit lightly.

"This is all my fault," admitted Audrey. "I'm not

turning out to be a very good companion for her, am I?"

Arthur munched thoughtfully on a crust. "You know," he began after a while, "Madame Akkikuyu is a lot more independent than she was when we set off – haven't you noticed? I don't think she needs you any more Audrey. I do believe she's settled in here better than we have."

"I ought to be relieved," sighed his sister. "It's funny though – I feel just the opposite, as if I've betrayed her."

"Don't be soft," Arthur told her. "You came all this way, didn't you?"

"Well, let her down then," argued Audrey. "I haven't been much of a friend to her have I? She thought we were best friends – I think I failed her in that."

"Pah!" declared Mrs Scuttle. "Rats and mice being friends! I never heard of such a thing!"

They waited for Audrey to finish nibbling her breakfast, then Elijah came puffing back.

"It's all fixed and sorted," he informed Arthur. "We put our heads together such as they are an' we come up with the answer."

"So I can still be a sentry?" asked Arthur.

"Aye lad, you can be a sentry for as long as you likes – till you goes home."

"Great!" shouted Arthur, dancing around. "When can I start?"

"Right now, if you're willin'. Mr Woodruffe's a-waitin' on you."

So, with great excitement, they all went over to the wicker-throne where the King of the Field sat with his staff of office on his knee.

"A blessed Eve to you," he smiled warmly.

They all bowed and curtseyed to him and Audrey contrived to whisper into Mrs Scuttle's ear, "Eve?"

"Midsummer's Eve, child," Gladwin murmured back.

"So Master Brown, you wish to become a sentry and guard our Hall from enemies. Is this so?" said the King of the Field.

"Yes Sir," said Arthur keenly.

"Majesty!" hissed Twit.

"Yes Majesty," corrected Arthur.

"Who presents this mouse to the King of the Field?" asked Mr Woodruffe solemnly.

"I do Majesty," chirped Twit. "He is a friend of mine and a braver lad you never did see." He found it hard to stifle the chuckles as he described Arthur to the King. He had to follow the correct procedure which had been unchanged for countless years.

"Now you must swear loyalty to me, your King, and the land of Fenny."

Arthur nodded to show that he understood.

"Raise your right paw, Art," prompted Twit. "Now hold this hawthorn leaf."

"The hawthorn represents virtue and honour, Master Brown," explained Mr Woodruffe. "But it is also the sacred tree of the Green Mouse and we shall name him as a witness. Are you ready to be sworn in?"

Arthur's lips had gone dry and he swallowed a lump in his throat. He wished his father was alive to see this. "Yes Majesty."

"Repeat after me," commenced Mr Woodruffe. "I, Arthur of the brown mice, visitor from the grey town, do most solemnly swear by holy leaf and in the Green's name to protect the Hall of Corn from any evil, though my life should fail in the attempt, till by His Majesty's leave I am released from service."

Arthur breathed a sigh of relief as he finished the last sentence.

Elijah nudged his wife. "That's the bit we put in," he told her proudly.

"Now young sentry," began the King briskly, "you may go about your duty. Have you been taught all the signals and alarms yet?"

"Why no, Your Majesty."

"See to it William Scuttle," ordered Mr Woodruffe with a twinkle in his eye.

They all bowed and curtseyed again and as they were leaving Twit said to Arthur, "They're real simple when you knows 'em. Blackbird cries and funny whistles – that sort of stuff. We usually use them to tell each other when it's dinner time though. Mind you, the most important alarm of all and one you must never use 'cept in the direst need is to yell *Fenny* at the top of your voice."

Audrey resumed her conversation with Mrs Scuttle. "Will you be celebrating the Eve tonight at all? We do in the Skirtings."

"I remember, yes we have a bit of a party. This afternoon all us mums and all the girls are going to make some bunting. There's a lovely group of rose trees over by the hedge and we thread the petals onto a string. It does look jolly."

"Could I come along?" asked Audrey. "I can't imagine anything more boring than watching my brother climb a stalk all day long. I haven't a clue why he wants to do it."

"Hah," said Gladwin. "You sound like you've lived in Fennywolde all your life. We can't understand why the menfolk love it either. Anyway, you'd be most welcome dear. Oh there'll be such a time tonight! In the excitement of William returning and the Hall-making going on I clean forgot all about the Eve myself till Elijah asked about it last night."

The sun was climbing higher in the brilliant sky.

The heat hammered down and Audrey felt dizzy.

"Is there somewhere cool I could sit, Mrs Scuttle?" she inquired, wiping her forehead.

Gladwin tutted and scolded herself. "Why, there I go, forgetting myself again – when I first came here I was limp as a lettuce for weeks. House mice aren't used to all this sunshine. Mind you, I can't remember it being quite so hot as this before." She gazed around at the merry families with their plump, pleasant wives and red-eared husbands. This is what she had given up her old home and family for and she had never once regretted it. Suddenly she clicked back to the present and looked at Audrey sheepishly.

"Oh dear," she flustered, "there's me wandering off again. You want to get cool don't you dear – well the best place I used to go when I felt a bit off with the heat was the still pool."

"Yes," said Audrey, "Arthur told me that's where you get all your water from."

"Now the ditch has dried up we have no choice. You should see poor Grommel trying to carry a full bucket of water with his bad back – poor thing."

Mrs Scuttle eventually pointed to where the pool was. "Just follow the ditch and you can't miss it."

Audrey set off. She went through the great doors of the Hall and walked straight into Jenkin Nettle.

"Hello miss," he grinned.

"Oh," muttered Audrey, blushing. "Good morning Jenkin," she added lamely.

"You looks nice this mornin' miss," he said, enjoying the situation.

Audrey giggled and thanked him. "But I always try and look this nice for Arthur." And she sauntered out of the field with Jenkin's eyes following her admiringly. The younger children were playing dust slides near the elm roots.

"You'll catch it when your mothers see you," laughed Audrey.

The grubby children considered her for a moment, wondering whether they ought to say anything in reply but cleaner, older sisters grabbed them by the paws and dragged them away whispering at them.

"No Josh you mustn't – you know what Mam told you 'bout that one."

Audrey was taken aback. Evidently, Mr Nettle's outburst yesterday had been the chief topic of Fennywolde gossip. Audrey was surprised that so many had actually believed his ridiculous accusations.

"Still," she shrugged, "it takes a long time to make friends and time is something I'll have plenty of here."

She carried on along the ditch, past the elms and the winter quarters and an entrance where the sound of Mr Nettle hammering on the mouse-brasses rang out in time to his deep voice booming out hymns to the Green Mouse.

Soon she found that she had wandered into a patch of dismal shade and she shivered to herself. Rearing high above her was the lonely yew tree, the frightening tree of death. Its branches poked out like bony fingers and sharp claws. She hurried on, past that place – it was much too eerie and dark for her liking. No grass grew in its shadow and no birds sang in its branches.

The floor of the ditch began to get softer. Instead of dry choking dust it had become a rich brown mud, which yielded under her little pink feet like a dark fruit cake that had been cooked too quickly. The surface was crusty yet underneath it was still gooey and spongey.

It was a sign that she was not far from the pool.

Soon her footprints began to fill up with water as she passed. She pushed through the trailing leaves of an ivy creeper and found herself staring into the still pool. It was as if she had crossed the threshold into another world, a cool, silent place where magic was almost visible. The harsh sunlight was filtered through the layers of bright new leaves and dappled the water with great splashes of shimmering green, which in turn were reflected back and bounced around once more. Dragonflies in their polished emerald armour flashed over the water's surface chasing gnats. Fine trails of bubbles slipped through the water then burst silently, too small to make a ripple. The still pool was a beautiful place.

Audrey stared, not even daring to breathe in case everything should disappear – so much did it look like a fairy grotto. The edge of the pool was fringed with plants: water-plaintains, horse-tails and yellow-rattles grew there. Behind one clump a husky voice began to speak.

"Alison Sedge – you are the loveliest thing in creation."

Audrey looked up, startled.

"You are lovelier than the flowers in your hair. Just look at you. That hair, the goddess would be proud of it."

Audrey put her paw over her mouth. She wanted to laugh. It was a girl's voice that spoke.

"Those eyes – they're luscious they are. A boy could drown in those."

Audrey crept round the plants to see who it was – it didn't sound like any of the girls she had met the day before.

"Those lips – don't you want to eat them up lads? A finer cherry red pair of lips there never were, won't someone pick them?" Now there came a sound of pretend kissing.

Through the leaves Audrey saw Alison Sedge. She was gazing at herself in the water, enchanted by her own reflection. Her thick hair hung down either side of her face nearly touching the water. This was the reason Audrey did not recognise the girl immediately. She decided that it was rude to stay there without letting the mooning fieldmouse know she was there so she coughed politely.

Alison Sedge whipped round and stared in horror at Audrey, embarrassment, shame and surprise all registering in her beautiful eyes.

"I'm sorry for intruding," said Audrey. "I'm Audrey Brown – a friend of Twit. I don't think we've met." And then she remembered, this was the girl who had glared at her that first night when Madame Akkikuyu chased away the owl.

Alison composed herself and groomed her pony tails back behind her ears.

"Saw you other day," she said mildly.

"Oh, when?" asked Audrey, not seeing the trap.

"When that rat woman made you look real stupid," Alison tittered.

"Oh!" was all Audrey could find to say.

"Your brother know Dimsel's after him?" asked Alison, her subtle mind moving on to a different subject.

"Erm . . . no," replied Audrey, trying to keep up with the shifting conversation.

"Not much of a catch – either of them," remarked Alison outrageously.

Audrey choked and spluttered. How rude this girl was. She could find nothing to say in reply. When she did manage to recover her wits, Audrey caught Alison running a critical eye over her dress and collar. This was better; Alison's plain frock was no match for them. The other girl sniffed and looked away.

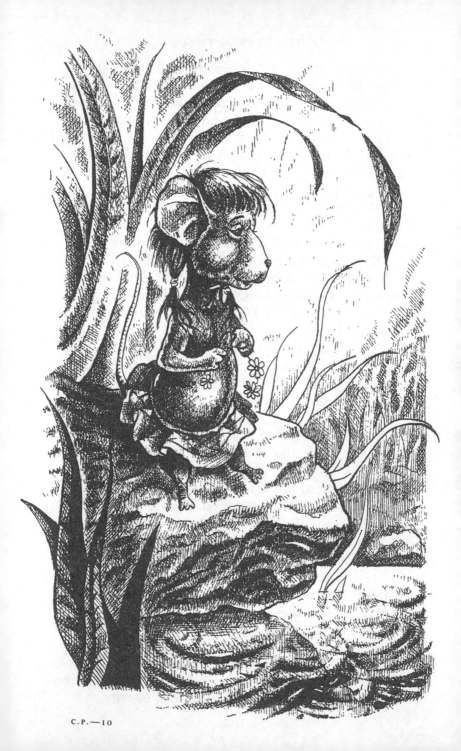

"Oh no," thought Audrey and she gave her tail a slight flick. The silver bells tinkled sweetly.

Alison jumped in surprise and stared at them coldly. Then she smiled and fiddled abstractedly with her mousebrass – it too tinkled: maybe not as sweetly, but it was enough to draw Audrey's eyes to it. She recognised the sign of grace and beauty and rolled her eyes heavenward.

"You not old enough to have a brass then?" queried Alison.

"I did have one," said Audrey, "but I lost it."

"Careless," the other observed coolly.

Audrey did not feel like explaining about the altar of Jupiter to Alison so she said nothing.

"Young Whortle's better now." Alison changed the subject again.

"Yes," said Audrey – this was another dig about her foolish display yesterday morning. Well, she thought, if that's all you can throw at me, go ahead.

"Skinny Samuel's gettin' better too," resumed Alison.

Audrey decided to join in this little game. In an innocent voice she said, "That Jenkin's a nice boy isn't he?"

The hit went home and Alison scowled. Through clenched teeth she managed to say, "The Nettles are all barmy. I'd have nowt to do with 'em."

"Oh I don't know," sighed Audrey demurely. "Jenkin's always sweet to me."

"He's like that to all the common sort," spat Alison. She didn't like it when someone got the better of her and was not used to her remarks thrown back with added sting. "I had to tell him to stop pesterin' me," she added.

"Said I looked nice this morning and always calls me 'Miss'." Audrey held out her paw to examine her nails – something she never did usually.

Alison pursed her lips, then her eyebrows arched craftily and said, "His dad's loony too – wonder how he knew 'bout your daft dolly though?"

Audrey understood at once, and for her the game ended.

"Can be dangerous livin' in the country if'n you're not used to it," droned Alison. "And try an' take what don't belong to you."

"Oh I'm quite safe," said Audrey defiantly and with an edge to her voice. "You see I don't scare easily – if I come across a snake I don't run away."

"Really?" Alison sounded bored and unimpressed. "You'd get bitten then."

"Oh no," Audrey assured her calmly. "You see Madame Akkikuyu and I are best friends. I'd get some of her potions and shrivel that snake up." She brought her face close to Alison's and added darkly, "Either that or I'd choke it with my bare paws just for the fun of it."

Alison backed away – she did not like the look in Audrey's eyes. She tossed her head and said, "I can't waste my time here all day."

"Yes," smiled Audrey, "I saw you wasting your time before."

Alison huffed and flounced off.

Audrey shook her head. So that was Alison Sedge! Lily Clover was right – she did have claws; it might not be wise to get on the wrong side of her but it was too late now.

Audrey lay back and enjoyed the tranquil magic of the pool in peace.

*   *   *

The morning turned to lunch time. On sentry duty, Arthur's stomach began to growl. He looked over to Twit and signalled that he was about to climb down.

Twit waved back cheerily but made it clear that

he was quite happy to stay on duty a little longer.

Arthur scrambled down the stalk and went in search of food.

A narrow path veered away from the main corridor and he wondered if it was a short cut to the Hall. It seemed to go in the right direction so he took it and began to whistle one of Kempe's songs.

He stopped in his tracks, something was wrong – he could feel it. Cautiously he continued further along the path. What was that in the way up ahead?

"Oh no," muttered Arthur under his breath. He ran over to the dark lumpy shape which sprawled awkwardly over the ground. At his feet was the body of a mouse.

For a couple of minutes Arthur could only stand and gape, shock freezing his limbs. Then he knelt down and bravely laid his paw on the sad little body. It was stone cold. The mouse must have been lying there for hours. Gingerly, he turned the body over, and squealed in fright. It was Hodge. He recognised him at once. But it was not just that which upset him. Hodge's face was ghastly to look on. Like a mask of horror, the eyes were popping out, and the mouth was fixed in a wild and silent scream. It seemed almost as if Hodge had died of some terrible fright. But Arthur could see savage marks on his throat and his neck looked pathetically thin and squashed.

Slowly it dawned on him. Hodge had died of strangulation – someone had murdered him.

Now the corn stems seemed to hem Arthur in and the whole place took on a sinister aspect. His skin began to crawl. He gulped and gazed round fearfully. What if the murderer was still there somewhere, hiding and watching him? What if even now it was coming to get him?

Arthur yelped as panic got the better of him. Never before had he been so frightened. "I've got to get out!" he squeaked and ran up the path again, stumbling and falling in his haste.

"FENNY! FENNY!" he cried out desperately.

Voices were raised at once in answer to the urgent call. Arthur picked himself up from the ground, took no heed of his bleeding knees and ran straight into Jenkin. The fieldmouse stared at Arthur's terrified face and gasped.

"What is it?"

Arthur hid his eyes and began to shake all over.

Jenkin shook him urgently. "Tell me Arthur, what is it?"

Arthur pointed up the path. "Hodge," he said thickly, pointing back up the path.

Jenkin dashed to see. "Don't look at him," cried Arthur after him. It was too late. Jenkin cried out in horror.

Other sentries came running. Twit was the first. He stopped in surprise when he saw Arthur's expression.

"Art?" he began curiously."What is it? Why, you're tremblin' all over."

A group of sentries gathered round. Arthur would not let them pass. They were all anxious to know why the major alarm had been used.

Eventually Jenkin came staggering back – his face matched Arthur's and he was weeping.

The sentries murmured and looked at one another nervously.

"It's Hodge," sobbed Jenkin. "He's dead."

The sentries opened their mouths and shook their heads in disbelief. Twit looked fearfully at Arthur who was trying to say something.

"No!" he shouted violently. "He's been murdered!"

*   *   *

A grim, silent group made its way to the Hall of Corn. Mourners lined the corridor and the sound of lamentation was heard everywhere in Fennywolde.

Jenkin, Young Whortle, Todkin and Figgy carried the body of their friend on their shoulders. A white cloth had been placed over Hodge's face by Jenkin so that no-one would have to look on that grisly horror again.

Grommel and the other guard opened the great doors and let the group in. Word had spread quickly through the field and the grief of Hodge's parents was terrible to hear and to see.

Elijah came and took Arthur to one side. Twit disappeared into his nest and brought out the flask given to him by Thomas Triton.

"Here Art," he said gently, "drink some of this."

Mr Woodruffe held up his staff of office and cried angrily, "What creature has done this? We must not rest till the fiend is captured. Summon everyone into the Hall at once!"

For those who had not already heard the tragic news, Jenkin placed a piece of straw between his thumbs and blew hard. A high screech echoed over Fennywolde and all who heard it clutched their mousebrasses fearfully and ran to the Hall. Isaac Nettle dropped his hammer and abandoned the forge.

Soon everyone was there except Audrey. The Hall was buzzing with grief and anger as the mice held on to their children tightly and called for the murderer to be found.

Isaac learnt from his son what had occurred and turned to the King furiously.

"See," he raged bitterly, "now do you see what happens when you turn your back on the Green's holy laws. He has been swift to show His anger."

"Silence, Nettle!" stormed Mr Woodruffe. "I will not have you say such rubbish in front of Hodge's parents."

"Thee must all pray – pray hard and beg the Green's forgiveness for having allowed the heathen into our midst." He whirled round and pointed an accusing finger at Arthur. "Where is thy sister – the blasphemer?"

"Isaac!" roared the King before Arthur could answer. "I will not allow you to turn this into one of your prayer meetings! I have a search party to organise and you could attend to Hodge there."

Mr Nettle calmed a little and regarded the body grimly. "Verily – I shall order the service."

As Mr Woodruffe despatched fieldmice to search the field, Arthur turned to Twit and said, "I wish I knew where Audrey was. This is another thing for Mr Nettle to jump down her throat about. Did you see the faces of some in the crowd? They were agreeing with him!"

"Here's Akkikuyu, Arthur," Twit warned as the rat strode into the room.

"What goes on?" she asked. "Who make all the noise and hullabaloo? They wake Akkikuyu." Then she saw Hodge's body and tutted sadly. "Poor mouselet – he beyond Akkikuyu's help."

"He was strangled," said Mr Woodruffe gently.

"Who did so?" she asked in astonishment. "I give *them* a throttling."

"We are about to try and find out," said the King gravely.

"Poor, poor mouselet," she sighed. "No more cheeses for you."

"Arthur," ventured Twit, looking at the fortune-teller, "you don't think?"

"What . . . Akkikuyu?" said Arthur. "No, she was too shocked when she saw Hodge just then. I don't

169

think it was her . . . good grief, no, it couldn't possibly have been."

Alison Sedge watched everything in horror. She could not take her eyes off the body. That lifeless thing had once been a boy she had flirted with and lured into the meadow. Now the thought of it made her ill.

The painful wails of Hodge's parents were unbearable to her. She stumbled to her nest and bit her nails nervously. A dreadful thought had come to her. She recalled Audrey's words at the still pool: "I'd choke it with my bare paws just for the fun of it."

Alison was scared – should she tell someone or would the town mouse punish her. She wondered what Hodge had done to warrant his horrid reward.

The ceremony was held that afternoon in a shady area kept tidy for such purposes. As the body was lowered into the ground Mr Nettle intoned, "Receive this innocent soul, Almighty. He is beyond our care now. Take him to thy bosom and cherish this small servant of yours. Mould to mould, body to Green."

Arthur's head felt thick and fuzzy. The search parties had found nothing unusual – only Audrey asleep by the pool. Now she stood looking down into the grave next to him.

Hodge's parents cast a hawthorn leaf and his favourite flower into the grave. Then Mr Woodruffe led them away in silence.

"We'll have to double the sentries," said Jenkin as they walked away. "If some maniac is still out there we don't want him to strike again. And don't you go off on your own again miss," he said to Audrey.

"I shan't," she answered. It had been a nasty

shock to wake to a different Fennywolde, one full of grief, anger and fear. She could feel the whole atmosphere of the place had changed.

Gladwin Scuttle linked her arm in Elijah's and went home. No-one felt like celebrating the Eve of midsummer now and the rose petals that had been gathered were left to rot.

Madame Akkikuyu looked back to where Isaac was filling in the grave. Night was drawing closer and she rubbed her ear thoughtfully.

10

MIDSUMMER'S EVE

Audrey stared out of her nest and up into the gathering dusk. Everyone in Fennywolde had gone to bed early, trying to blot out the tragic day with sleep. Even so, Audrey could hear the sound of weeping. She lay back on her moss bed and reflected on the death of Hodge and its implications. Was it now dangerous to walk alone in the field? Was the murderer of Hodge still at large out there? And what manner of creature was it anyway? Some of the fieldmice had come to the conclusion that the beast had been a wandering rogue whom Hodge had surprised. But after all the searching the general feeling was that whoever had done this atrocious deed had undoubtedly escaped and was now far away.

"Ain't been nowt like it since that old owl was around," Old Todmore had observed gravely.

The mood of the fieldmice was one of unease. Audrey had noticed that now – more so than before – the simple country mice shied away from her and looked quickly at the ground if she smiled at them. It was almost as if they thought that she had brought this tragedy down on them. She wondered if they pointed at her in secret and muttered nonsense about jinxes and the like. It was certainly good fuel for Isaac Nettle's sermons on the importance of prayer to the Green Mouse. Audrey found all this too tiresome and worrying to dwell on, so she turned her thoughts to other things.

Was Piccadilly safe in the city? She wished he was here; he'd give Mr Nettle something to make him sit up and scowl at. She almost laughed as she tried to imagine what Piccadilly would have said, but the smile faded on her lips with the thought that the grey mouse must surely think badly of her. She had been too horrible to him for him to think anything else.

Audrey shifted uncomfortably and tried to redirect her thoughts. An image of Jenkin sailed brightly before her eyes. It was hard to believe that he was the son of sour-faced Mr Nettle. What a fine young mouse Jenkin was! In some ways he reminded her of Piccadilly. Audrey fell asleep with the two mice filling her thoughts.

The night stars wheeled over Fennywolde. Silvery moths flew up and rode the secret breezes. The hedgehog waddled out of a leaf pile and roamed along the ditch searching for more mouth-watering delicacies. The moon rose full and bright and somewhere in a patch of deep shade Nicodemus muttered to Madame Akkikuyu of potions and spells and their mysterious ingredients.

Audrey stirred in her sleep and gradually became aware of a faint sound pulling her awake. A distant lilting music caught her ears, and, despite its faintness, her heart yearned to follow it.

She opened her eyes and rubbed her brow drowsily. It was an achingly beautiful melody hovering just on the edge of hearing. Audrey tilted her head and wondered where it was coming from. It haunted and enchanted her, beckoning with sweet invisible fingers.

Audrey quickly determined to find the source of the music. She slipped out of bed and turned to look for her dress. She paused and blinked: from her bag of clean clothes and personal treasures a dim light was shining.

Apprehensively, Audrey pulled open the neck of the bag and peered inside. A creamy glow at once illuminated her face and she gasped in wonderment and surprise. She put in her paw and drew out the sprig of hawthorn blossom that Oswald had given to her, back in Deptford. Tonight it was a thing of magic. The petals of the blossom, which for many weeks now had been so dry and yellowed with decay, were as fresh as the day they had been picked – only now they shone with a clear and supernatural light of their own.

Audrey could only stare at it in amazement. Yet it seemed to be the most natural thing in the world – for tonight was the Eve of Midsummer and almost anything was possible. A thrill of expectation ran through her body as, holding the blossom before her, she left the nest and clambered down the ladder.

In the Hall of Corn nothing stirred. The nests which lined its long walls were dark and their entrances gazed at her blindly. The moonlight cast weird shadows all around her, and the breeze moved them so that the black shapes waved mysteriously in the gloom.

The thought of poor Hodge and his unknown assassin crossed Audrey's mind but she managed to suppress her fear. She just had to follow the strange music. It seemed to tug her along and she noticed that the light of the hawthorn blossom grew brighter if she went in a certain direction. Using this as a sort of magical compass Audrey passed out of the Hall and into the wild tangle of corn stems. Through the field it led Audrey and along the ditch, a will other than her own driving her feet towards the source of the music.

She crossed the ditch and made for the still pool. It seemed that the tune was coming from there, and as she looked a twinkle of light glimmered from behind the surrounding hawthorn bushes.

She hesitated, breathing softly. This was it – the source of the wonderful sound. The light of the blossom in her paw welled up suddenly like a star fallen from heaven. Audrey felt a pang of fear; now she was there she wondered what lay beyond the hawthorn bushes. What would she see when she drew back the branches?

Audrey bit her lip and for a moment wanted desperately to run back to her nest, but it was too late for that now. Slowly, she pulled the branches to one side.

There in the hawthorn grotto were all the mice of Fennywolde. They were arranged in a semi-circle around Mr Woodruffe and all were silent and bowed. Audrey glanced up and saw why they were all so hushed and reverent. She fell to her knees and cried out in surprise.

Floating above Mr Woodruffe, like a dense cloud of growing things was the Green Mouse.

He was at the height of his midsummer power and mightier than when Audrey had seen him in the spring. His fur was lush and green as grass, and on his brow he wore the crown of wheat. Here and there, fiery mousebrasses blazed out from his coat of leaves. Indeed, Audrey could not tell where his coat ended and the hawthorn thicket took over for little green lamps had been hung all around and they increased the wondrous quality of the place.

The Green Mouse was smiling kindly at his subjects, his long olive-green hair cascading down like a lion's mane, and sparkling mousebrasses kindling a green fire in his noble eyes.

Audrey bowed her head. When she dared to look up she found that the Green Mouse was looking straight at her.

Those eyes which she had never forgotten now shone on her once more. Slowly, the Green Mouse beckoned to her and timidly Audrey moved towards him. He held out his great paw and she kissed it.

"We are pleased with you little one," came the huge voice. Audrey flushed and hung her head. "There are still dangers you must face," the Green Mouse told her. "Be brave, my brassless one. I shall take care of you while I can, for spring and summer are mine to command. Remember that the green fails in autumn and is dead for the winter." He furrowed his immense brow and shook his great head. "Let us hope my protection will not be needed in the bleak months to come, and the summer will end as we pray it will." The Green Mouse smiled and it seemed as if it was daytime. The lamps blazed back at him and Audrey realised that they were not lamps at all but shining leaves. The more he smiled the brighter they became, and the more others began to shine. Soon the entire grotto was filled with a blinding glare of green.

"Now," the Green Mouse addressed all the Fennywolders, "be not sad in heart, for verily I know your grief. Let peace fill your troubled hearts! Forget the pain of your sorrows." He raised his paws and his voice resounded round the grotto: "Tonight is the Eve, when I am in full glory, so let my light dispel your shadows."

The fieldmice cheered and began to dance in time to the music. Audrey looked around her and noticed Arthur and Twit. She rushed over to them. They were staring at the Green Mouse in wonder.

"Oh me," sighed Twit heavily.

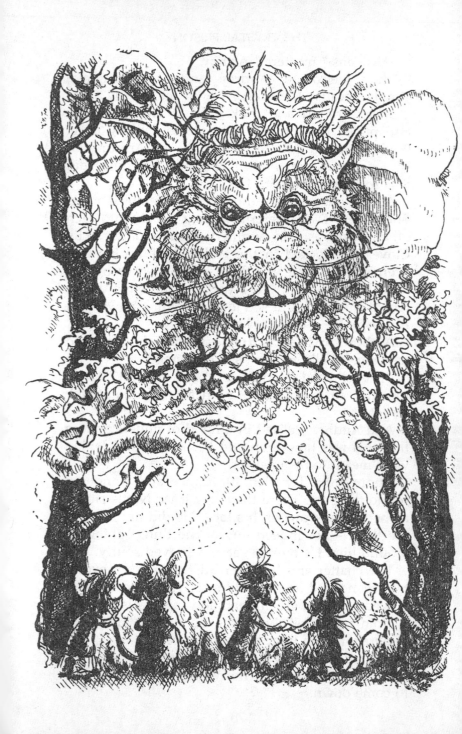

"Heavens," muttered Arthur.

They welcomed Audrey and then laughed, simply because they felt so light and giddy. Twit pranced around and took hold of Audrey's paw and pulled her into the rest of the dancing mice. Shyly, Dimsel Bottom sidled up to Arthur and smiled up at him. Arthur coughed nervously but was soon dancing with her.

Audrey glanced around at the assembled mice. There were Twit's parents staring deeply into each other's eyes as they whirled about sedately. Lily Clover was locked in the embrace of Todkin and even Samuel Gorse was there, completely recovered from his mauling by the owl. At the edge of the crowd Audrey could see Jenkin holding paws with Alison Sedge – then he kissed her!

Audrey was so surprised that she stopped dancing. "Well I never!" she exclaimed.

Twit followed her glance, "Aye, tonight they're together. In the magic of Him all resentments are forgot."

And Audrey realised in a flood of understanding that this was how it should be. Alison and Jenkin were meant to be together.

Audrey and Twit left the dance and wandered round the pool. There they saw Isaac Nettle sitting alone with a scowl on his face. He did not seem to see them – nor indeed any of the things going on around him. He merely sat and prayed sourly.

The chatter and laughter hushed and an expectant silence fell on the fieldmice. The Green Mouse bowed his great green head and raised his paws.

"Join us Lady!" his voice boomed. "Grace our celebration with your holy presence."

Audrey looked up, holding her breath. The Green Mouse was beseeching the White Lady of the moon to come down.

In the sky above, through the fluttering, glimmering hawthorn leaves, the silver moon shone out brightly. A slight wind sighed through the branches as a faint mist flowed down to the earth and threaded its way past the fieldmice. Those it touched gasped and felt refreshed. A rich perfume came with it and here and there tiny moon beams twinkled and glowed in its depths.

"Oh my," said Twit as the mist reached him and tears rolled down his little face.

The White Lady floated round the gathering and the Green Mouse lowered his eyes.

Audrey stared at the milky mist in disbelief. Now and then the wind moved it and she saw glimpses of something within. There was a fold of dress revealed for a moment, richly encrusted with pearls, and the toe of a silken slipper. The White Lady said nothing to the fieldmice but the mist shifted in what might have been a bow to the Green Mouse. He too bowed, then pointed to the water of the pool. The mist rose up and curled round in a wide arc then it poured down onto the pool's surface and vanished. The Fennywolders saw only a reflection of the night sky and the creamy circle of the moon shimmering in it.

"Drink," the Green Mouse instructed them.

The fieldmice cautiously went to the water's edge and cupped their paws together.

"It's like wine," shouted Young Whortle excitedly and all the mice gasped in wonderment as they drank the moon mead.

Twit smacked his lips thoughtfully, "You know," he declared, "that beats old Tom's rum paws down."

Only Audrey did not drink the magical water. She sat at the edge of the pool staring into its dark mirror and fancied she saw shapes swirling amongst the stars. Slowly the shapes turned to pictures: she saw a long dark tunnel with bright lights at the far end of it and there, running for all he was worth was a familiar grey figure – it was Piccadilly. Audrey cried out in surprise. Piccadilly was being pursued by a horde of rats! Another image took over; it was all white, a landscape of frost and ice. Stretching far and wide the snowy wasteland moved beneath her as if she were a bird flying. Something dreadful was in the sky but she was unable to make out what it was. A glittering spear shot down at her and the white ground lurched below and sped up towards her. Audrey felt herself hurtling down, the ribbon was snatched out of her hair and she hit the ground with a tremendous crash.

*　　*　　*

Another hot, beautiful day began.

Audrey found herself curled up in her nest. For a moment she stared up at the woven ceiling blankly. She was unable to remember how she had got there. The previous night was all still so vivid in her mind that the bright sunlight confused her. The sprig of hawthorn was lying next to her – dry and brittle once more. Audrey picked it up and held it against the light trying to remember how the blossom had looked the night before.

It was the uncomfortable heat that made Audrey finally lean out of her nest.

"It's hotter than yesterday," Arthur's voice came up to her. Audrey waved lazily down at him. The Scuttles were having their breakfast. She dressed quickly and descended the ladder eager to discuss the marvels of the Eve.

"Wasn't it magnificent?" she cried running to them.

Elijah Scuttle gazed at her dumbly. "What were, missey?"

"Last night, of course, Mr Scuttle! Wasn't the Green Mouse wonderful?"

Elijah and Gladwin exchanged puzzled glances.

"The Green Mouse, dear?" asked Mrs Scuttle.

Audrey looked surprised then laughed. They were teasing her. "Yes," she persisted excitedly, "when the Lady came down and everyone drank the magic water."

There followed a painful, embarrassed silence broken only by Arthur coughing nervously. Twit began to giggle and tickled Audrey mischievously.

"What you on about Aud?" the little fieldmouse chuckled happily. "You been at old Tom's rum?"

Audrey stared at them. So they weren't teasing her after all! They did not remember a thing about last night. She opened her mouth to argue but saw Arthur giving her a warning glare from behind his breakfast.

Irritated and confused Audrey quickly drank her milk. The terrible heat did not help her growing bad temper, and she pressed her forehead with her fingers, saying thickly: "I'm sorry, it's too hot for me here. I must go to the pool – I feel dreadful." She wanted to get away from them so she could be alone and think this through – last night seemed too real to be a dream so why did they know nothing about it? She got up to leave.

"Poor dear," tutted Mrs 'Scuttle, "it does take some getting used to."

Arthur crammed the last of his porridge into his mouth, mumbled to the others and ran after his sister.

"Well I never did," remarked Elijah, highly amused. "That girl do take the biscuit for fanciful ideas. Hob-nobbin' with the Green Mouse an' all.

You'm got some quaint fr..ends, Willum."

But Twit was staring after the Browns with concern.

*   *   *

"Wait Sis," Arthur yelled, puffing behind Audrey.

She stopped and turned to wait. When he reached her he took hold of her arm and stared hard.

"Look, are you really feeling okay?"

"Yes Arthur," she answered simply, "it's just the heat. I can't stand it."

He scratched his head and pressed his lips together. Finally he burst out, "What was all that rubbish back there then?"

Audrey looked at her brother for some moments and shook her head. "You really don't remember anything at all?"

Arthur pulled his "don't try that on me" face and said crossly, "Don't be daft, there's nothing to remember. We went to bed early last night: that's all that happened – not this Green Mouse stuff."

"But he was there, Arthur," she insisted passionately. "He was there – larger than life – and so were you and everyone in Fennywolde. I'm not going bonkers, believe me."

"Oh Sis," he sighed sadly, "how can I? If it's what you want to believe then fine, but just do me a favour and don't mention it to anyone else. You'll end up embarrassing you, me and the Scuttles. So just keep a lid on your fairy stories eh?"

Audrey was too angry to say any more. She spun round and strode away. How could they all have forgotten about it? A disturbing doubt crept into her mind. What if she was going barmy after all? In this stifling weather maybe even that was possible.

She made her way as fast as she could to the still pool. With her heart in her mouth she pushed through the hawthorn and entered the dappled shade.

There was no sign or trace of anything which might reassure her and prove that the Green Mouse had been there. Audrey sat down heavily and stared at the water. She was glad that Alison Sedge was not here today.

*   *   *

Arthur and Twit left breakfast to go on sentry duty. Arthur was excited as he would have to stay up all night on watch.

Twit nodded to Grommel as they passed through the great doors. "How do," he said.

"Mornin' Twit," greeted Grommel as they went by. "Watch this," he called after them and proceeded to bend down and touch his toes. "It's me back," he explained, seeing their puzzled faces. "That Madame Ratlady gave me an ointment to rub on and I feels brand new."

They congratulated him and continued on their way. "Can she get any more popular?" asked Arthur.

After a short while Twit ventured. "Arthur, what did Audrey mean before?"

Arthur shrugged, "I think Audrey had a dream, that's all. Where are we going to start today?"

But Twit would not let the matter drop. "I dunno 'bout dreams – ain't too impossible – her seein' the Green Mouse. She done so afore you know."

"So she says, but if you expect me to believe all that claptrap . . . why she's always making things up!"

Again Twit persisted. "And our Oswald – when I was sittin' with him, he said summat 'bout seein' the Green Mouse in Jupiter's chamber."

"Oh pooh!" scorned Arthur. "Oswald wasn't well, he was saying all sorts of daft things. I'm not interested in Audrey's silly stories and I'm surprised at you – don't go encouraging her, for heaven's sake. Look, there's Jenkin. Let's go join him."

The matter seemed to be closed. Twit chewed the inside of his cheek thoughtfully then ran after his friend. The watch began.

*   *   *

Madame Akkikuyu waded through the deep leaf piles near the oaks. Her bag was stuffed full with fresh herbs and wild flowers, the ingredients for a special potion. Nicodemus had instructed her to collect them the night before but there were some things which Madame Akkikuyu had trembled at the thought of getting. Nicodemus had been very persuasive.

"Listen Akkikuyu and remember well," he had told her. "I shall tell you how to free me from the black limbo where I am imprisoned. There must be a great spell to unfetter me and bring me back. Look how the land needs me. It is dying, Akkikuyu! When I am released I shall cause the rain to fall and restore the water to the thirsty land and heal its burns."

Madame Akkikuyu had thought that was a very admirable thing, so she had asked him, "Tell Akkikuyu what she must do to release you."

"There must be a potion," Nicodemus had begun quickly, "and it must be the distillation of many things – but are you ready for this Akkikuyu?"

"Yes Nico," she had stated firmly.

"There will be herbs and flowers which only bloom on moonless nights," the voice on her ear had continued, "and other things which are necessary but you may find difficult to gather."

"Akkikuyu get anything," she had claimed hastily.

"Good," Nicodemus had declared, "then fetch me

a frog and boil away the flesh till only the white bones are left."

"No," the fortune-teller had cried appalled. "Akkikuyu no kill poor froggy – she good and kind."

"Believe me, Akkikuyu," the voice had wheedled, "it is only because this is so urgent that I would ask this terrible thing of you. If this is not done then no rain will fall and all the frogs are sure to perish – better one die than all."

Madame Akkikuyu had been forced to agree with his reasoning and Nicodemus had told her to find him a frog the very next day. She looked down at her bulging bag and grimaced; there was no frog in there yet – she still demurred at murder, and had collected all the plants instead. She wondered if Nicodemus would scold her when night fell. Everything seemed muddled when he was not there to reassure and guide her and everything seemed so less important in the daylight.

She trudged up the dell and wandered about the roots of the oaks, wiping her face with her shawl.

"Too hot," she moaned to herself. She squinted at the tattoo on her ear but it was still. "Hah, old Nico – he not like the heat. He not see me in daytime."

She surveyed the leafy world around her and spotted some strange chalky looking objects scattered about the base of one of the oaks. She went over to examine them.

"Hmm," she mumbled, prodding one with her claw. It was grey and dry and broke open at her touch. "Hooty cough ups," she remarked with disdain.

They were owl pellets, tight little bundles of bone and fur that had been swallowed greedily by the owl as he devoured his prey, only to be regurgitated later when he had been unable to digest them.

"So owly still here," muttered the fortune-teller. She looked up at the trunk of the tree and saw the dark hole in its trunk. "Just you stay away from my mouseys," she threatened, shaking her fists, "or Akkikuyu come pluck you again."

She thought she heard a frightened hoot in response and was satisfied. It was time to find a shady place to sleep. Her nightly lessons with Nicodemus were leaving her with no energy for the rest of the following day. Madame Akkikuyu yawned widely and lumbered off to rest.

11

MAGIC AND MURDER

As the afternoon wore on, the fieldmice gathered in the Hall of Corn to discuss the unusually hot weather.

"Tain't natural," remarked Old Todmore, squinting at the sky. No rain fer weeks now. Mark my words, young uns, there's summat very wrong 'bout all this."

The ground had become like stone and here and there long cracks had begun to appear. The corn in the field looked dry and some of the stalks were withered and sickly – an omen that did not go unnoticed by the anxious mice.

Waves of disquiet now coursed through Fennywolde, building on the unease left by Hodge's death. The tired and anxious Fennywolders took to looking nervously over their shoulders at the slightest noise.

Isaac Nettle, accustomed to the great heat of his forge peered out over the field and declared to those willing to listen, "The fires of the infernal are at work here. Repent ye and crave pardon from the Almighty Green." And Mr Woodruffe was too tired and overheated to stop him.

Some mice swooned in the swelter and all throats were burned by the hot breeze. Many spent the day by the still pool, leaving a large space between themselves and the strange town mouse who had brought the odd weather with her.

Eventually, the day burnt itself out and the early stars pricked the evening sky. The fieldmice clambered into their nests, relieved that the long, uncomfortable day was over and worried about the next. They cast themselves on their beds and fell into exhausted faints rather than sleep.

From some of the little round nests plaintive voices were raised in prayers for rain. "Please oh Green, deliver us from the sun. Bring down the rain."

Madame Akkikuyu passed through the field with a satisfied grin on her face. She had been nosing around the top end of the ditch where the mud was still spongey, and after much searching had found a dead frog.

It was a bit old and whiffy but Madame Akkikuyu felt very pleased with herself. She had managed to keep her promise to Nicodemus without killing anything. How clever she felt! He would be very pleased with her – no need to mention how it was acquired. She hurried along, eager to put the grisly object into her pot so that the skin could be boiled away ready for the night's instruction.

As she was walking through the Hall of Corn a voice called down to her from one of the nests. Hastily the fortune-teller thrust the frog into her bag and glanced upwards.

Young Whortle's father came scurrying down and stood beside her.

"Forgive me dear lady," said Mr Nep apologetically, "but I have a . . . well . . . er . . . something to say to you."

Madame Akkikuyu narrowed her gleaming black eyes and closed her claws tightly over her bag.

"Akkikuyu listen," she said at last.

Mr Nep first looked down at his feet, then twiddled his thumbs and wiped his face in embarrassment. Finally he blurted out, "Can you make it rain?"

It was not what Madame Akkikuyu had expected and she was dumbstruck for a few moments. But Mr Nep babbled on:

"Oh . . . we're so desperate! You've shown yerself to be wise in the craft of healing, so some of us set to thinkin' that mebbe you had other . . . skills. There, I've said it."

The rat considered him for a while and said, "You want rain magic? Akkikuyu no witch or cloud-dancer – she healer."

Mr Nep looked aghast. "Oh, I have offended you. Please, no such insult was meant. It's just that even the pool is getting low in water now and well – we're getting very worried."

Madame Akkikuyu smiled. She liked it when the fieldmice came to her for assistance. A warm tingle shot up her tail and she puffed out her chest. She rubbed her tattooed ear thoughtfully and told Mr Nep, "Akkikuyu try – no promise."

"Oh thank you," he said, his face relaxing "I'll tell my Nellie, she'll be so relieved. We don't know what we'd do if it weren't fer you." Mr Nep scampered back to his nest.

"A difficult promise to keep," came a soft whisper.

The rat jumped in surprise.

"What are you going to do about it?" her tattoo continued.

"You . . . you heard Nico?" ventured the fortune-teller nervously.

The voice of Nicodemus mocked her. "Oh yes, I heard. You want to help these little creatures by bringing rain to them." The voice suddenly changed and became full of anger. "How dare you give such promises! Who are you to offer them the power of nature? The power of life-giving rain is not yours to give, it is the province of we land spirits."

"Akkikuyu only want to help poor mouseys," she whined.

The tattoo snarled back, "Don't bother to lie, I know you Akkikuyu – perhaps better than you do yourself. I can see into your soul, and you wish to rule these poor fieldmice."

"No," she protested immediately, "I likes them."

"Twist and turn all you like but you cannot escape the truth. You want them to become dependent on you – to run to you for the slightest thing until they are your subjects, enslaved to your evil will."

Madame Akkikuyu sobbed. "That false. I not like that, mouseys know – they love Akkikuyu; she their friend."

"You have no friends," snapped Nicodemus savagely. "Put your trust in me alone. The mice are using you – can you not see that? They take from you all the time, what do they give in return? Nothing."

The fortune-teller fled from the Hall. But at the edge of the ditch Madame Akkikuyu sat down and wept. "I like mouseys," she blubbed through her great salty tears.

"Then give them the rain you promised," muttered Nicodemus.

"I can't," she wailed unhappily. "Akkikuyu not powerful enough. Mouseys will laugh at me and say I cheap trickster."

"You should have thought of that before," scolded the voice.

"Nico," she began, "Nico, can you not make it rain? Only tiny bit, not much?"

"But I have already told you," said Nicodemus sternly, "until I am freed I can do nothing. My powers are useless!"

"Then Akkikuyu is washed up – mouseys not believe in her any more."

The soft voice in her ear whispered to itself and the painted eyes closed meditatively. "There may be a way," the voice began slowly. The rat sat up, excited and eager.

"Tell me quick," she insisted. "Akkikuyu will help, best she can."

Nicodemus sounded uncertain. "Are you ready though?" he asked doubtfully. "What is required might make you tremble."

"Akkikuyu not afraid," she affirmed and to prove it she flourished the dead frog from her bag. "See, I bring this, like Nico ask."

"I asked for it yesterday, Akkikuyu, yet this creature has been dead for more than three days. Do you think you can trick me?"

"No . . ." she answered feebly, letting the dried frog clatter down the steep bank and smash on the stones below.

"I must have absolute obedience, Akkikuyu," demanded the voice. "Absolute! Do you understand?"

"Yes Nico!"

"Then swear – on your soul, to obey me in all things."

"I . . . I . . ."

"Swear!"

"Akkikuyu . . . Akkikuyu swear – on soul." She hung her head and said no more. The tattoo smiled an unpleasant, triumphant grin.

"Excellent," resumed Nicodemus, "now we may proceed. The essence of rain lies in the invocation of two elements, air and water. As I am trapped you must work the spell for me. I shall tell you what to do and let us hope some rain will fall." The voice dropped to a low whisper as Nicodemus said, "For these elements we must use symbols to call upon the necessary forces – if I was there I could do it myself."

"Symbols?" asked the fortune-teller detecting something sinister in the whispered tone. "What symbols?"

"Something which represents the elements," said the voice. "For water a fish will be most suitable."

"And for air?"

"A bird," declared the tattoo wickedly. "At the bottom of the field in the hedge you will find a blackbird's nest. Bring the bird back here."

"Alive?" asked Akkikuyu hopefully.

Nicodemus just laughed at her.

Madame Akkikuyu set off for the hedge in misery. Would her triumph in getting the rain to fall be worth the life she was about to take? At the hedge she peered up into its dark, brambly depths. It was quite difficult to see anything in there at all at night time, but eventually she discovered it. Gingerly the rat squeezed through the thorns and began to climb.

The blackbird was still and silent, its feathers were fluffed out and the tiny bead-like eyes were firmly closed. Only its gentle heart beat stirred its breast.

Madame Akkikuyu pulled herself up and looked at the bird fearfully. She thought about what she had to do and her heart beat faster. The bird looked so peaceful that tears sprang to her eyes again.

"I cannot," she whispered hoarsely.

"You must," came the voice in her ear. "One swift blow and the creature will be dead. It will feel nothing! Think of your mouse friends and the rain you can bring them."

So Madame Akkikuyu slowly raised a quivering claw and shakily drew the bone out of her hair. Then, closing her eyes tightly she brought it crashing down on the nest.

At the ditch she lit a fire under her pot and pushed the feathery body into the bubbling water.

"And now, a fish, Akkikuyu," ordered Nicodemus, not letting her think too long about what she had done.

So the fortune-teller went to the still pool and stared long at the dark water, taking no notice of the grim reflection that gazed back at her with accusing eyes. Suddenly a string of tiny bubbles rose to the surface. With a great SPLASH she smacked her claw down and scooped out a spout of water. Within it a little fish was wriggling. As she caught it in her other claw Nicodemus said to her,

"Well done – but listen Akkikuyu, do you hear?"

The fortune-teller stood still and waited. A faint croaking was just audible amid the rustle of the hawthorn leaves.

On Nicodemus's instruction she crept round to a clump of water iris in time to see a small brown frog leap into sight and hop away from the pool.

"Catch it!" screamed Nicodemus. "We still need one and this will be fresh."

Madame Akkikuyu ran after the little frog and pounced on it.

Breathlessly she made her way back to the ditch and her bubbling pot. Hurriedly she dropped the fish into the boiling potion and repeated the spell after Nicodemus.

"Here me, folk that dwell in the spaces between the stars," he began. "I abjure all light, darken the sky, bring down the rain – in the name of Nachteg I command it, for you know who I am."

There was a silence and the rat looked up expectantly. But the tattoo said, "Now you must kiss the frog Akkikuyu and the spell shall be complete."

Grimly Madame Akkikuyu returned to the edge of the ditch and picked up the limp, slimy body. She gritted her teeth and kissed its head.

Nicodemus sighed and the first spots of rain pattered down.

In the Hall of Corn the fieldmice were disturbed in their sleep. They nuzzled and snuggled deep into their moss beds but could not escape the incessant drumming overhead. One by one the mice were roused from their beds and popped their heads out of their nests to see what the noise was.

"Rain!" they cried out with glee. "It's raining! Hooray!"

They abandoned their nests and danced around in the Hall with their faces upturned.

Mr Nep gasped in wonder at the miracle, woke his wife and went down to tell everyone. "It's the ratlady! I asked her to make it rain and she has! What a marvel she is. We must go and thank her." The fieldmice joyously trouped out of the Hall to find Madame Akkikuyu. The door guards went with them.

Sleepily, Audrey leant out to see what the fuss was. A large drop of rain fell with a *plop* on her nose. She wiped it off and looked into the drizzling sky.

"Hello dear," said Mrs Scuttle, descending the ladder close by. "My, what a wonder! Everyone's saying that your ratwoman has made it rain. They've all gone to find her – imagine. Elijah and I are going to follow them – I don't think I'll sleep any more tonight and it will be light soon." She let the rain fall on her gladly. "Oh it seems like years since the last drop we had. Are you coming?"

Audrey shook her head. Here was another feather for Madame Akkikuyu's cap. Wearily she sighed, "Give her my regards – but I'm going back to bed."

"Oh well you know best dear."

*   *   *

At the ditch they found Madame Akkikuyu beaming broadly. Her potion pot was now empty and the fire was out.

"Mouseys," she welcomed, throwing open her claws. "Akkikuyu bring rain as promise."

"Astounding," cried Mr Nep shaking her by the claw vigorously, "truly wondrous – well done." Everyone joined in to praise her, until Madame Akkikuyu flushed with pleasure.

But the celebrations were short-lived. The rain suddenly stopped.

"Won't be no more rain out of that sky," said Old Todmore, examining the heavens.

He was right. The magic rain shower had finished and Madame Akkikuyu shook her head in dismay – it certainly wasn't worth the murders she had committed that night.

"That spot o' water won't have done much good at all," observed one mouse sorrowfully. "Ground's too dry to soak it up. It's not long afore sunrise an' all that rain'll steam off soon. Bah – darned waste o' time."

The Fennywolders tutted sadly. All their high hopes had been dashed. Now they felt more flat and miserable than ever. All agreed however that Madame Akkikuyu had done her best, better than any of them could have done, but this didn't get them anywhere.

Madame Akkikuyu glanced at the tattoo on her ear but Nicodemus was silent – it was too near daybreak for him. She wondered if he had known how short the shower would be. She left the mice and sat by herself on the steep bank and cried regretfully.

* * *

Young Whortle was making his way through the field when dawn's grey light crept over Fenny-wolde. He was a heavy sleeper and was surprised to find himself alone in the nest that morning. He knew nothing of Madame Akkikuyu's rain-making and none of the others had returned yet.

He had gone through the great door wondering where Grommel and the other guard had got to.

"Funny," he said to himself, "where they all gone then?" He put his paws behind his back and began to hum a jolly tune. He felt much better now and his shoulders only gave him an occasional twinge. Secretly he hoped that he would have scars like Mr Scuttle, as proof of his bravery.

A mist was rising as the meagre rainfall turned to vapour. It was thick and white and soon, without realising, Young Whortle wandered out of the main corridor.

"Oh curse this fog," he muttered crossly. "I wish Sammy was here with me." He rubbed his shoulders for they had begun to ache in the damp mist. He looked up suddenly. He ought to be out of the field by now, but the white, swirling mist billowed round him. He was hopelessly lost.

Something moved in the corner of his eye. He turned quickly and the mist pressed round closely. "Hello?" he called brightly, "someone there then?" There was no reply, only the rustle of the corn stems. Young Whortle shrugged and put the movement down to the swirl of the mist. He set off again in no particular direction, knowing that sooner or later he'd come across some familiar landmark. The mist grew thicker and flowed over his plump face.

"This is a daft nuisance," he muttered and began to whistle a tune that Hodge had taught him. The tune died on his lips as he remembered his dear friend. He had been found murdered in this very field . . . Something rustled behind him – and it wasn't just the corn stems. Young Whortle walked a little faster. He wanted to stop and take a look. But what if it was something horrible waiting for him with long sharp teeth and pointed claws? Young Whortle shivered. He knew he was giving in to panic.

The rustling sounded again – only this time it was on his left. He yelped and stared wildly around him. Suddenly he broke into a wild, panic-stricken run, deeper and deeper into the field, not caring where he went just so long as he was away from the horror which lurked in the suffocating mist.

He crashed headlong through the dense stems squealing out loud. Sharp stones bit into his pink feet till they bled and coarse leaves razored through his paws. "Oh no," he whimpered as he felt his breath rattle in his chest, "I can't go on much further."

His legs crumbled beneath him and Young Whortle lay panting on the hard ground. He was a small, frightened animal, totally alone in a turgid sea of mist. He had never felt so forlorn. Even when the owl was after him at least he had known what he was up against. But this was different. Here the danger hid out of sight, waiting to strike when its victim least expected.

He strained his ears for some minutes but could hear nothing.

"Wait till I tell Sammy this," he told himself in a voice louder than he had intended. "He won't half laugh! 'Things you get yourself into, Warty' he'll say."

Young Whortle got to his feet, his legs still a bit wobbly. He scratched the top of his head and tugged the little tuft of hair that grew there. Then he froze.

Thin, long fingers appeared out of the mist and came for him. As he yelled for his life he felt something tighten around his neck.

"FENNY!" he screamed desperately,"FEN . . ."

Only the corn stems rustled in reply.

* * *

Arthur looked up. He was sure he had heard something. He and Twit were the only sentries left on duty – the others having gone to see Madame Akkikuyu with the rest of the fieldmice.

Arthur looked across at his friend who was swaying happily on a corn ear. "Did you hear that Twit?" he shouted.

The fieldmouse gazed over with a blank look. "What be the matter, Art?" he called back.

"I'm not sure . . . but I think I heard the alarm."

Arthur tried to pierce the low mist with his eyes. He felt ill at ease. Something dreadful was happening down there – he was certain of it.

"I'm going to raise the alarm myself," he told Twit decisively. "I don't like that mist down there – it could hide anything. It's creepy." He cupped his paws round his mouth, keeping a tight hold on the stem with his legs and tail, and called out "FENNY!" as loud as he could. Twice he repeated the cry, then both he and Twit climbed down.

"Should we wait fer the others?" asked Twit anxiously. Now he was on the ground the mist was up to his chest and writhed over him like a living thing. In the dark places of the field the mist looked deeper.

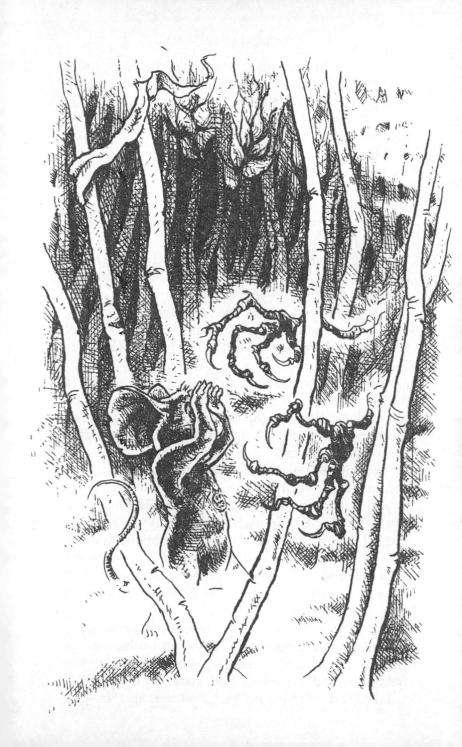

"No time," said Arthur firmly, "come on."

They left the corridor path and plunged into the wild places of the field.

"Is it Hodge's murderer, do you think?" asked Twit quietly.

"Might be," answered Arthur gravely. "We should have brought a stick or something just in case."

"Here," Twit pressed a stout staff into Arthur's chubby paw. "Thought they might come in handy," he explained.

"Good thinking," praised Arthur, greatly cheered. "The two of us should be able to handle whoever it is."

"Or whatever," added Twit timidly.

Arthur gulped. "Well," he said, trying to sound brave, "we've fought off a band of bloodthirsty rats before now."

"Yes, but there was five of us then and only three of them," observed Twit glumly. Arthur brandished his stick before him like a sword, cutting through the dense mist only to have the gaps fill up again thicker than before.

"We'll be all right," he said aloud, but his feigned confidence fooled no-one. "Just don't think of anything frightening, Twit. What would old Triton say if he could hear us, eh? Something like 'Lily-livered land lubbers' I bet. And what about Kempe? Why don't we sing one of his bawdy songs to make us feel better and get rid of all this gloom?" Arthur cleared his throat. "Rosie, poor Rosie . . . why aren't you singing, Twit? Twit?"

Arthur spun round, but his friend was gone. Only the mist met his gaze and closed in on him. From far away – or so it seemed, he heard the little fieldmouse call his name anxiously.

Twit had stumbled over a stone and in that

instant had lost his friend. The mist poured in around him and he was alone.

"Arthur!" he shouted meekly. "Where are you, Arthur?" But the fog swallowed his tiny voice greedily. His cries dwindled to murmurs and then into silence. Twit was afraid. The stick he held trembled in his paws as he tried to make his way through the corn. He was totally lost. For all he knew he was going round in futile circles. Then he began to hear the noises.

The fieldmouse paused and waved the stick about him in a frenzy. "There . . . there's five of us here matey, so clear off sharp!"

The stems crackled and snapped to his right. He ducked and darted off to the left. Now it was in front of him, rustling and scraping, coming ever closer. It was going to get him – to murder him as it had done with Hodge. Twit turned to flee again, but the noise seemed to be all round him now. His courage left him and he stood still and howled sadly, "Please no!" but the thick milky mist muffled his voice.

Long twig-like fingers emerged out of the fog like ghosts. Twit tried to fend them off but it was all in vain. A plaited loop was pulled over his ears and caught him round the neck.

"EEEK! HELP! FENNY!" he squawked as the loop began to tighten and strangle him.

"Help . . . Fenny . . . Help . . ." Twit choked on each word and scrabbled at his throat. It was no use. The loop continued to throttle him and Twit fell senseless to the ground.

"Twit!" bawled Arthur smashing through the stems. "Twit!" He thrashed the air with his stick but could see no-one. The fiend had slipped silently away.

"Twit," moaned Arthur as he knelt by his friend's

side. "Oh Twit, don't be dead." He cradled his friend's head in his paws and listened for a heart beat.

A faint murmur fluttered in Twit's chest, and Arthur wept. Slowly, the mist began to disperse.

Gradually Twit came to. His breathing was laboured and he touched his neck tenderly. There were big black bruises forming all round his throat. He grinned at Arthur shakily.

"Reckoned I were a goner then, Art," he croaked.

"You'll be fine now," assured Arthur. "We ought to get out of here while we can. Look, the mist's thinning." He helped Twit to his feet and they staggered off.

"Did you see who it was?" asked Arthur, curiously.

Twit shook his head slowly. "No Art . . . but it were uncanny. All I saw was something that looked . . . looked as if it were made totally out of straw."

12

HUNTERS IN THE NIGHT

When Arthur and Twit hobbled into the Hall of Corn, they found a throng of mice waiting for them. The Fennywolders had heard Arthur's alarm call but had had no idea where to go, so they had assembled in the Hall and waited.

Arthur breathlessly explained what had happened to him and Twit, and Mrs Scuttle hurried over to help her son.

The fieldmice shook their heads, stunned that this could happen again. Mr Woodruffe stepped onto the throne and raised his staff for silence.

"Now we know," he declared, "the creature – whatever it is, is still at large. We must search the field once more."

As the fieldmice went to find weapons, Mr Nep came rushing out of his nest with a pale, frightened face. "My son," he cried, "my son has gone."

"Has anyone seen Young Whortle?" asked Mr Woodruffe grimly. All the fieldmice shook their heads and a chill entered the Hall. "Then we must look for him also," he said, "and let us hope he has only gone exploring again."

A large party of strong husbands set off through the field, wielding sticks and cudgels. Arthur was too tired to join them – he had been up all night and desperately wanted some sleep. He even declined the offer of breakfast.

A group of wives who had been left behind chatted together dismally and clutched at their mousebrasses. All were fearful.

Suddenly one small child asked its mother, "Are we all going to die, Mam?" Nobody answered. But the tension was broken and a hysterical mousewife burst out, "Who is doing these things? What have we done to deserve this?"

Just then, Mr Nettle came into the Hall followed by Jenkin. "Perhaps the villain is amongst us!" he shouted above the hubbub.

This was too much for the worried mice. A ripple ran through them, and they looked at their neighbours suspiciously. Why, it might be any one of them.

"What do you mean, Nettle?" asked Mr Woodruffe sternly.

"All I say is that though ye search ye will find nought. Maybe the foul one is one of our folk, play-acting behind a fair mask."

The crowd stirred uneasily and murmured to each other.

"Now just wait a moment," said Mr Woodruffe. He feared that something nasty could happen if Isaac was allowed to go any further. He did not want the fieldmice to be at odds with one another. "You're talking out of your hat, Nettle," he said. "We were all at the ditch with Madame Akkykookoo when this happened, so it can't be any of us."

The crowd sighed with relief.

Isaac Nettle shook his head and gazed upwards. "Were we all present, I wonder?" he said loudly.

Everyone followed his glance and the murmurs

began again. There, climbing out of her nest, was Audrey.

"I think perhaps one was not with us," uttered Isaac darkly.

Arthur sprang forward in spite of his fatigue. He saw what Mr Nettle was driving at. "Rubbish!" he growled angrily. "Not even you believe that."

Mr Nettle's face was stony and the crowd's mutterings grew louder.

Jenkin stepped up to his father. "Dad," he pleaded, "you know Miss Brown's not to blame."

Isaac turned on his son and struck him violently across the face. "What dost thou know of yon painted sinner?" he bellowed, but Jenkin merely glared back at him with a face full of anger, then turned and walked away.

Isaac strode after his son.

"Listen to me all of you!" boomed Mr Woodruffe, commanding their attention again.

"If there are any among you who are foolish enough to listen to old Nettle's rantings then I warn you now. There are stiff penalties for those who disobey the King of the Field. Let none of you lay a paw on our guests from the town. Now go about your business or wait for your husbands to return; only clear the Hall."

The crowd shuffled away grumbling and whispering.

Audrey had watched all this curiously. She had not the faintest idea of what was going on but caught several hostile glances aimed at her from the crowd. The fieldmice moved away from her when she passed them as though terrified of what she might do to them. She quickly made her way to the throne and asked Arthur, "What's going on? What's happened?" Quickly Arthur told her about the creature that had tried to choke Twit.

"Arthur," she said when she had made sure that Twit was all right, "I don't like it here – these mice don't like me. They think I'm some sort of devil – and quite frankly they give me the shivers too. You wouldn't believe some of the stares they were giving me then. I felt as if they would tear me apart given half a chance."

Mr Woodruffe put his arm around her shoulder. "Now lass, don't you fret none. They're a friendly lot in Fennywolde really. It's just that right now they're scared, what with the weather and Hodge's murder and now poor Twit this morning. They need to feel safe, and if that means they have to stick the blame on some outsider then that's what they'll try and do. Don't worry though, I'll not let them – I've a cooler head than most, but it's a tricky job with old Isaac sticking his tuppence in. He knows how to get them riled, he do, and it's a shame, but he don't like you, and once he's got summat in his mulish bonce that's that."

Audrey was not comforted. The day was another scorcher but she stayed away from the still pool for fear of confrontations. Instead, she helped Mrs Scuttle with small tasks and jobs that did not really need to be done, but it kept her busy and out of folk's way.

Arthur and Twit slept all day so Audrey had no-one of her own age to talk to. She felt bored and lonely, and the Hall of Corn began to feel like a jail. Once she spotted Iris Crowfoot carrying a bowl of water for her mother. Audrey waved but Mrs Crowfoot scolded her daughter for daring to smile back. How could anyone think that she was connected with the murder of Hodge? It was too ridiculous for words! Audrey would have laughed at their silliness if she was not so worried and afraid.

*　　　*　　　*

Alison Sedge sat in the meadow weaving a necklace of forget-me-knots. As she worked, she mulled over her suspicions. She hated Audrey with all her heart. She wished that Mr Nettle had struck her instead of Jenkin – Alison would like to see Audrey's lip swell up like a blackberry. That would spoil her fairy looks! She cursed the ill-fortune which had brought the town mouse to her field – just when she was having a bit of fun with the boys too. It had been a good start to the summer, she had been admired by everyone, and had flirted with everyone.

Suddenly Alison shuddered. A horrible thought occurred to her. One of her suitors now lay under the earth: if she had been nicer to him on that fateful day would Hodge still be alive now? Young Whortle was missing as well – she hoped he was safe. If things got any worse there would be no boys left for her to flirt with.

The meadow grass rustled close by. Alison sprang to her feet and backed away nervously.

"Who's there?" she asked.

"Oh, is that you, Alison Sedge?" It was Jenkin's voice and he sounded none too happy at meeting her.

Quickly Alison sat down again and struck her most casual and alluring pose. "Over here Jolly Jenkin," she invited huskily.

He came into sight through the silvery flowering grasses, and Alison beckoned him over. His eye was purple and the lip was bleeding again.

"Oh Jenkin," she cried in alarm. "You look awful, this is a real baddun this time. You rest there," she added kindly. "I'll go fetch some water to bathe that eye in."

But Jenkin wouldn't have it. "I'll be aright in a

bit," he explained.

"Is it very sore?" she asked. His eye was an angry bluey purple and she could actually see the lip throbbing. Alison wanted to throw her arms about him and make it all better. This was what she wanted, and at that moment she realised that all her flirting had simply been a waste of time. Time that should have been spent with Jenkin.

"Oh Jenkin," she said moving closer, "Your dad's horrible to you – p'raps it's time you left him an' built a nest of your own in the Hall."

With his good eye Jenkin regarded Alison coolly. Her creamy hair brushed against his arm and her breath smelt of wild strawberries. There had been a time – not long ago, when he had prayed for her to be near him like this, but not now. He stood up and moved away.

"Were my fault these," he said meaning his bruises. "I oughtn't a mentioned Miss Brown – my dad don't like her."

Alison was slightly vexed. He had interrupted her just as she was about to kiss him. "I don't like her either," she snapped. "She ain't right in the head an' I think she's got summat to do with Hodge."

"Pah," snorted Jenkin, "you'm just jealous. Not even my dad really believed that rubbish, he just said it to make her look bad."

"But Jenkin," protested Alison. "She told me, she said that she'd choke anyone what got in her way."

"Shut it Alison, don't bother." Jenkin turned and looked away. "Y'see," he confessed shyly, "I likes Miss Brown a heck of a lot and nothing you can say will change that."

He left Alison on her own. She twisted her fingers round the necklace she had just made and tore it off. In a cascade of tiny blue petals Alison Sedge wept bitterly to herself.

*　　*　　*

Audrey lay in her nest staring at the starry sky. Everyone had gone to bed – everyone except for Arthur and the other night sentries. Twit was not allowed to join them till he was fully recovered. His throat was still sore and his voice was hoarse and croaky.

Audrey wondered how much longer she could go on living in Fennywolde if the hostile atmosphere continued. Her job as companion to Madame Akkikuyu was more or less over now – she had only seen the rat briefly that day at lunch but she was so popular with everyone that they had only said a few words before someone grabbed the rat and invited her to join them.

There was one thing that really puzzled Audrey. Madame Akkikuyu looked different. For some time she had not been able to put her finger on what it was. Then she realised. The fortune-teller was no longer black – her fur was changing colour! Now she was a sleek chestnut and it seemed to get lighter with every day. It was most peculiar, but the Fennywolders believed that it was the country air and sunshine that was the cause.

Madame Akkikuyu certainly looked very different to the pathetic creature Audrey had seen in the Starwife's chamber. She had grown strong and if not fat then well-padded.

Her thoughts were interrupted by a small, polite voice whispering under the nest entrance.

"Miss Brown," it said.

"Who is it?" she whispered back.

"It's me – Jenkin."

"Oh," Audrey was surprised, "what do you want?"

"To talk to you – meet me down here when you're ready."

Quickly she pulled on her clothes and tied up her hair with her best ribbon. What could Jenkin want at this time of night? It had to be very important. She climbed down the ladder and stood before him. Even in the pale moonlight she could see the marks left by his father's hard paw.

His eyes lit up when he saw her. "You always do look nice," he said.

"Thank you," she blushed. "What is it you want?"

Jenkin looked round furtively. "I can't tell 'ee here," he said shyly. "Can we go somewhere a bit private-like?"

"Yes, all right," she consented, extremely curious. Jenkin led her out of the Hall of Corn by a small side entrance, taking care that the sentries did not see them.

"Why all this secrecy?" she asked him.

"My dad's forbid me to see you," came the reply in a hushed voice." He says you're a town heathen who don't know good from bad."

Audrey felt that there was quite a lot she could say about Mr Nettle but for once she held her tongue and let Jenkin continue.

"He tells me you ain't worth a crumb, that you're wicked all through an' that since you've come here we ain't had nowt but misery an' death."

This was quite enough! Audrey felt herself near to exploding. "If that's all you've got to tell me I might as well go back now. I've got a brother who can tell me all that and more besides, thank you very much. In fact, if I don't go now you'll find yourself with another black eye."

To her astonishment he laughed. Not an unkind, mocking laugh, but a gentle good-humoured chuckle. "Reckon you could do it too," he said. "But don't go yet – not till I've had my say. Look, we're all right here now. There ain't no-one to listen."

The moonlight fell on his fine hair, and for the first time Audrey noticed that he had combed it. He swallowed hard and began.

"I told you what my dad thinks," he lumbered on awkwardly, "cos that don't matter to me no more. I'm never goin' back to him or our winter quarters – I've left."

"Good for you Jenkin," said Audrey, not yet seeing what he was driving at. Was that berrybrew she could smell on his breath?

"Tomorrow I shall start a-buildin' a nest round the Hall," he told her proudly, the stars sparkling in his round, excited eyes. "What I'm sayin', Miss Brown – Audrey is . . . well, I'd like you to share that nest with me. Cos I loves you and wants . . . to wed you . . ." He stared at her hopefully, then uttered something under his breath, "Darn I forgot!" and quickly he knelt down on one knee. "You don't have to answer straight away like – think it over."

Audrey was bewildered. A proposal of marriage was the last thing she had expected and it took some time for it to properly sink in.

"You really want to marry me?" she sounded shocked and slightly amused.

"More than anything – that's the Green honest truth." He watched her intently with wide, trusting eyes like a baby.

Audrey's heart went out to him. The plain truth was that she did not love him, but a strong desire to see Piccadilly again grew in her.

She knelt down beside Jenkin and took his paw in hers. "Oh Jenkin," she said slowly, "I'm sorry, I don't want to hurt your feelings but I can't accept. I'm extremely flattered but no – you see I now know that I love another. I never realised it before."

Jenkin hung his head. Audrey felt so sorry for him but she remembered the Eve of Midsummer and knew that Alison was meant for him.

"There is someone who cares for you very much," she said, trying to break through his barrier of sullen silence.

"Who's that then?" he asked miserably.

"Alison Sedge," Audrey replied and she squeezed his paw tightly.

"Tuh," sniffed Jenkin, "she don't care for no-one but herself," he answered thickly.

"Was she always like that?"

"No – there was a time when me an' Alison went around together quite a bit but then she got her mousebrass an' everything changed."

"Then it can change again, Jenkin," urged Audrey, "forget about me – I'm just getting in the way of the two of you. I know that you and she are meant for one another. Truly."

There was such a ring of certainty in her voice that Jenkin looked up at her and for a second caught a flash of green fire flicker in her eyes.

He gasped and Audrey kissed his cheek. "You just wait," she said, "you'll be the one giving her the run around, only don't make her suffer too much – I've already made that mistake."

"Have I made a fool of myself?" asked Jenkin bashfully.

Audrey smiled. "Not at all – it's nice to know that not everyone in Fennywolde thinks I'm a monster." But as she said it the hairs on the back of her neck tingled.

Suddenly the corn stems were thrust aside and something crashed towards them.

Audrey could not believe her eyes and Jenkin fell back in fear. The corn dolly she had made was lurching towards them! No longer was it the trim, neat figure she had woven but a mass of tangled, twisted stems – bent with hatred and evil spells. The arms which had been pretty corn ears had grown long and wild with spiky fingers which clutched at the air greedily and waved around full of menace.

The nightmare figure staggered towards them, its twiggy fingers outstretched, ready to catch them.

Jenkin acted quickly.

He grabbed Audrey's paw and dragged her away just in time. "Come on!" he yelled.

Audrey snapped out of her trance and they stumbled off through the field, the figure pursuing them closely. It scraped its untidy skirt over the stony ground and flayed the air with its thin arms, groping for them. Its plaited loop head twisted from side to side, seeming to sense rather than see where it was going.

Jenkin and Audrey ran in blind terror with the papery crackling sound rustling close behind. She slipped and quick straw fingers grasped at her heels. "Aaarh!" she squealed as they dragged her back and the figure loomed over her, lowering its plaited loop purposefully.

Jenkin beat the straw with his fists and the fingers released Audrey and grabbed him. The loop slipped over his head but he ducked and nipped off with Audrey.

"Not far to go till we're out of the field," he called to her, "then we should be able to go faster."

Audrey leapt over stones and dodged the stems which blocked her path. Her tail bells jangled wildly as the clutching fingers searched for her hungrily.

"Quick Audrey, hurry!" Jenkin had reached the edge of the field and turned round to help her.

She glanced over her shoulder and cried out. The corn dolly bore down on her, sweeping over the stony ground at a terrific speed. It raised its spindly arms and brought them knifing down.

Audrey felt herself yanked backwards. Jenkin had hold of her and he carried her clear of the field.

"Look Jenkin," she gasped, "it isn't following us."

Jenkin put her down and stared back. The corn dolly remained within the confines of the field, its arms upraised.

"Why isn't it chasing us?" asked Jenkin nervously.

"Maybe it can only live in the field," suggested Audrey. "Perhaps it needs to be amongst the growing corn to come alive."

"It's horrible," said Jenkin shivering. He frowned; the thing seemed to be waiting for something to happen. It reared back the loop head as though sensing another presence. Jenkin moved his eyes from the straw figure, up to the tops of the dark elms and out into the starry sky . . .

"Get down," he yelled and roughly pushed Audrey to the ground. It was too late to save himself.

A pale, silent ghost slipped out of the night sky and snatched him up. Jenkin squeaked in pain as Mahooot scooped him up in his vicious talons. He saw the ground disappear below him and heard the owl cackle to itself wickedly.

"Foood, foood, lovely mooouses."

Audrey saw the owl swoop into the darkness over the meadow and heard Jenkin's frightened voice fade away.

Then Audrey screamed.

The corn dolly rustled its pleasure and slunk back into the shadowy cover of the field.

On sentry, Arthur recognised his sister's voice and soon everyone in Fennywolde was awake and lighting torches. They ran in a blazing line to see why she was making that fearful noise.

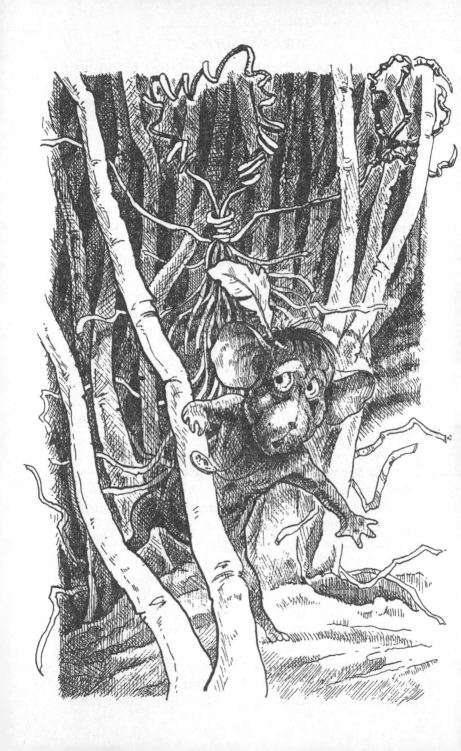

Audrey was on her knees when they found her, staring across the meadow with big dark eyes that were dreadful to look on. Arthur shook her to stop the piercing screams.

"What is it Aud?" he asked wildly.

Without seeing him she pointed out into the sky and said weakly, "The owl! The owl has got Jenkin."

The fieldmice cried out in dismay, but from their midst, one figure stepped forward into the circle of torchlight. It was Jenkin's father. None dared look at him. His face trembled with emotion and his lips turned white.

"Jenkin lad," he said, sounding as if he had been stabbed. He turned on Audrey and his eyes burned at her accusingly. He raised a quivering finger and pointed. "You have done this, you!"

Before she could reply, out of the crowd stepped Madame Akkikuyu. The rat took a torch from one of the fieldmice and held it above her head.

"So," she shouted and all looked to her. "Mousey boy got by owly. What you do?"

"What can we do?" asked Arthur bitterly.

"Go fight the mangy bird!" she cried, whirling the torch around. "Come mouseys, we go to save him!"

The fieldmice cheered her as she led them down the banks of the ditch like a general. Mr Nettle followed like a sleep walker.

Arthur and Audrey were joined by the Scuttles. "Arthur," Audrey whispered to her brother, "Jenkin and I were chased out here by a terrible thing! It was . . . it was my own corn dolly, Arthur! It must have killed Hodge! It tried to kill us too! What can I do?"

Arthur gulped. There was no use doubting her. Twit had been attacked by something made of straw that morning. "Look," he said, "don't mention this to anyone yet – you're in enough trouble already. What do you think they'll do if they find out your figure has come to life and murders people?"

They hurried after the lights of the rescue party. Twit took Audrey's paw and patted it.

In the empty glade near the field only one mouse was left. It was Alison Sedge. She watched the torchlight dwindle in the distance and shook her head. Her sobs were silent and her heart broken. She ripped off her mousebrass and flung it away.

*   *   *

Madame Akkikuyu led the fieldmice through the dark meadow. She whooped and shouted challenges to the owl and the fieldmice took heart at her courage. They came to the oak trees and the rat thrust her torch into the earth.

"Stay here mouseys," she told them. "I go to hooty!"

"Find my boy!" begged Mr Nettle.

"Kill the owl," chanted the fieldmice, and Arthur and Twit were alarmed to hear them. They spoke, not as individuals but as a great, many-headed creature with a hundred fiery eyes eager for blood. Only Twit's parents and Mr Woodruffe did not join in. They hung back and put their paws to their mouths fearfully.

Madame Akkikuyu began to climb the tree. It was easy for her. Her claws sank into the soft bark and she ascended swiftly.

"I get you hooty," she snarled angrily. "I tell you leave my mouseys be."

She pulled herself up to the hole in the trunk and announced herself.

"Hooty. Akkikuyu here again."

"Whooo?" came a hollow voice.

"Akkikuyu – the owl rider and neck plucker. I

have mattress need stuffing!" she laughed and pulled the bone from her hair.

Sounds of agitated scrabbling issued from the black recess. Mahooot was trapped and he knew it.

"Ha!" bawled Akkikuyu, springing across the threshold and stabbing the bone in front of her.

Mahooot had been lying in wait for her, intending to bite her head off as soon as it poked through the hole in the tree trunk. He darted forward, but she brought the bone crashing down on his open beak. It crunched and chipped, and Mahooot hooted in agony.

In a foul temper he shot out a deadly talon and snapped it tight around the fortune-teller's neck. She wailed in surprise and dropped the bone as he dragged her into the darkness.

"Not so fast hooty," she yelled and kicked the owl in the stomach.

"Oooof!" moaned Mahooot as the air rushed out of him and he collapsed wheezing on the floor.

Madame Akkikuyu shrieked with laughter and disentangled herself from his clutches.

She retrieved her bone and brought it smashing down on the talon that had gripped her. The sharp claws splintered into a thousand bits.

Mahooot roared in his pain and Madame Akkikuyu crowed with delight. Then she dealt the other foot a devastating blow and danced about.

The owl lunged at her in a mad rage. He knocked her off balance, so that she stumbled and fell backwards. Then Mahooot beat her down with his powerful wings until she was overwhelmed by his feathery bulk. His body crushed her and he bent his flat head to nip with his damaged beak. He pulled out a quantity of her thick hair until Madame Akkikuyu squawked shrilly. That was it! This owl was getting above itself.

"Enough hooty," she said, spitting feathers out of her mouth.

Mahooot cackled and continued to squash her. She thrashed her tail from left to right so he bit it and the blood oozed out. Madame Akkikuyu gnashed her teeth. He had gone too far.

"Dooown yooou doxsie!" he hooted, revelling in her suffering. "Mahooot is yooour dooom!"

Madame Akkikuyu blew a muffled raspberry underneath him and managed to pull an arm loose. With one swipe she punched Mahooot savagely under his beak. He staggered backwards and she was free.

Nimbly she stepped out of the dark hole and ran along the branch outside.

"Nyer nyer," she taunted him, waggling her bottom at the hole. "Come out hooty, Akkikuyu thrash you good an' proper."

In a cloud of soft white feathers Mahooot left the hole. He spread out his enormous wings and reared himself up to a towering height.

"Die!" he boomed in a chilling voice.

"Oho," chuckled the fortune-teller, "not yet owly, Akkikuyu not ready to snuff candle – you play her game now." She slipped her claw swiftly into the bag slung over her shoulder and pulled out a small cloth pouch.

Mahooot made a ravaging dive at her. The rat flung the pouch at him and a poisonous concoction exploded in his face.

She smartly stepped to one side as Mahooot floundered past. His eyes were stinging and he could not see. The smell of burnt feathers fouled the air.

"Ooow!" he screeched in panic as he fumbled along the branch on his broken talons. "Mahooot is blind, ooow."

Madame Akkikuyu poked and teased him mischievously, until he could bear this monstrous rat-woman no longer. The owl flapped his wings and rose shakily into the air.

The fortune-teller let him go unmolested.

Mahooot spiralled round, unable to see where he was going. Then with a dull thud which smashed more of his beak he flew into a tree trunk. Mahooot fell to the ground bouncing off the branches.

"A fine sight to see," said a voice in the fortune-teller's ear. "What a heroine you are. The darling of Fennywolde."

"Nico," she welcomed, "I thought you not come tonight."

"I have been busy elsewhere," said Nicodemus, "but come, we must talk, you and I, for it is time you learnt of the spell which will release me."

"Wait," said Madame Akkikuyu as she remembered Jenkin, "I have mousey to find."

"The lad is dead!" said Nicodemus coldly. "Now step into the owl's hole Akkikuyu and I shall tell you what must be done."

* * *

As Mahooot came crashing down out of the high branches the fieldmice who were waiting below cheered wildly and rushed forward.

"Stop, wait!" ordered Mr Woodruffe but they surged past him like a river and began to hurl stones at the dazed owl and beat it with their sticks.

"This is obscene," shouted the King of the Field. But they did not hear him. They only heard the gasps and cries of Mahooot as they tore at him.

"They've gone mad," said Arthur appalled.

Mr Woodruffe turned and hid his head in disgust, then threw down his staff of office. "They will not listen to me any more and I want nothing more to do with them. They are not mice tonight – they are the nastiest kind of rats."

"It's far worse than it ever was at home," said Audrey. They walked away with Mr and Mrs Scuttle. Fennywolde had become an evil place to live.

*　　　*　　　*

In the owl's nest Madame Akkikuyu listened as Nicodemus began.

"It is a mighty spell which we dare to attempt Akkikuyu," he said. "Are you brave enough for it?"

"Yes Nico."

"Then this is what we need. You must build a fire and feed it with the herbs I shall tell you to gather. Around this fire you must say the words of release and cast into the flame a mousebrass."

"A mousebrass Nico – why so?"

"All this shall become clear to you, yet it must be a special mousebrass, it must be made in hatred and be a sign of destruction and death."

"Where I get such a dangler?"

"That also I shall tell you. All has been arranged. Wheels have been set in motion Akkikuyu, and the time for the ritual is soon. At the time of the ceremony however I must be protected from the heat of the fire for I shall be vulnerable for a while. I must project my essence to a place of safety. Look in your bag – there you will find a vessel suitable for me."

Akkikuyu rummaged around inside her bag until she found what Nicodemus meant.

"You mean this, great one," she muttered, reluctantly taking out her most prized possession. The moonlight curved lovingly over the smooth glass ball that the fortune-teller had brought with her from Deptford.

"Excellent," he crooned delightedly. "That is most suitable! Have it with you at the fire's edge – only remember Akkikuyu, that once the spell is complete you must smash your prize to release me. I do not want to spend another age imprisoned in there."

"I promise Nico," she said with regret as she stroked her beautiful crystal ball.

"And one more thing, Akkikuyu. There must be an exchange of souls or the spell will be useless."

The fortune-teller trembled. "Souls? What am I to do this time?"

"There must be a sacrifice to the flame," Nicodemus whispered. "My essence will cross over to your world, and a soul must cross back in return. We must cast into the fire one who is not protected by a mousebrass."

"Who you think of?" she asked warily.

The reply was snarled back at her: "The one who has abandoned you, Akkikuyu, the one who spurned your friendship and tried to make a fool of you in front of everyone."

"No," cried the rat in dismay.

"Yes!" hissed Nicodemus. "She is unfettered by the Greenlaws and bound to no-one. It must be her. You are sworn to obey me – throw Audrey Brown into the fire!"

"Mouselet!" Akkikuyu wailed miserably.

13

A WITCH AND
A FOOL

The sun rose over Fennywolde to announce yet another feverish day.

Twit rose and leant out of his and Arthur's nest. The Hall of Corn was unusually quiet – but not calm. He could almost feel dark forces surging through the field like evil water and a half-forgotten memory awakened in him.

"Blow me," he said to himself.

Behind him, in the sweet mossy darkness, Arthur's drowsy voice mumbled, "What is it?"

The fieldmouse scratched his head and said, "I just remembered summat, Art."

"If it's about last night I don't want to know," came the weary reply.

"Well it has summat to do wi' last night," admitted the fieldmouse, "but really I was just thinkin' of those bats back in Deptford."

"Oh, Orfeo and . . . who was it?"

"Eldritch."

"That's right – what made you think of them?"

"Well, when they took me a-flyin' through the roof an' into the sky they showed me some wild critters – they were 'orrible and mindless. I only just recalled that Orfeo askin' me if there were any of the – how did he put it – any of this 'untame breed' in my field. I said as I didn't know of any."

"So?" Arthur was baffled. "What made you think of that now?"

Twit turned a worried face to his friend, "Don't you see Art? The bats knew. They was warnin' me!"

"What, against wild cats here?"

"No," said Twit gravely, "against my own folk here. Last night, Art, they weren't mice – Mr Woodruffe said so, they were just like that 'untame breed' in the city. Horrid beasts with no thought 'cept killin'. I'm afeared for Fennywolde. What'll happen next?"

*   *   *

Madame Akkikuyu looked down into the ditch and prepared herself. Her task today was not pleasant, but she had sworn on her soul to obey Nicodemus. She mopped her brow with a corner of her shawl and set her jaw determinedly. She hated the idea of what she had to do, but Nicodemus would not be pleased with her if she failed him today.

She marched from the edge and strode to the elm trees where she hoped to find Mr Nettle. A mousebrass was needed and he was the only one who could make it. Her problem would be persuading him.

Isaac Nettle, grim and steely-eyed, was hammering a piece of metal in his forge. The ruddy glow of the forge fire shone on his fur and glinted off his drooping whiskers. But that was the only light in the gloomy place. Even in Isaac's heart there was darkness. Only grief and loss filled him. He pushed himself into his work passionately, smiting the red hot metal with his hammer, trying to blot out his sorrow with the effort. Fiery sparks flew and scorched his skin, but he was thankful for them. He wanted to feel pain and be punished: for Jenkin, the shining joy of his sour life was gone, plucked out of existence.

The ringing of his hammer was so loud that he did not hear the knocking at the door. He continued to beat the yellow metal till it was flattened, then, with a pair of tongs, he plunged it into a bucket of cold water. It was only when the steam had cleared that he noticed the ratwoman standing quietly by the door.

Madame Akkikuyu nodded at him. "Morning," she said.

Isaac grunted. He did not want to talk to anyone this day – or any other for that matter. He turned back to the fire and raked the embers together.

"I say morning," the fortune-teller repeated.

Isaac looked at her with unfriendly eyes. "Leave me!" he growled.

She shook her head. "You lose boy last night. You need talk – get it off bosom, Akkikuyu good listener, she hear your woe."

For a moment his face was impassive, but suddenly he broke down. Like a wall of glass his defences shattered. Mr Nettle wept openly.

"Jenkin, Jenkin, I've lost you, my son. I loved you and I never told you – not once."

Madame Akkikuyu took Mr Nettle in her arms and patted him gently on the back. "There, there," she soothed, "that right, let it out. Tell Akkikuyu."

"Oh Meg!" he cried. "Look after our boy, he's with you now."

"Meg?" asked Akkikuyu, "She your wife, yes?"

Isaac nodded feebly. "Meg died when Jenkin was born. I always blamed him for that – I loved her so. And now I've lost him too. I don't know what I'm going to do. I'm so sorry, lad, if you can hear me. Forgive your father!"

"Shhh," hushed Akkikuyu, pushing him gently

onto a stool, "in the great beyond all things are forgiven – he knows now."

Mr Nettle calmed down. When his last sniffs were over he thanked the rat shyly. "Verily, thou art a messenger from the Green, come in my darkest hour. And last night also – you did what no other dared, you tried to save my son. I thank thee for that. Truly thou art blessed!"

Madame Akkikuyu shrugged off these compliments, "Yes, I try, but was too late. What a shame your boy out last night. Why he not here safe with you?"

Isaac's face tightened and he became stern and grim once more. "It was the town mouse!" he spat bitterly. "It was she who lured my son away." He had forgotten now that it was his beatings which had driven Jenkin away from him.

"Aaahh yes," muttered the fortune-teller, "Miss Audrey! Tell me Nettley, why did your boy meet her last night outside the field? And why she not there when Hodge was found, and where is the other boy?"

Mr Nettle rose and scowled. "It is she!" he declared. "Ever since she came here there has been nought but pain and death! She has brought it!"

"Quite so," agreed Akkikuyu. "And tell me this! That mousey is of age, so why she no wear a mousey dangler?"

Mr Nettle looked at her wildly. He had never noticed that, and he the mousebrass maker. "She should have one," he gasped. "Every mouse receives a brass when they come of age."

Madame Akkikuyu rushed in with her explanation. "Maybe Green Mouse think she not worthy of such a gift."

"My Lord!" Isaac exclaimed staggering back. "Where were my wits? Why had I not thought of this? She must be evil indeed for the mighty Green to deem her unfit for a mousebrass. What manner of creature can she be?"

"A witch!" snapped Akkikuyu. "Why else your corn wither in the ground and mouseys die young? What black powers she brung to your fair field, Nettley?"

Isaac was incensed. "What can we do? We must confront her and cast her out."

"No," said the rat hastily. "We must pray to the Green, see what he thinks." She narrowed her eyes and peered at Isaac through their narrow black slits. "Maybe," she began, as though working out a plan, "maybe you should make a special mousey dangler that will bring ruin on the mouselet. Make it with curses and surely the Green will hear you."

Isaac looked doubtful. He took his position as mousebrass maker extremely seriously. He considered the suggestion but declined.

"I will not presume upon my Lord," he explained. "I will not anger him by making a brass of my own design. I must know it to be his will."

Madame Akkikuyu sighed, but there was one more trick up Nicodemus's sleeve. He had been prepared for Isaac's piety and had instructed her to take him to the owl tree and wait there.

"Nettley," she said, "it hot in here, I go for walk. Come join me, leave your danglers and talk with Akkikuyu."

Isaac was unwilling: others in Fennywolde might see him and he did not want that. As if she understood this, Madame Akkikuyu added, "We not go to Hall, we walk in meadow!" Mr Nettle agreed and he followed her out of the forge.

As they walked Madame Akkikuyu pointed out plants and reeled off their good – or bad qualities. Mr Nettle tried to listen and pay attention but his mind was elsewhere. Inside, he was seething. The thought of Audrey Brown, that odious town mouse who had wrought so much grief and harm inflamed him and his fingers itched for his hammer. What could be done with her? Her crimes were too great to go unpunished. If she was a witch then there was only one way to deal with her. He wondered if the Fennywolders would agree with him.

When Mr Nettle next looked up they had left the meadow and he drew a sharp breath. Madame Akkikuyu had steered him towards the oaks and the sight of them brought the pain of his loss back to him.

"Why are we here?" he questioned her with a faltering voice.

"Oh me!" said Akkikuyu, trying to sound shocked that she could have been so thoughtless and unsympathetic.

"Silly Akkikuyu – her head not screwed on today. Come Nettley we go from here." She moved back a few paces and observed Isaac keenly. He seemed to have seen something near one of the roots and he made no attempt to follow her.

"Look!" he said, "There's a shining thing over yonder. What can it be?"

Akkikuyu squinted in the direction he was pointing. The fierce light of the sun was reflecting off something down there. Isaac walked up to the great root cautiously.

"Oh no Nico," she breathed to herself, "not this – he suffer enough."

When Mr Nettle reached the great root he fell to his knees and shrieked. Madame Akkikuyu ran over to him and looked over his quaking shoulder.

There on the dusty ground was an owl pellet, one of those tight little bundles of fur and bones. Sticking out of it was Jenkin's mousebrass.

The sign of life blazed in the sunlight as Mr Nettle wrested it free of the pellet. Then he turned his face on the fortune-teller and cried, "I shall make that brass, and may eternal damnation fall on that town mouse. For every stroke of the hammer shall be a curse and malediction – may she suffer for the agony she has given to me and my son."

Madame Akkikuyu smiled soberly – Nicodemus would be pleased.

*   *   *

The morning passed and the afternoon crept up. The rings of Mr Nettle's hammer sang over Fennywolde.

The atmosphere in the Hall of Corn was terrible. Arguments broke out for the slightest reason. Old Todmore yelled at the children who were pestering him for a story and told them he had better things to do. One of the young boys kicked his stick and ran away.

"Come back 'ere Abel Madder," fumed Old Todmore, "I'll clout you one!"

Dimsel Bottom and Lily Clover were seen quarrelling and they had to be separated when plump Dimsel flew at her friend in a shocking fit of rage.

Josiah Down kicked the family nest to pieces while his wife called him a no good Cheddar head.

All this was watched in fearful silence by the Scuttles and their guests. They kept well away from the rest of the fieldmice and looked at one another in disbelief. What was happening to everybody?

Audrey decided to go to bed early that night. She sat in her hot nest with her knees tucked tight up under her chin. She was frightened. Several times that day she had heard her name mentioned in high, disapproving voices and when Mr Nep went by he actually spat on the ground when he saw her.

* * *

Alison Sedge was restless. She did not want to go to bed. All day she had lain in the shade by the still pool, thinking of Jenkin. She remembered their happy days together before she had received her mousebrass, but that was gone now and good riddance. She wore no flowers around her neck any more and had not once gazed at her reflection. Her hair was forgotten and neglected in two untidy plaits. She had not eaten all day.

Twilight came. Reluctantly, Alison picked herself up and ducked under the hawthorn branches. She passed over the ditch and entered the field. The corn was silent. No wind rustled its ears or rattled its stems. Their long black shadows fell on Alison like the bars of a prison. She became increasingly uneasy. The field was an eerie place. She had never noticed how impenetrable those dark shadows were before. Alison gulped nervously as she remembered the murderer that hid in here throttling unwary mice who wandered around alone. How could she be so stupid?

A noise startled her. The corn moved behind and a crackling rustle moved towards her.

Alison did not wait to look. She ran deeper into the field towards the Hall of Corn but the rustling grew louder. It was ahead of her now and she could see dim shapes before her. Alison wheeled round and sped back towards the ditch, missing the path in her haste.

Suddenly she tripped and stumbled. She put out her arms to save herself but landed on something soft.

Panting heavily Alison lifted her face – and stared into the blank eyes of Young Whortle. She had fallen on top of his discarded body. Alison leapt up and screamed at the top of her voice.

In the Hall of Corn the fieldmice were once more disturbed by the alarm call. What could be the cause this time?

They lit their torches and fled out of the great doors.

"What is it?" asked Audrey, as Twit slid down past her nest.

"Another alarm," he answered, "we must all go – come on Aud!"

They followed the other mice. Arthur had been on duty and slid down a corn stem as they ran by. "Wait for me!" he puffed.

The fieldmice ran along the ditch, fearing the worst. Had another tragedy occurred? Then, crashing out of the field came Alison Sedge. She ran to her mother's arms and squealed.

"It's Young Whortle – he's dead. I found his body in there."

Mr and Mrs Nep held onto each other for support. "Where is he?" cried Mr Nep, preparing to enter the field.

"No, don't go in there," shouted Alison, "there's something after me – it nearly got me."

The fieldmice made angry noises and lifted their torches high above their heads. "We must find it!" they declared. "We must put an end to this murder!"

Before any of them could move, there came a splintering and rustling sound. Out of the field, silhouetted against the sky, was the evil corn dolly.

Its looped head jerked from side to side as if it were sniffing the air. Then it began to advance stiffly towards them.

The fieldmice gasped and staggered back in horror.

"It's that doll thing!" some of them muttered. "How is it moving like that? It is bewitched."

Isaac Nettle came out of his quarters and beheld the scene with a mixture of horror and satisfaction. The straw figure was truly an abomination, yet surely now there would be no doubt that the town mouse was to blame for everything. Here was the proof of her witchcraft.

The corn demon marched awkwardly on and the mice fell back before it. Its wild arms were raised and its twiggy fingers twitched eagerly.

From the dark shadows near the ditch Madame Akkikuyu observed the scene with interest. "See how I let the mice do our work for us," whispered Nicodemus. "We shall see what they do with Miss Brown."

The demon struck out with its arms and caught hold of Dimsel Bottom. She squeaked with fright as it drew her near its lowered head.

Isaac raced up to the thing and dealt it a savage blow with his hammer. The corn dolly buckled as the hammer plunged into the straw but it reared itself up again immediately and with one powerful arm swept Mr Nettle off his feet and flung him to the ground.

"Save us Green Mouse!" he wailed.

The thing was unstoppable. It placed its head over Dimsel's and the plait began to tighten. Arthur rushed out and pulled the hideous thing off and Dimsel sped away.

The fieldmice were driven back terribly afraid. "Where is that town mouse?"some began to ask and the call was taken up by all of them. "Where is the town mouse? Where is the town mouse?"

At the rear, Audrey held Twit's paw in terror. Out of the crowd Mr Nep saw her and cried, "There she is. Bring her forward."

Feverish paws grabbed Audrey and pulled her away from Twit and the Scuttles. Through the mass she was dragged and shoved until she was pushed out in front of her creation.

Audrey could not escape. She tried to turn back but angry paws and bodies barred her way. Arthur tried to help her but found that his arms had been grabbed and the mice were holding on to him fiercely.

The corn dolly swept up to Audrey and lowered its head again. Audrey screamed, "Stop. Stop."

The figure jerked up quickly and lowered its arms. Then to her everlasting horror it bowed before her and fell lifeless to the ground.

The crowd stared at it with wide eyes and then Mr Nep said, "It obeyed her."

"Witch," hissed the mob, "witch, witch witch!" They circled round Audrey menacingly.

Try as he might, Arthur could not struggle free and at the back, Twit could not break through the crowd.

Isaac Nettle came striding forward booming, "The town mouse is a witch. She has insulted the Green Mouse by weaving idols, and conjured spirits to give life to her hellish work. Three of our folk have died because of her. What do we do with a witch?"

"Burn her," cried the crowd.

"No," whimpered Audrey as they tied her paws behind her back. "I'm not a witch!"

But her voice was drowned out by the cries of the angry mice.

Isaac picked up the motionless corn dolly and cast it down into the ditch. Then he hurled a blazing torch after it and the figure immediately burst into flames. The loop head blackened and withered into a wisp of oily smoke.

The fieldmice pushed Audrey to the edge of the ditch and the glowing ashes rose up and curled round her ankles.

"Burn, burn!" They repeated excitedly. Two strong husbands lifted her up and swung her out over the flames.

Madame Akkikuyu covered her face with her claws and trembled. Nicodemus laughed triumphantly. All was going wonderfully.

"STOP THIS!" Mr Woodruffe wrestled forward angrily. "You must all stop this!" He pulled Audrey out of the mice's paws and she clung tightly to him.

Isaac thundered in and whirled Mr Woodruffe round. "Go back to your nest Woodruffe. You are not our king now. Let us do what must be done. The witch must die!"

"But you can't burn her, Isaac. It's unspeakable!" He appealed to the crowd, "Surely you cannot have sunk so low to allow this. Never has a mouse been burned in Fennywolde. As for you, Nettle, I'm surprised. This has the smack of paganism in it."

The fieldmice looked anxiously at their leader. Mr Woodruffe was right, they had never burned a mouse before. "But what are we to do with her?" asked a frightened Mrs Nep.

Isaac snarled and yanked Audrey from Mr Woodruffe's grip. "Then she shall hang!" he proclaimed. "Let her choke, just as her creature choked Hodge and Young Whortle." He signalled to the crowd and they swarmed along the ditch, with him at their head and Audrey stumbling at his side.

"We've got to do something," said Arthur when his captors released him. "Will they really hang her, Mr Scuttle?"

"'Fraid so lad," he answered in dismay. Gladwin wrung her paws together.

"We're not done yet boy," said Mr Woodruffe. "Come on!" They ran after the angry crowd and

234

pushed their way through.

Twit remained behind. He had never felt so useless in all his life. He was too small to do anything useful. He wished that Thomas Triton was there – he would have shown these mice a thing or two with his sword. But the midshipmouse was not there and there were far too many fieldmice to fight against anyway. This needed a cool head and lots of wits. Twit, the simple country mouse, had neither. He was the one with "no cheese upstairs", the butt of every joke. Now the life of a friend was in danger and he could think of nothing to help.

Suddenly he gasped. "Could I?" he asked himself. "Would it work?" There was only one way to find out. He rushed forward.

At the yew tree a tight circle of mice had formed. In the centre were Mr Nettle and Audrey. Her wide eyes were rolling in terror and their whites were showing. A straw rope had been slung over the "hanging branch" and a noose had been tied in one end.

Mr Woodruffe barged in followed by Arthur. "This must not happen!" he cried. "Execution must only be as a result of a trial and only then if the accused is found guilty."

"We know she'm guilty," yelled Mr Nep. The crowd roared their agreement.

"This is against the Greenlaws!" continued Mr Woodruffe.

Isaac held out a trembling paw. "Thou knowest full well the respect and honour I hold for the mighty Green. I would not do this thing if the law did not permit. It is you who have forgotten the law, Woodruffe. Did not Fenny himself declare that all witches must be put to death?" The mob roared again and waved their torches. "Bind their paws so they may not interfere!" commanded Isaac.

Both Arthur's and Mr Woodruffe's paws were tightly bound and strong arms were clenched about their necks.

"No, no," wailed Arthur. "My sister's not a witch – believe me."

Madame Akkikuyu left her place of shadow and moved towards the yew. "Quickly Akkikuyu," said Nicodemus. "I must see! The girl must not die by hanging, she must be alive when the flame takes her. If you can cut her down before she is dead we may still be able to perform the spell. But hurry, and keep away from those torches, the heat of them is agony for me." The fortune-teller hurried forward, a confusion of loyalties whirling round her jumbled head.

Mr Nettle put the noose round Audrey's neck and pulled the knot down tightly. Then he took hold of the other end and began to draw it down. Arthur closed his eyes.

Yelps and squeals broke out of the crowd and the mice jumped as something bit and clawed its way through. It was Twit. He didn't care how he got past. He ran into the ring and before anyone could stop him he had slipped the rope from Audrey's throat.

"Leave her be!" roared Isaac, looming over him with his paw raised.

A smouldering green fire seemed to issue from Twit's eyes and Isaac faltered. "I come to claim her!" Twit shouted at the top of his voice. "I claim her in the name of the Green."

"How dare you blaspheme!" growled Mr Nettle. "She is for the noose."

"Do you forget your own laws, Nettle?" Twit barked back at him.

"What laws?"

"The law of the gallows," snarled Twit.

"The gallows law," repeated everyone in astonishment – surely Twit was not that stupid.

Mr Woodruffe reminded Isaac as he stood, searching his memory. "The gallows law runs thus," he said. "Any may invoke the law of the gallows – if a willing spouse can be found beneath the hanging tree then the accused, whatever the crime, will be reprieved."

"A spouse!" mocked Isaac. "Who would marry a witch?"

"I will," said Twit proudly. "I invoke the law and offer my paw in marriage to Audrey Brown."

The crowd rippled in discontent and Nicodemus hissed in Madame Akkikuyu's ear.

"No! The girl must not marry – it will bind her up in the Greenlaws and she shall be useless to me. Stop this now."

The fortune-teller entered the circle, but instead of obeying Nicodemus she said, "Mousey must marry – follow the law of your Green. Join the two before you feel his anger." In the centre of all the fieldmice the tattoo dared not move on her ear but it glared at her venomously.

"Imbecile!" it whispered harshly.

Isaac stared at the rat in disbelief. He had made a brass for the destruction of Audrey at her request. Why was she changing sides now? "But she is to blame!" he said blankly. "Are you telling me now that she must go free?"

"She must, it is the law!" demanded Twit. "I call on the Green Mouse to witness all that goes on here. He shall know who disobeys him."

The crowd murmured. There was no getting away from it. If Twit married Audrey then she could not be hanged.

"No," cried Mr Nep as he sensed their doubt. "We cannot let her go unpunished. My son is dead."

It was Isaac who answered him. "Silence Nep. The way has been shown, though it grieves me no less than you. We must obey the law or we ourselves are guilty. But hear me, tomorrow we shall drive Twit and the witch to our borders and banish them. Then if any find them crossing our lands they have the right to do with them as they see fit. They are outcasts." He turned back to Twit and Audrey.

"Now, take the witch's paw in yours, William Scuttle," said Mr Nettle.

Twit looked at her. She was much calmer now and she stared back at him with gratitude. "Do you mean to go through with it?" she asked him.

"If'n I don't marry 'ee Aud they'll lynch yer," he replied.

"I don't know what to say," Audrey mumbled.

"Just say 'yes' an' save yer neck," advised Twit.

"Kneel ye," ordered Isaac, "and humble thyselves before the Green Mouse." Audrey felt someone cut the ropes which bit into her wrists and she dropped to her knees beside Twit.

"Dost thou, William Scuttle, take unto thyself this mouse, Audrey Brown? To cherish through the winter and revel with in the summer? Forswearing all others until the grass grows green over you both?"

"I does," said Twit.

"Who blesses the husband?" asked Isaac. It was usual at mouse weddings for both the bride and groom to receive a blessing. This could not come from their families. It was usually friends who performed the task, but at this torchlit marriage everyone wondered who would dare bless the union of a witch and a fool.

"I do," said a solemn voice and Mr Woodruffe shook off his guards. He wriggled his paws free of the ropes and stood before Twit.

"May the Green bless and protect you," he said with feeling and he placed his right paw on Twit's shoulder.

"Thank 'ee," replied Twit gratefully.

Then it was Audrey's turn.

"Dost thou, Audrey Brown," intoned Isaac bitterly, "take unto thyself this mouse William Scuttle? To cherish through the winter and revel with in the summer? Forswearing all others until the grass grows green over you both?"

Audrey tearfully thought of Piccadilly. Sobbing she uttered, "I do."

"Who blesses the wife?" Isaac looked around. No-one said anything. He smiled. There might be a hanging yet, for no marriage was complete without the two blessings, and he who blessed the groom could not bless the bride as well.

Arthur gazed at the fieldmice pleadingly. "Please, someone, anyone, don't let Audrey die." But the mice shuffled their feet and hung their heads.

Isaac chuckled and was about to pronounce the ceremony void when a figure stepped up to Audrey.

"I bless mouselet!" declared Madame Akkikuyu. Isaac glared at her but the fortune-teller came and knelt before her friend and said tenderly, "May his mighty Greenness bless and protect you for always, and may you forgive Akkikuyu. Remember that she love you and want you to be happy in summer light – it's all I ever wanted, my mouselet." She leaned over to kiss Audrey's forehead.

"Thank you," she wept.

A big tear streaked down Akkikuyu's nose. "Ach! I always blub at weddings."

Isaac concluded the ceremony.

"May the Mighty Green join these two together, through winter, harvest, youth and age. Let no creature come between them for now they are under the Green's great mantle." He sucked his teeth and said, "Rise Scuttle and Scuttle."

"You better be gone before midday tomorrow," shouted Mr Nep, "or I swear I'll hurl you both into the fire myself. The crowd began to disperse, and drift back into the field.

Twit's parents rushed forward and hugged their son and daughter in law. Gladwin was tearful, but Elijah was proud. "There's another Mr and Mrs Scuttle round here now," he beamed.

"Not for long though Dad," said Twit. "Aud may be my wife but I don't 'spect her to stay wi' me." He turned to the new Mrs Scuttle and said softly. "'S all right Aud. I know you aren't keen on me in that way so p'raps it's best if'n you go home tomorrow eh?"

"What about you Twit?" Audrey asked. "And I can't go home anyway – what about Oswald and the Starwife's bargain?"

"Let's go and have something to eat," suggested Arthur, "then we can decide what to do."

Under the yew tree Madame Akkikuyu stood alone, snivelling into her shawl and drying her eyes.

"You fool," rebuked Nicodemus. "You interfering cretin! We might have had the girl if you had not blessed her. My plans are ruined now – Audrey Brown has been tied to the Greenlaws, the spell cannot work."

"Mouselet name Scuttle now," checked Akkikuyu sadly, "and I glad you not use her – she my friend. Akkikuyu not have many friends, mouselet only one."

The tattoo writhed with frustration. "Curse you – you Moroccan ditch drab. The spell I have prepared needs a female sacrifice, one who is of age but has

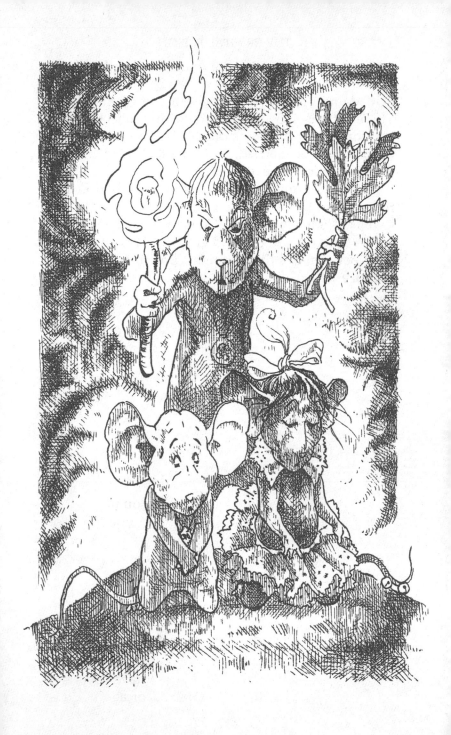

no mousebrass. Am I to be marooned in the abyss till the end of time?"

Madame Akkikuyu stared out along the bank. There sat Alison Sedge, miserable and dejected. She had longed for Audrey's death and now her enemy lived and was married. With Jenkin dead, Alison knew she would never marry.

Akkikuyu frowned as Alison stood up. No mousebrass hung from her neck.

"Nico," she whispered. "Akkikuyu find another."

The tattoo stared out and grinned. "Excellent. We shall perform the ritual tonight. Prepare the girl for sacrifice."

14

THE SACRIFICE

Alison Sedge kicked the tufts of dry, scruffy grass and turned to follow the others back into the field.

"Hoy, mousey, wait for I."

The rat's voice startled her. Crossly she waited for Madame Akkikuyu to come out from under the yew tree.

"What you want?" asked Alison rudely. She did not like Madame Akkikuyu – she blamed her for bringing Audrey to Fennywolde in the first place.

The fortune-teller approached, smiling sweetly. "Let me help poor mousey," she said. "Ah, but mousey has lost pretty dangler. Where it go?"

"I got rid of it!" snapped Alison. What business was it of the rat anyway? "What do you mean you could help me?" she added in a sullen tone.

Madame Akkikuyu walked round the girl and sprinkled fragments of yellow leaves over her. In a secret, low whisper she said. "I have spells mousey, bring disaster on your enemies."

The mouse regarded her through the screen of fluttering leaves. What was she up to? wondered Alison. "What enemies?" she asked stubbornly.

The rat moved closer. "Those who rob you of suitors – those who get in your way sweet mousey. Jumped up girls not as pretty as you."

"You mean that town mouse?" she interrupted.

"Yes, I don't like her, but if you hadn't blessed the marriage back then she'd have danced the gallows jig. What are you going on about now, you barmy so-and-so?"

"Akkikuyu stop hanging yes, because that too quick and easy for her. She too evil! She put spell on Jenky boy to make him fall for her. She led him into open and let Mahooot make him owl bait."

Alison exploded with rage. "Is this true? I ought to go and tear her apart! All that butter-wouldn't-melt routine. I hate her. I knew my Jenkin didn't really fancy her. Tell me what I can do."

The fortune-teller grinned. Alison Sedge had been an easy fish to catch. It would be easy throwing her on the fire – how could she loathe her mouselet so much?

"Akkikuyu will cast spell. You help, go get wood for bonfire."

Alison hurriedly ran to collect some sticks.

"Well Nico," the rat began, "what you think?"

"She is perfect Akkikuyu," gloated the voice, "did you feel her spite and anger? They are strong, raw emotions. Her life essence will be most eagerly received by the gate keepers of the abyss. Tonight I shall be free again."

Akkikuyu cleared a space on the high bank. She gathered some stones and arranged them in a circle, leaving it incomplete so that she could enter. She waited for Alison to return, then, once all the wood they needed was within, she sealed the ring with them inside. "Now mousey," she said, "we must not break through the stones till spell complete." She began to build the bonfire. From her bag she pulled out the skull of the frog she had killed and placed it at the heart of the framework. Then around it she sprinkled the magical herbs and flowers that she had carefully gathered at night. At last the fortune-teller announced that all was ready. She stood back and admired her handiwork with Alison. It was a tall pyramid of dry branches and twigs, a satisfying result to her labours.

"Light it," urged Alison, "cast your spell."

Nicodemus chuckled to himself. "Give her the crystal," he muttered to Akkikuyu.

The rat brought from her bag the glass globe and caressed it lovingly with her claws. "Stand there and hold this!" she told Alison.

Alison took the smooth globe in her palms and gazed at it wondrously. What a marvellous mysterious object! How lovely it was with those swirls of colour in its centre.

"What is it?" she gasped.

"It is my delight – my peace," Akkikuyu replied sadly, "and soon it must smash."

"Will you light the fire now?" asked Alison. She was feeling impatient and wanted to get on with the ceremony.

Akkikuyu nodded. "Yes, I light fire, but first my Nico must be safe from heat."

"Nico?" asked Alison suspiciously. "Who is Nico?" She stared around her, trying to see who Akkikuyu was talking about.

"I AM NICODEMUS!" cried the tattoo triumphantly. Alison whirled around, then stepped back in alarm.

"The face! The face on your ear – it moved, it spoke!" she spluttered aghast.

Nicodemus mocked her: "I move – I speak. Hah hah hah."

Alison had had enough. She turned, and tried to run from the circle of stones but a wall of invisible force prevented her escape. She howled in dismay but Nicodemus laughed all the more.

"Mousey not leave now ring complete," tutted Akkikuyu. "You not listen mousey. Now, Nico we must begin yes?"

"Truly," said the voice still chuckling as Alison twisted and turned round the circle in vain. "I shall project my essence into the heart of your crystal, there shall I be safe from the heat of the fire. I hope that I shall still be able to talk to you, but my powers will be much weakened by the glass." The tattoo screwed up its ugly face and became quite still.

A black cloud moved over the stars. Alison stared at the crystal in her paws and saw a pin prick of cold blue light glimmer there. Slowly it began to pulse. The light grew and filled the globe until the crystal shone like a star fallen to earth. The glass became freezing to the touch yet Alison could not let go. Breathlessly and with great difficulty the voice spoke again, it was nearer yet somehow it echoed hollowly. "Quickly Akkikuyu," it said with an effort, an edge of fear creeping into it, "light the fire now! The spell must be completed soon or the keepers of the gate will draw me back and bind me ever stronger. I have but a little time here unless the exchange is made." Akkikuyu lit the bonfire.

The wood was so dry that it kindled easily, and soon the flames leapt up greedily. The heat singed her whiskers and scorched Alison's face but the crystal remained icy to the touch.

"Aaagghh," said the voice, "even here I feel the fire! You must hurry. Throw in the mousebrass, Akkikuyu."

The fortune-teller fished out the brass that Isaac had made for her. It was a twisted, ugly thing, made in a spirit of hatred and vengeance. She cast it into the white hot heart of the crackling flame.

"Hear me Arash and Iriel," cried Nicodemus. "I send you a soul in my stead. A female unprotected by the Greenlaws. Accept her and let me go free."

A deep rumble boomed in the night. Thunder was

approaching. On the horizon, fingers of lightning zig-zagged down between heaven and earth. A freezing gale blew up, but protected by the circle of stones, the bonfire remained unaffected. Madame Akkikuyu threw some powders into the blaze and a ball of blue flame burst into the darkening sky.

"Prepare the vessel Rameth so I might live again." Nicodemus screamed above the clamouring storm.

Akkikuyu hurled more powder into the flame. A blue column of smoke shot up into the air. The fortune-teller was frightened. She had not expected anything like this at all. If it carried on the fieldmice would come soon to see what was going on. She winced and clutched her stomach. Something was happening to her . . . something dreadful . . . A terrible pain ripped at her insides. She doubled over in agony, and as she did so, she caught sight of her own body, and cried out in horror.

Her fur was changing colour. Instead of being a sleek coat of black, it was now a bright marmalade orange with dark stripes. The secret, closed doors of her mind were forced open and she bellowed with fear as she remembered the past, and saw through Nicodemus's disguise.

Nicodemus laughed amid the thunder and as he did so his voice changed – it became deeper, more sinister and absolutely evil. He crowed his triumph with insane jubilation.

"Yes Akkikuyu," sneered the great deceiver, "it is I, your master returned. JUPITER has come back from eternity."

"No!" she yammered plaintively. "You Nico-demus, spirit of field – Jupiter dead."

"Ha ha – I am the father of lies, Akkikuyu, you know that. You have helped to release me, I shall not forget. I intend to reward you with the highest honour that is mine to give."

"What honour?" she asked in horror.

"You have opened the door of death, Akkikuyu," he congratulated her, "but my old body has been destroyed. *You* shall be the new host for my dark spirit."

"Nooo!" Akkikuyu tore at her hair and tried to flee, but like Alison she could not break out of the stone circle.

"You cannot escape," tutted Jupiter. "Do you not listen? Continue with the spell!"

"Never," she cried and slumped to the ground in a desperate heap, cringing from that terrible snarling voice. But unseen forces gripped her and the rat was dragged to her feet. Her claws were forced into her bag and a will outside her own guided them to the next ingredient. The powders were thrown into the flame.

"Hear me Ozulmunn – bind her to me."

Akkikuyu's eyes stung and their black orbs trembled. A thin film of gold closed over them until only narrow slits were left. Her ears were pulled out of shape and she felt her tail grow thick stripey fur. Jupiter's evil spells were changing her into a cat!

She threw open her mouth to scream but all that came out was a pitiful "Miaow". Madame Akkikuyu clapped her ginger claws over her mouth to stop the terrible noise.

"Now, Akkikuyu, throw the girl into the fire, then smash the globe!" commanded Jupiter.

The rat's feet dragged themselves towards Alison.

The mouse had witnessed everything with incredulous despair. She cried for pity as the striped ginger rat lurched towards her. But there was nowhere to escape.

"Throw her in, Akkikuyu!" Jupiter ordered

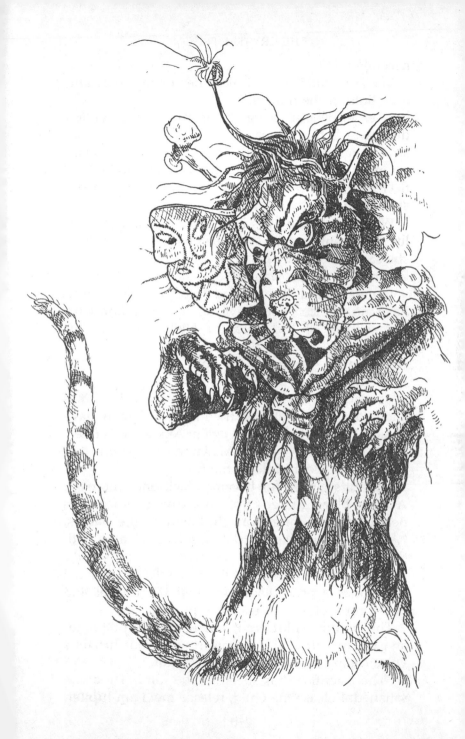

severely.

Madame Akkikuyu blinked her tawny eyes and took hold of the mouse.

"Please, please!" begged Alison as the rat pulled her towards the flames.

The lightning flashed and crackled overhead. Thunder shook the ground and Jupiter laughed.

"Please don't throw me in," pleaded Alison, "please, have pity on me!"

With her golden eyes it seemed to Akkikuyu that for a moment Audrey stood before her. "Mouselet," she said. "Go, run free."

"I can't," Alison wailed.

Jupiter heard them and scoffed. "You girl, have no choice. You have an appointment with the keepers of the gates of Hell. Dispatch her Akkikuyu."

Madame Akkikuyu thought of the eternal torment that lay before her should Jupiter take possession of her body. She let go of Alison and shouted, "Mouselet my friend! It is I who have choice. I will not serve you again! Akkikuyu is free!" With one terrific leap, Madame Akkikuyu cast herself into the middle of the fire.

The rat's ginger fur became black once more . . . As the blaze roared up, Akkikuyu's voice was heard one last time from the heart of the flames, "Akkikuyu tried so hard mouselet . . ." and with that she died.

A bolt of lightning struck the circle and blasted the stones apart. Alison dropped the crystal and fled through the gap, escaping into the field.

The bonfire spluttered, the flames leapt higher and the tumult of the storm drowned out Jupiter's voice calling from the glowing crystal.

"The sacrifice has been made and They are satisfied. Release me child, release me. I am Jupiter,

Lord of all Darkness! I command you to break open the globe!" Without his tattooed eyes he could not see that there was no-one to hear him.

Bright, fiendish sparks shot out of the fire and fell within the cornfield.

Before long, the corn was ablaze.

The terrible spirit within the globe called out in pain as the fierce heat scorched the glass. The bonfire toppled over and fell with a flurry of burning ashes on top of the crystal. Jupiter's furious cries were muffled.

* * *

In the Hall of Corn, the Scuttles, Arthur and Mr Woodruffe had decided that Audrey and Twit should go back to Deptford to tell the Starwife what had happened.

The rest of the fieldmice were mumbling and talking to each other in low voices. Some of them were repenting their hasty actions whilst others were sorry the town mouse had got off so lightly.

Suddenly a cry made everyone turn round. All the sentries were in the Hall; none had seen Alison Sedge crashing through the field. She burst into the Hall of Corn and shouted. "It's the ratwoman – she's working for a devil, *she* is behind all this."

But before anyone could question her further, another voice yelled out, "FIRE!"

All heads turned again. The sky was aglow and black plumes of smoke blew towards the Hall. Hot ash started to rain down and the Fennywolders squeaked in panic.

"To the still pool!" declared Mr Woodruffe, jumping onto the throne. "Fly as fast as you can. Save yourselves."

The fieldmice streamed out of the great doors and through the corridor. They were met by the ravaging fire devouring the corn at a terrifying rate.

The Fennywolders could not escape that way – they were beaten back into the Hall of Corn by the blaze and with a splintering "Whoosh" the great doors collapsed behind them.

"We're trapped!" cried the mice.

It was getting difficult to breathe, as the air was sucked up by the flames.

One of the nests caught fire and began to burn furiously.

"Over here," bawled Arthur, "it hasn't reached here yet." Everyone ran to the Scuttle's area and Twit guided them out through a narrow channel of choking smoke. It was so thick and hot that it burned the eyes and filled the lungs. Old Todmore coughed and spluttered in the blackness.

"Where we goin', you daft lad? I can't see," he wheezed.

"I knows this way in me sleep," Twit called back to him.

The ears of corn above burst and spat down fiery missiles.

"Come on," shouted Arthur, trying to sound calm, "nearly there."

The babies gagged and cried, turning their tiny pink faces away from the glaring flames. Elijah and Gladwin clutched each other's paws tightly as they crouched beneath blazing arches.

The heat was furnace hot and the tips of tails sizzled, whilst delicate ears roasted.

A few times Twit hesitated, doubting the way. His whiskers smoked, but the noise of the inferno coupled with the lightning confused him.

"This way," he decided, crossing his fingers. He dived through a wall of smoke and found himself in the glade. "C'mon," he shouted.

Soon everyone was there and they hurried over to the hawthorn bushes and dived into the pool.

"Hang on," said Arthur, "Where's Audrey?"

"Not with me, Arthur," said Gladwin, getting worried.

"I think she was with Mr Woodruffe," Elijah muttered.

"But I haven't seen him either," Arthur cried.

"Then she must be still in there," said Twit looking back at the field. The fire was out of control.

"Nothing could live in that," murmured Arthur grimly.

"Oh Aud," said Twit.

When the fieldmice had left the Hall, Audrey and Mr Woodruffe heard a faint cry. They hurried back and found Isaac Nettle lying on the ground. He had been overcome by the smoke.

"Get on yer feet Nettle," snapped Mr Woodruffe. He pulled the mouse up and slapped his face firmly.

"Let me be," whined Isaac miserably. He sagged down again. "Let me rest."

"Oh no Nettle, you've done too much harm this night to fizzle out now you old goat," said Mr Woodruffe hauling him away.

"Will he be all right?" asked Audrey anxiously as she looked desperately round at the burning Hall.

"Aye lass, if we can get him out in time. Now come on Nettle, use yer legs."

"No," cried Isaac suddenly. "The brass, my son's brass, it was in my paw. Where's it gone?"

"It must be back there," said Audrey.

"Leave it Nettle."

"I must have it, I must. Jenkin, my lad!" He struggled wildly with them.

"If you go back in you'll suffocate," shouted Mr Woodruffe. "Stay here! I'll go."

"No," yelled Audrey.

Mr Woodruffe charged through the thick clinging

smoke and searched for Jenkin's mousebrass.

There came a fierce roar as a line of burning nests crashed down behind. They formed a fence of fire between him and the others. He was trapped.

"Mr Woodruffe!" called Audrey.

"Go child, while you can," he yelled. "You can't save me. Take Nettle out of here."

More nests tumbled between them and Audrey fled tearfully away.

Mr Woodruffe made it across to his wicker throne and sat on it just as the blazing walls caved in on him. The king died with his field.

Audrey tugged furiously at Isaac who was singing in a mad voice. The way was practically impassable now. Terrifying sheets of fire raged on either side of the path.

"Glory to the Green," raved Mr Nettle insanely. "See his blossoms grow."

It took all of Audrey's failing strength to make him follow her, and the ground scorched her feet badly as she dragged him to safety.

"Please, this way Mr Nettle," she implored.

"What flowers are these?" Isaac asked, staring up at blazing corn stems. "Come Jenkin, see this fair garden. What wonders have we here?"

"Please Mr Nettle," she cried, yanking at his paw.

The flames swallowed the path behind them.

"With red roses and orange blossom – how bright they are," marvelled Isaac. He coughed painfully.

Audrey pushed him further along. Her hair smouldered and she discarded her lace collar so she could breathe.

They came to the end of their journey. A massive wall of flames reared up before them. Audrey sobbed: they could go no further. They were cut off.

"Praise be to Him who makes the flowers," ranted Isaac.

Audrey fell to her knees. The fire roared on every side and blazed overhead. She looked round dizzily and gave up. Audrey fainted.

"Blessed be the new leaves of the hawthorn," rejoiced Mr Nettle.

Thunder split the sky and the clouds were rent apart. Heavy rain teemed down with torrential force. The pool filled and flooded into the ditch while the blazing field hissed and seethed.

*   *   *

Audrey opened her eyes. There was a low, rough ceiling over her head and she was in a small bare room. It was the Scuttle's winter quarters.

"Hello Aud!" Twit was sitting by her side.

She smiled at him, "How did I get here?" she asked. "There was fire everywhere. I thought I was done for – what happened to Mr Nettle?"

"He's sleepin'. We found him an' you when the rain put the fire out. We all thought you were dead but you were only in a swoon. You was lucky this time Aud."

"Yes," she pulled her fingers through her singed hair and remembered. "Mr Woodruffe, did you find him?"

Twit looked at the floor sadly. "He didn't make it Aud. And we found summat else," The little fieldmouse fidgeted with his toes.

"What else?"

The fieldmouse raised a pale face. "Akkikuyu's dead – she burned in her own bonfire."

Audrey shook her head. "Poor Akkikuyu – are you sure?"

He nodded hurriedly. "Ain't no doubt there."

Audrey burst into tears. She had started out hating the rat but had grown fond of her funny ways. The memory of last night's wedding ceremony and Akkikuyu's blessing flooded back.

"Oh Akkikuyu I'm sorry," she wept.

Twit patted her hand. "Least ways you're free of that bargain now Aud. You can go home. Oswald is safe."

"Yes," she sniffed, "the bargain is over." She stared at Twit and said, "But you're my husband now Twit. I can't leave you."

Twit reassured her, "Now don't be daft Aud," he said, "we both know I only married yer to stop yer gettin' hanged. I told 'ee you don't have to stay. Go back to Deptford – it's where you belong."

"And you?"

Twit shrugged. "A fieldmouse belongs in a field," he told her. "I'll stick around, providing my banishment's been lifted, and help with the clearing up. A nasty mess – very nasty."

"You know," whispered Audrey, "you're not as cheeseless as folk make out, William Scuttle. You're a very wise mouse indeed. I'll miss you." She kissed him.

"Aw," he puffed, turning bright red and twisting his tail in his paws. "I reckons I'll come back one day to see me wife an' have a chinwag with old Thomas over a bowl of rum."

Gladwin Scuttle bustled in. Her hair was tied up in a scarf and she wore a white apron. "Oh you're awake Audrey," she said, "well that is a relief. I'm just on my way to help with the clean up. Half the tunnels are flooded by the rains and it's still pouring. No, don't you get up, young lady. You stay there for at least a week. You hear me?"

Audrey laughed.

It took nearly a week for the clean up to end. The tunnels had been flooded with sooty water and this left everything grimy and unpleasant. One of the first things the fieldmice did was start redecorating. They stained the walls with berry juice and decked flowers everywhere. The drab years had passed and in his sickroom Isaac Nettle, recovering from his madness, accepted the way of things. He even strung nutshells together and painted them bright colours. He was a changed mouse. Many of the children were ill with smoke sickness and Samuel Gorse left his room to visit them and cheer their spirits by acting out, with Todkin and Figgy's help, the story of Mahooot the owl. Figgy played the part of Young Whortle who was sorely missed by them all.

Arthur arranged the burials of Mr Woodruffe, Young Whortle and Madame Akkikuyu's remains.

It was the first time Audrey was allowed out of doors and she was stunned at what was left of the field.

All was charred and ugly. The corn had disappeared leaving unlovely, spiky stubble poking out of the ground. Rain puddles were coated with ash and everything was drab and dismal. It seemed that the whole world had turned dark and grey.

The King of the Field was buried on a drizzling morning near the rose trees. The fieldmice raised a mound over him and Isaac carved a beautiful crown of hawthorn leaves from a single piece of wood. Into it he inscribed the words, "We have lost our King whose light shone on our darkness."

He laid the monument on the top of the mound and fresh flowers were placed there every day.

Young Whortle was laid to rest next to Hodge. Mr and Mrs Nep mourned the loss of their son for the rest of their lives.

The Fennywolders could not decide where to put Madame Akkikuyu. Some thought that she ought not to be buried at all, but be thrown to the birds. Most fieldmice though remembered her eagerness to please and the bravery she showed with

Mahooot. So it was decided to lay her to rest under the hawthorn around the still pool. There it was hoped she would find peace at last. Audrey, swallowing back her tears, insisted that the remains of the fortune-teller be placed in a patch of ground that the sunlight touched. So the branches were cut back, and as the earth was piled over her grave the sun appeared in the wet sky and a pale, slender ray shone down upon the last resting place of the fortune-teller.

"It's all she ever wanted," wept Audrey.

The still pool became known as "the witch's water" and in years to come youngsters would go there to cast offerings into it and beg for wishes. And sometimes, on certain summer evenings, when the last flickering beams of the setting sun touched a particular spot – wishes did indeed come true.

In Fennywolde the clear up finished and Audrey began to think of going home.

Arthur was upset at the thought of leaving. He had gained everyone's respect and now they knew that Audrey was innocent the mice had warmed to her too. A veil seemed to have been lifted and they became the good-natured creatures they had always been.

Finally the day dawned when it was time to leave.

Audrey kissed Elijah and Gladwin goodbye.

"Tell my sister to stop poking her nose in where it's not wanted – she did that when she was a child you know."

"Fare'ee well lass," said Elijah.

It was time to say goodbye to Twit. "I'll miss you William," she said thickly, her eyes brimming with tears. "I'll never forget you."

"See you Aud," he replied brightly, but the twinkle had left his eye for ever. "Say hello to

Oswald for me, an' thank Thomas for his rum. Take care now."

"I will. Goodbye." She kissed her husband for the last time.

Arthur said his farewells briskly. "Cheerio," he said, waving to everyone who had come out to see them off. Dimsel Bottom slunk away and stared after him sorrowfully.

Brother and sister set off. Twit raised his paw but his voice croaked hoarsely, "Bye!" He tried to wipe the tears from his eyes but they would not stop. "I did love 'ee Aud," he whispered.

Arthur Brown and Audrey Scuttle became two specks on the horizon, making for the river. When the farewell cries of the country mice had finally dwindled into nothingness, the two town mice looked back for their friends, but they had already travelled too far. All they could see as they gazed back towards the corn field were the elms rising high above the ditch and the yew tree spreading darkly behind them. This picture stayed in their minds long after. But although they both vowed to return one day, neither ever saw the land of Fenny again.

SUMMER'S END

It was the last day of summer. The breeze was fresh and cool, the sun was a pale disc in the sky. The leaves of the elms were past their best and had that tired, old look which suggests the coming of autumn. Some of them were already curling up and turning gold.

Alison Sedge sat on the edge of the ditch lost in thought. She no longer took great care of her appearance. Her hair needed brushing and she let it fall in tangled, untidy knots over her face. Her dress was shabby – but why should she care? In her mind she was with Jenkin. They laughed together and smiled at one another in a dreamworld she greatly cherished. Alison lived for such dreams now. She no longer tossed her head or flashed her eyes, and she never listened to compliments from boys. In fact such compliments had ceased. Alison did not bother about that, for in her mind's eye she was the way Jenkin liked her.

She turned the black thing over in her paws. She had found it buried in a pile of ashes and cinders. Her find was scorched, blackened and pitted but not broken. She raised the crystal of Madame Akkikuyu up to the sun but it was too black and opaque to allow her to see within.

It was some months now since the town mice had left Fennywolde and returned to Deptford. Alison had kept out of their way. How fickle everyone was to begin liking that horrid girl after everything she had done. But no, it was the ratwoman who had caused all the evil wasn't it? Alison was confused. Her thoughts were really too full of Jenkin to dwell on other subjects for long. But there was something about this globe – it had something to do with . . . oh she could not remember any more.

"Curse you Audrey," she spat and discarded the black sooty ball. It began to roll down the steep bank . . .

Alison struggled to her feet and walked away. She was oblivious of the light noise behind her, and did not hear the glass crack and then smash on the sharp stones at the bottom of the ditch.

Unwittingly Alison had completed the spell that had caused so much suffering. Whilst she dreamed of a time long before when she and Jolly Jenkin had been happy together, a hideous great shadow rose up from the ditch behind her.

Jupiter soared into the sky – free at last from the crystal prison.